ONE HUNDRED YEARS OF PROGRESS

The History Of Veterinary Medicine In Minnesota

By

John P. Arnold
D.V.M., M.S. and Ph.D.

and

H.C.H. Kernkamp
D.V.M. and M.S.

Edited By

Thomas H. Boyd
M.A. and J.D.

FOREWORD

"100 Years of Progress

The past 100 years have been a period of great change for the veterinary profession in Minnesota. How this change came about is a story that needs to be told. Thanks to the dedicated efforts of our good colleagues Dr. John Arnold and the late Dr. Howard Kernkamp this story has been told in this fascinating book. Having lived through much of this period of progress I certainly was pleased to finally see this story in print. The veterinary profession will be forever indebted to these dedicated historians for recording this story for posterity.

One hundred years ago, in the late 1800's, the Minnesota veterinary profession was made up of a small group of individuals often referred to as "Horse Doctors." Formal veterinary training in the late 1800's consisted of two or three years of training at a private veterinary college. The training focused on the basic sciences, animal husbandry and basic therapeutic information known in that period. These veterinarians were handicapped by the lack of the drugs, biologics and medical techniques that are readily available today. Despite these limitations, our veterinary predecessors were able to serve the health care needs of the horse industry which played such an important role in farming and transportation in that era.

Today, 100 years later, our Minnesota veterinary profession has made extensive medical progress. The profession is now made up of several thousand highly trained, technically capable professionals who are highly esteemed members of the animal health care delivery system. They have at their disposal a vast array of medications, biologicals, instruments and therapeutic equipment of great complexity and utility. With the medical interventions and surgical procedures available today few livestock health problems are not amenable to successful treatment.

How did these extensive changes occur? Therein lies the motivation behind this book which has been written to document the progress made during the last century by our profession and the role played by Minnesota veterinarians in this progress. Many of our veterinary colleagues have long since passed on. However, their contributions to our profession progress still remain. Veterinarians with names such as Boyd, Brimhall, Coffeen, Cotton, Fitch, Flannery, Flint, Fenstemacher, Ghostley, Higbee, Hohn, Jensen, Kitchell, Kerr, Magnusson, Mack, Mather, Pint, Pomeroy, Prtichard, Schwartzkoff, Trump, Thorp, West and on and on, who made so many contributions must not be forgotten.

As you read this book, remember the veterinary profession is where it is today because of the blood, sweat and tears of our predecessors. This book is dedicated to them.

Dr. Walter J. Mackey, President
Minnesota Veterinary Historical Museum

ERRATA

Page 40 – Date on photograph – 1950s instead of 1850s.

Page 105 – EXHIBIT 4 – 1990, Kenneth Greiner instead of
Michael F. McMenomey.

INTRODUCTION

The veterinary profession in Minnesota began in 1872 when Dr. Bernhard Lambrechts established a veterinary practice in Willmar, Minnesota. Dr. Lambrechts was a graduate of the Royal Agricultural and Veterinary College at Copenhagen, Denmark. Prior to 1872, and for many years thereafter, veterinary services were also performed by non-graduate, self-styled and self-trained veterinary practitioners.

During the pioneer period, from 1872 to 1900, a private veterinary college that graduated veterinarians was established in Minnesota. A veterinary curriculum was subsequently listed in the University of Minnesota catalogue. The Board of Veterinary Examiners and the Minnesota Veterinary Medical Association was also established during this period.

The development of veterinary medicine in Minnesota continued to advance in the 20th century with better trained veterinarians, improved pharmaceuticals, the development of bacterins and vaccines, and the advent of preventative medicine programs.

In 1952, Dr. Preston Hoskins, editor of the Journal of the American Veterinary Medical Association, asked Dr. H.C.H. Kernkamp to write a history of veterinary medicine in Minnesota.

Dr. Kernkamp was a native Minnesotan who had joined the faculty of the University of Minnesota in 1913. After working in serum production and on disease problems of all species, Dr. Kernkamp subsequently became a swine specialist. He was acquainted with many of the pioneer veterinarians due to his work on disease problems. Dr. Kernkamp also appeared as an expert witness in court cases through the state. He was active in professional organizations, and served as both secretary and president of the Minnesota Veterinary Medical Association.

At Dr. Hoskins' request, Dr. Kernkamp collected information and began to write the manuscript of this book. Simultaneously, he also published articles in the 1965, 1966 and 1967 issues of the Minnesota Veterinarian on the history of the College of Veterinary Medicine at the University of Minnesota.

I began to work with Dr. Kernkamp on the book in 1970. In 1974, while I was visiting Dr. Kernkamp at his apartment, he pulled a box from under his bed that contained the manuscript he had prepared. He asked me to complete the history of veterinary medicine in Minnesota.

I was raised on a farm in central Minnesota. My father was an objector to the testing of cattle for tuberculosis who signed petitions in opposition and took part in legal efforts to stop testing. Notwithstanding this opposition, he never interfered with veterinarians who performed the testing. After receiving my D.V.M. degree, I entered a large practice in southern Minnesota where the farms were well kept and there were large numbers of livestock. I later practiced north of the Twin Cities where the farms tended to be smaller and the livestock was less productive. I also took part in area tests for tuberculosis and brucellosis. In 1950, I joined the staff of the College of Veterinary Medicine at the University of Minnesota. I have been active in professional organizations and served as president of the MVMA and the Minnesota Academy of Veterinary Practice. I have also been acquainted with many of the pioneer veterinarians in Minnesota.

Over the years, I have added additional information and material to the original manuscript that Dr. Kernkamp presented to me in 1974. Material for this book has been gathered from many sources, including the records of the Minnesota Veterinary Medical Association, Board of Animal Health, State Board of Health, University of Minnesota Regents, Board of Veterinary Examiners, Minnesota Legislature, and College of Veterinary Medicine, as well as countless newspapers, veterinary periodicals, oral histories and interviews.

A considerable amount of the information for the book originates from the authors' personal experiences and knowledge, or from experiences and knowledge of others that have been communicated to the authors. The authors have endeavored to confirm this information through other sources. However, errors may nonetheless have crept into the book. If errors are present, they are unintentional and the most sincere apologies are offered in advance.

Many people have contributed valuable assistance in the preparation of this book by giving interviews, providing information, reading drafts, and offering suggestions and encouragement. Those who have read pages and offered encouragements include: Drs. Martin Bergeland, Stan Diesch, Gary Duke, Jack Flint, Bee Hanlon, James J. Hanson, George E. Keller, Walter Mackey, Glen Nelson, JoAnn Schmidt O'Brien, Barbara O'Leary, Harry Olson and Roland Olson.

Dr. Benjamin S. Pomeroy has read the entire manuscript and rendered invaluable assistance in the preparation of the section on avian diseases; Dr. Dale K. Sorenson assisted in the section on the history of the college; Dr. Walter Mackey helped prepare the section on the Board of Animal Health; and Dr. Terrance O'Leary spent much time reading the manuscript and offering kindly suggestions and needed encouragement. My daughter, Mary Parenteau, has also rendered valuable assistance.

The staffs at the Archives of the University of Minnesota, Board of Animal Health, Minnesota Veterinary Medical Association, Board of Veterinary Examiners, College of Veterinary Medicine and Minnesota Historical Society were very helpful in making information and photographs available.

Michelle Mero Riedel, the College of Veterinary Medicine photographer, was very helpful in providing photographs. The fine work of William Pletsch of Schering-Pletsch Studios is evident in the class photos.

I would like to acknowledge the contribution of Winthrop & Weinstine, P.A., attorneys and counselors, in providing the editing and typing of the manuscript. Without this assistance, the book never would have reached the stage of publication. The tremendous undertaking of typing the drafts of the manuscript was capably performed by secretaries of Winthrop & Weinstine, P.A. under the excellent leadership of Ms. Kathy Petrie and Ms. Elizabeth Mulvaney. Thomas H. Boyd cannot be thanked enough for his labors in editing the manuscript.

Dr. Walter Mackey deserves much recognition for his efforts in making the publication of this book a reality. He took it upon himself to see that it was published, spent endless hours raising funds, and helped resolve the many problems that arose in preparing the book.

The publisher, James Mealey, was very helpful with suggestions and did a commendable job in publishing the book.

Lastly, Dr. Kernkamp and I owe much to our wives, Edna Kernkamp and Margaret Arnold, for their understanding when we were not good companions but were instead buried in a corner working on the manuscript or covering tables with material for the book.

John P. Arnold, D.V.M.
White Bear Lake, Minnesota
September 1993

FINANCIAL CONTRIBUTORS

The Minnesota Veterinary Historical Museum and the authors are most grateful for the private contributions that have made the publication of this book possible. In particular, we thank Dr. Herbert Hohenhaus for his extremely generous personal contribution. American Cyanamide Company and Midwest Veterinary Supply have also provided significant financial support. Finally, the following individuals and organizations must be recognized for the generous contributions they made toward the publication and sale of this book:

Dr. Sam Allen
American Cyanamide Co.
Dr. Larry Anderson
Dr. Robert K. Anderson
Dr. Wesley Anderson
Dr. John & Mrs. Margaret Arnold
Dr. John Baille
Dr. Milton and Mrs. Betty Bauer
Mr. Thomas Boyd
Dr. Dennis Brewer
Buffalo Veterinary Clinic
Dr. Les Butman
Dr. LeRoy Christiansen
Dr. Carlos Contag
Dr. Paul Cox
Dr. Robert and Mrs. Mary Ann Dietl
Dr. P.M. Eppele
Dr. James Flanary
Dr. Tom Fletcher
Dr. J.G. Flint
Dr. A.E. Follstad
Dr. Peter Franz
Dr. Donald and Mrs. Isabelle French
Dr. Ken Griener
Dr. James Gute
Dr. Milo H. Hagberg
Hanlon Research Fund
Dr. Griselda (Bee) Hanlon

Dr. and Mrs. James O. Hanson
Dr. Rodney Hanson
Dr. Warren Hartman
Dr. Stanley E. Held
Dr. Stanley Hendricks
Dr. Herbert Hohenhaus
Dr. Elmer Hokkanen
Dr. Duane Jacobs
Dr. Leslie Jacobson
Dr. Doug Jensen
Dr. Hans and Mrs. Kathy Jorgensen
Dr. James N. Karcher
Dr. George Keller
Dr. John F. Larson
Dr. Donald Luchsinger
Dr. John Luther
MVMA Auxiliary
MVMA Foundation
Dr. Walter Mackey
Dr. William F. Maher
Dr. Donald and Mrs. Maxine Manthei
Dr. Robert Mersch
Dr. Arthur Magnusson
Dr. William F. Maher
Midwest Veterinary Supply
Minnesota Academy of Veterinary Medicine Practice
Dr. Ralph Molnau
Dr. George Morgan
Dr. Barbara O'Leary
Dr. T.P. O'Leary
Dr. Charles F. Parker
Dr. B.S. Pomeroy
Dr. Norm Purrington
Dr. Jay H. Sautter
Dr. C.B. Schmidt
Dr. L.K. Schwartz
Dr. Stanley Skadron
Dr. M.T. Szatalowicz
Dr. Edgar J.Taggatz
Dr. Lyle E. Trout
Dr. Hugh Williams
Dr. Paul Zollman

TABLE OF CONTENTS

(*Table of Contents Continued*)

CHAPTER I

Pioneer Veterinary Medicine in Minnesota

PIONEER VETERINARY MEDICINE IN MINNESOTA

In prehistoric times, when man first domesticated animals, animal health problems were addressed through instinctive and simplistic methods such as water immersion for a fever; exposure of stiff joints and contusions to the warmth of sun; removal of foreign bodies; and licking the wounds. Eventually, herbs and other plants were utilized in treating these disorders. Humans and animals generally received the same treatments. As time passed, some people were recognized as more adept than others in determining the appropriate treatment of a given condition. The first veterinarian recognized in literature was Salihotra in India who, in 2350 B.C., was mentioned as treating animals in Sanskrit literature. In 1900 B.C., veterinarians began to appear in Egypt and, later among the Romans. Veterinarians first located in cities and larger villages where there was more demand for their services. In sparsely populated areas, the inhabitants had to depend on themselves or neighbors to treat and care for animal diseases. This was the situation when the early European settlers came to Minnesota.

NEIGHBOR HELPING NEIGHBOR

No veterinary services were available when the first settlers with livestock migrated to Minnesota in the mid 1800s. Using common sense and rumored remedies, the settlers simply did the best they could in treating their animals themselves. However, as the animal population in newly settled Minnesota communities increased, so did the animal health problems. Since there were no graduate veterinarians in the area, information on animal diseases was sparse. Moreover, expertise in treatment was similarly difficult to obtain.

Farm magazines provided some assistance by reprinting articles on animal diseases that had been published in the eastern United States and Great Britain. These magazines also contained letters from subscribers on various animal health problems that were accompanied by comments from the editor. Alternatively, the magazine readers would offer their own solutions to a particular animal health problem. These proposed solutions would appear in subsequent issues of these magazines.

The Northwestern Farmer and Breeder was one such magazine. The following are examples of treatments contained in the Farmer's 1884-85 issues:

> For colic, a good charge of gun powder in a pint of good vinegar, or sometimes a good dose of saleratus [sodium bicarbonate] with milk well sweetened with syrup.

> For what may be botts, give one ounce of alum and in 15 or 20 minutes give raw linseed oil, from one pint to a quart, if botts it will remove them.

> [Hogs] die very suddenly [of quinsy inflation of the tonsils]. If you notice the first thing, the glans [lymph nodes] will swell and it will become difficult to swallow or breathe. The best remedy that I ever tried is to blister the throat with turpentine and give salt peter in teaspoon doses once every two hours until you give three doses.

The Farmer became such a major source of information for animal health matters that, in 1892, the magazine added a veterinary department and hired Dr. Robert White of St. Paul, Minnesota, to serve as editor.[1]

Additional sources of information on animal health problems were books available for purchase that discussed the diagnosis and treatment of sick animals. In 1882, the Farmer offered the following books for sale: Farmers Veterinary Advisor, $3.00; Diseases of the Horse and How to Treat Them, $1.25; American Cattle Doctor, $1.25; and Every Man His Own Cattle Doctor, $7.50.

The most common method for treatment of animal health problems arose out of neighbor helping neighbor. Necessity compelled the settlers to treat their own animals, and some of these pioneers were more adept and had greater success in such diagnosis and treatment than their neighbors. Eventually, these individuals' reputation grew and their neighbors would request

---

[1] The settlers also sent letters to the State Board of Health, which had been established to deal with human diseases. In its 1886-88 report, the State Board of Health reported that it had received 717 letters relating to diseases of horses, 221 letters regarding cattle, and 11 letters concerning health problems with other domestic animals.

them to treat their animals. Such requests were commonly granted and no remuneration was expected. The owner of the ailing animal would often repay the favor by assisting his neighbor with work on the farm or providing him with food and farm produce such as hay and grain.

THE EMERGENCE OF THE EMPIRICS

The reputation of some of these farmers became so widespread and the number of requests for their assistance increased so greatly that the treatment of animals began to take considerable time away from their farm or business. Consequently, they began to charge payment for their services. These individuals became known as empirics. Such men were very personable and not the least bashful about publicizing their accomplishments, whether real or imagined, in treating sick animals.

The empirics were never at a loss for a diagnosis. As a result, some strange but colorful terms for diagnoses were developed. "Hollow horn" or "hollow tail" referred to loss of flesh or debilitation similar to symptoms occurring in chronic diseases or malnutrition in cattle. The empirics treated hollow tail by making an incision in the tail and rubbing salt in the incision.

Another diagnosis was "loss of cud," which meant that the animal had stopped ruminating. Rumination is a normal process whereby a bovine regurgitates food in the form of a bollus or "cud" to more thoroughly masticate the food. Failure to ruminate is a symptom rather than a cause of illness. One of the popular treatments offered by empirics for this condition was to extract a bollus from the mouth of a healthy animal and place it in the mouth of the sick animal.

A popular diagnosis of certain horse ailments was "blind staggers." Originally, this term was applied to horses with a cerebral disturbance that resulted in blindness and a staggering gait. However, the empirics used this term as the diagnosis for any condition in which a horse evidenced a lack of coordination.

Empirics were also prone to use such terms as thick, thin, and bad to describe an animal's blood in connection with the diagnosis of a range of diseases.

While their diagnoses and treatments were primitive, it is important to recognize that many of the empirics were honorable citizens and made a genuine effort to increase their knowledge of diseases in animals by reading and studying the available literature. Some of these individuals eventually became recognized as nongraduate veterinarians. Moreover, a number of the empirics were accepted to full membership in the State Veterinary Association when it was organized in 1897.

VETERINARIANS ARRIVE IN MINNESOTA

In 1870, according to the U.S. census, the livestock population in Minnesota totalled 686,606 domestic animals. Only ten years later, this number had more than doubled to 1,573,355, including 257,282 horses, 9,010 mules and asses, 659,050 cattle, 267,598 sheep and 381,415 swine. At that time, Minnesota's farm products were valued at $59,500,000.

In the meantime, the cities of St. Paul, Minneapolis, and Duluth were rapidly growing, and smaller towns and villages were springing up in all parts of Minnesota. The population of the state was 708,773. These impressive figures reflect the fantastic growth and development that Minnesota had experienced over the previous forty years. Competent veterinary medical services were long overdue in Minnesota.

There are ninety-seven individuals who may be recognized as Minnesota's pioneer veterinarians (Appendix I). These individuals were graduates of legally constituted and properly accredited veterinary colleges who lived and labored in the state at one time or another during the years 1872 through 1900. Of these 97 graduate veterinarians, 39 received their veterinary degree from the Ontario Veterinary College, 32 from the Chicago Veterinary College, 10 from the University of Montreal (McGill), and one each from Denmark, England and Germany.[2]

Of the pioneer veterinarians, 51 migrated to Minnesota from other states and from other countries. Another 41 of these pioneers were native sons of Minnesota. However, with only a few exceptions, it was not until the 1890s that native Minnesotans who were graduates of veterinary college began to return to this state for the purpose of pursuing a career in veterinary medicine.

[2]   There was a great demand for degrees in veterinary medicine in the latter part of the 1800s. To meet the demand, 33 new veterinary schools were founded by 1900. Most were private institutions and many closed after a short period of time. Some only lasted for one year and did not grant a degree in veterinary medicine.

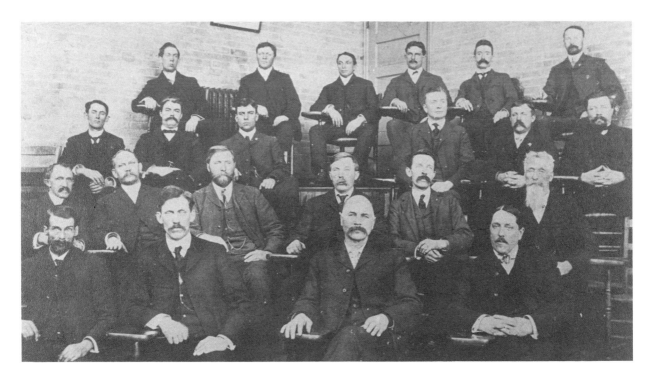

Veterinary Conference on St. Paul Campus, University of Minnesota, January 15, 1902; left to right, front row, Drs. J. Butters, E.J. Mckenzie, H.C. Lyon, Raymond LaPointe, second row, Drs. G.A. Johnson, C.C. Lyford, J.N. Gould, Anton Youngberg, M.H. Reynolds, third row, Drs. H.C. Peters, D.M. McDonald, C.A. Mack, J.M. Lambert, Frederick A. Illstrup, Bernard Lambrechts, fourth row, Drs. S.D. Brimhall, J.F. Annand, M.S. Whitcomb, C.N. Hackett, Arnold F. Lees, Mike Sexton.

For the most part, Minnesota's pioneer veterinarians possessed the strong qualities of leadership, foresight, perseverance, and a loyalty to their profession and to their community that mark all great pioneers. Their unceasing efforts to elevate the standards of the veterinary profession in Minnesota hastened the day when veterinarians became respected as professionals. The profession and the state owe much to the strength and dedication of these stalwart individuals.

VETERINARIANS IN COMPETITION WITH EMPIRICS

The early veterinarians in Minnesota tended to locate in larger urban areas where the owners of horses were more likely to use their services. During this time, horses were the most valuable species of domestic animals. However, veterinarians of that day treated all species and could be classified in today's terms as general practitioners.

Some of the early veterinarians located in smaller but progressive farming communities where their practice would involve a large number of good work horses and some of the better cattle. Work in such a community would provide a veterinarian with a good deal of practical experience before moving into the city. Some veterinarians chose to practice in smaller communities because of family ties in these communities.

When graduate veterinarians located in a new community, they would usually find that a number of nongraduate veterinarians and empirics already had established practices. The presence of these persons made it difficult for the new, albeit matriculated, veterinarians to establish their practices. To make matters more difficult for the new veterinarian, the public had no concept of a veterinary education. A diploma from a veteri-

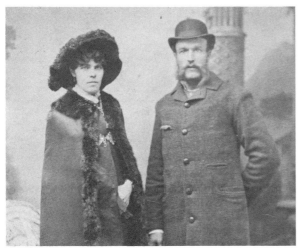

Pioneer Veterinarian, c. 1883 Dr. G.A. Dallimore with Mrs. Dallimore

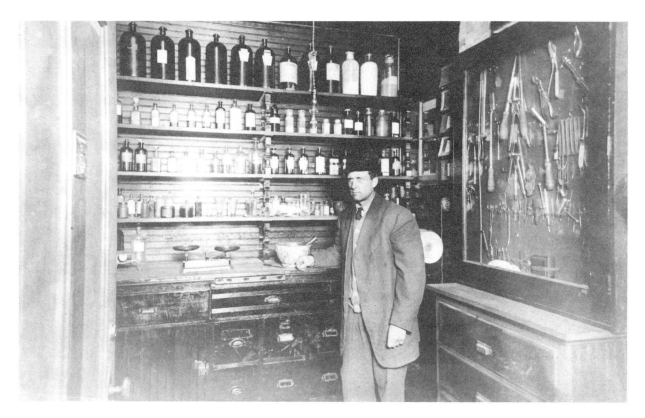

Dr. H.C. Williams in his New Richland, Minnesota office at the turn of the century.

nary college had little or no meaning to the early settlers of Minnesota. The public generally did not distinguish between graduate veterinarians and empirics, but instead collectively referred to all of these individuals as "horse doctors."

Townspeople tended to judge and compare graduate veterinarians with the empirics or "quacks" who had up until then provided all of the local livestock with health treatment. Thus, if the local empiric was held in high regard, the new graduate veterinarian would be more likely to gain the public's respect. However, when the local man was, for example, an alcoholic or slovenly in his habits, the graduate veterinarian would be presumed to also possess these same characteristics.

If the local empiric was indeed an alcoholic, his office would probably be located in the community's liquor store or saloon. Anyone who desired his services would simply transport the empiric from the drinking establishment to the ailing animals. Once the empiric had provided his services, he would then be transported back to town and given a bottle of whiskey in payment for his services. Although not all empirics were alcoholics, many had unclean habits and wore clothing that reeked with the odor of the drugs they used in treating their patients. Consequently, these individuals were, for the most part, social outcasts. Unfortunately, some of the early graduate veterinarians shared similar characteristics with the empirics, thus debilitating efforts to raise the public's esteem of veterinary medicine and the veterinary profession.

Livestock owners were reluctant to seek the services of an unknown and unproven veterinarian who would generally charge higher fees for his services. By and large, the public believed that skill in treating animals arose from natural talent and from extensive experience in applying the secret formulas and prescriptions for the treatment of diseases that had been made popular by the uneducated empirics.

Empirics were not only practiced in the art of self-promotion, but they were also effective in spreading stories and rumors regarding failures by graduate veterinarians. Empirics discredited what they termed "book learning," and maintained that they themselves enjoyed superior training in treatments that proved successful and effective through actual experience.

During this time, the referrals that graduate veterinarians received were generally limited to dying animals. In these cases, there was little the veterinarian could do to aid the animals. This limitation on referrals was generally considered a plot by the competition to ensure that the veterinarian would be blamed for the deaths of the animals.

Due to the hardships in establishing a practice in the early days, graduate veterinarians had difficulty generating sufficient income to meet their expenses. Thus, the veterinarians were obliged to supplement their income with odd jobs. Veterinarians accepted this employment with the understanding that when and if they received a call for medical services, they would be permitted to discontinue their work long enough to care for the animals.

EARLY FORMS OF CARE AND TREATMENT

The location of the pioneer veterinarians' office would vary from community to community. Some veterinarians would have an office in the same building as the pharmacy or local drugstore. This would facilitate the writing of prescriptions and, when the veterinarian was absent, the druggist was available to receive his calls and take messages. A number of veterinarians had their offices in the community's livery stable. Some of the early veterinarians would simply set up a clinic and office in their home.

Due to the primitive communication systems in rural areas during that era, veterinarians generally received requests in person or, in the alternative, animals were brought to their offices. In cases involving elective treatments, where it was not critical that the animal receive immediate attention, the owner would simply leave word of his request at the veterinarian's office or send the request through the mail. In such instances, the veterinarian would be requested to "stop in when out that way" so as to avoid incurring a mileage fee or to defray such a fee among the other patients on whom the veterinarian would be calling.

Unless the patient was within easy walking distance, the pioneer veterinarians' usual

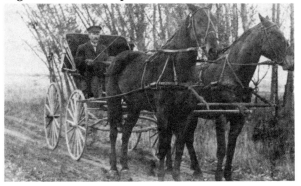

Dr. J.T. Jacobson on a call at Winthrop, Minnesota in the early 1900s.

means of transportation was by horse-drawn vehicle. He would travel by buggy when the roads permitted. During the winter, the veterinarian would use a cutter or a sled. Occasionally, he would travel with the aid of skis or snowshoes. When the roads were poor, the veterinarian might travel by horseback. The veterinarian would even travel by train in areas where the railroad system had been adequately developed.

During this era, veterinarians faced a host of contagious and infectious diseases. These ill-

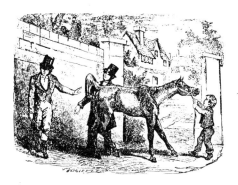

Tetanus (lockjaw) in a horse, from American Farmer's Stock Book by J. Periam & A.H. Baker, c. 1883.

nesses included glanders, tetanus, tuberculosis, malignant catarrh of cattle, actinomycosis or "a lumpy jaw," anthrax, hog cholera, and sheep scabies. Veterinarians were constantly worried about the potential for pleuropneumonia in cattle, and foot

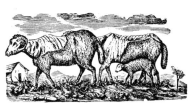

Scabies in sheep, From American Farmer's Stock Book by J. Periam & A.H. Baker, c. 1883.

and mouth disease in animals. Veterinarians also treated lameness, bloat, constipation, diarrhea, urinary problems, parturition difficulties, and abscesses.

Unlike today where veteri-

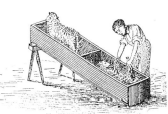

Dipping lambs for scabies, from Cyclopedia of Livestock by A.H. Baker, 1912.

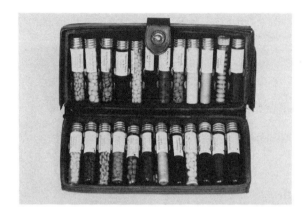

Medicine chest carried by an early veterinarian

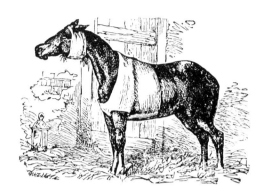

Mustard plaster, applied for bronchitis and pneumonia from American Farmer's StockBook by J. Periam & A.H. Bsaker, c. 1883.

narians have sulfonamides, antibiotics, bacterins, and vaccines, pioneer veterinarians had no drug to systematically combat infection. For surface infections, veterinarians used topical application of antiseptics in the form of ointments, solutions, and powders. The treatment for abscesses consisted of incising at the proper stage of development and dusting an antiseptic powder, such as iodoform, into the wound or irrigating with an antiseptic solution.

In treating disorders of the respiratory system, veterinarians often used steaming. In providing these treatments, veterinarians often used drugs such as creosote, turpentine, oil of pine, oil of eucalyptus, quinine, and carbolic acid. These drugs would be placed in a pint of water which was thereupon heated to approximately 140 degrees. This formula would then be placed in a position that would force the animal to inhale the vapors.

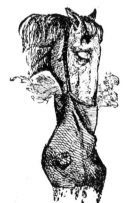

Nose bag used for steaming horses, bottom of bag was placed in a bucket of vaporizing medicine, from American Farmer's Stock Book by J. Periam & A.H. Baker, c. 1883.

Another treatment used by the early veterinarians as a counterirritant involved the application of a mustard plaster on the throat, neck, or thorax. A mustard plaster was made by mixing sulphur with water. This paste was then spread on newspaper and applied to the chest or thorax. The plaster was then tied in place with a rope and left there for at least a day.

For urinary problems, veterinarians would prescribe sweet spirits of nitre to increase the secretion of urine. When acute nephritis was diagnosed, a mustard plaster would be placed over the animal's loins.

Horses would often suffer from colic or abdominal pain. The objective of treatments of this disorder was to evacuate the digestive sys-

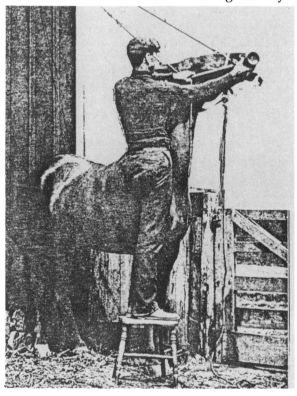

Drenching a horse in the early 1900's, source unknown

tem. Because stomach tubes were not commonly used with horses at that time, medication was given orally with a dose syringe or by drenching the animal. Long necked bottles, such as whiskey bottles, were used for giving the drench. The drugs administered orally included linseed oil, magnesium sulfate (epsom salts), castor oil, and aloes. Because some horses with abdominal pain assume the position of urination, owners believed that the animal's problem related to an inability to "pass his water." Thus, sweet spirits of nitre were sometimes prescribed.

Flatulent colic, or gas distension, was treated with a "trocar." A trocar is a large needle that was thrust through the abdominal wall and into the intestine to relieve the distension. At times, drugs such as turpentine were administered orally to reduce the amount of gas. Use of subcutaneous injections of eserine and pilocarpine were just beginning to receive attention in the literature and were not used commonly until much later.

Bloodletting—bleeding or venesection—was used by some veterinarians to treat cerebral disturbances, reduce temperature, and relieve acute congestion such as pneumonias and toxemias, and for other problems caused by "bad blood." To perform this procedure, a fleam was used to make an incision in the anterior vena cava vein or the jugular vein. The amount of blood taken would range from between two and six quarts according to the size of the animal and its diagnosed ailment.

Some drugs prescribed by the pioneer veterinarians existed in tablet form and were put into solution for subcutaneous injections. At the time, sterile water or saline solution was not available from supply houses. Thus, a common practice was to place some water in a shallow pan and boil it for five minutes. The tablet would be placed in a syringe and the required amount of dilutant was aspirated into the syringe.

While most empirics performed castrations and dehorning and were able to open abscesses, graduate veterinarians were able to perform a much wider variety of surgical procedures. In the late 1800s, there were

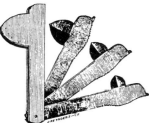

Fleam, used for blood letting, different size blades for different size animals, from John Reynolds & Co. catalouge, 1881.

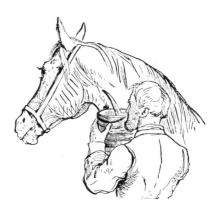

Bleeding a horse to remove "bad blood", from American Farmer's Stock Book by J. Periam & A.H. Baker, c. 1883.

some very competent veterinarians in Minnesota. It took time for them to be recognized nationally because of being located in a pioneer area. As they became better known, these veterinarians were invited to give papers at veterinary meetings.

The more important presentations at veterinary meetings were published in the American Veterinary Review, which later became the Journal of the American Veterinary Medical Association. The American Veterinary Review was the dominant veterinary periodical of that time. The level of development of veterinary surgery in Minnesota at the time can be judged by excerpts from two articles by Minnesota veterinarians during that period of time.

Dr. C. C. Lyford of Minneapolis wrote an article entitled "Radical Operation for Bursal Enlargements,"[3] in which he described the treatment and results of seven case studies. One of the case studies occurred in June of 1885 when Dr. Lyford saw a track horse with enlarged bursae on both front fetlocks. He aspirated the fluid from the bursae and injected tincture of iodine. Dr. Lyford's injection contained seven percent iodine, as compared to the two percent used commonly today. This was followed by the application of cooling lotions and three blisters.[4] The treatment appeared to be successful and the horse did some fast road work in the months of September and October of that year.

[3] A bursa is a tissue sac filled with viscid fluid and is situated at places where there is unusual pressure between a tendon or muscle and bony tissue.
[4] Blisters are irritants applied to the skin to produce an inflammation.

In November, the swelling had returned and Dr. Lyford again examined the horse. He surgically opened the bursae and injected tincture of iodine. This procedure was followed by daily injections of corrosive solution (bichloride of mercury) 1/500 and a wound dressing of marine lint[5] saturated with naphthalene. The parts were kept cool with wet bandages. This treatment continued for four weeks until the wound entirely closed. A strong blister was then applied every

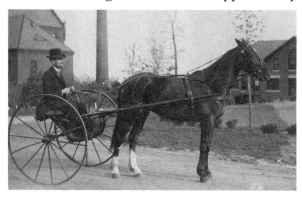

Dr. M.H. Reynolds with driving horse and cart; often used on veterinary calls.

fourteen days for six weeks. "At the end of two months the horse was apparently in good shape and returned home in January, 1886. He was immediately given road work and used for speeding on ice." In spring the owner reported the horse showed no signs of returning trouble and that he was intending to put the horse on the track. Unfortunately, the owner died and Dr. Lyford lost contact with the horse.

Another article that appeared in the American Veterinary Review in 1895 was written by Dr. M. H. Reynolds. At the time few dogs were being spayed in Minnesota. Dr. Reynolds' article was an effort to bring veterinarians up to date and encourage greater use of the operation. In preparation for the operation, Dr. Reynolds recommended the dog should be placed on a liquid diet of water or milk and given "a generous dose of oil twenty-four to thirty-six hours before the operation to rid the intestines of a variety of germs, and their toxins with the faeces, this cleaning out the intestines and securing more nearly an intestinal asepsis."

Dr. Reynolds recommended sedating the animal with morphine injected subcutaneously.

Preparation of the operative site included washing the animal's abdomen with 1/2000 solution of bichloride of mercury. Another bowl of bichloride of mercury of the same concentration was heated until it was hot. This solution was used to sponge the wound during surgery. A midline incision was made through the abdominal wall. Then a finger would be inserted into the abdominal cavity to hook a horn of the uterus and bring out the ovary. "The ovaries may be removed with a pair of scissors, in the case of young subjects that have never been in heat, and with an ecraseur,[6] torsion forceps or, better still, by a strong and clean finger or thumb nail." Surgical gloves, of course, had not yet come into common use.

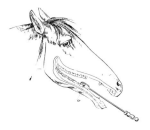

Floating (filing) horse teeth, source unknown

Three sutures were used to close the incision. Dr. Reynolds listed wire, silkworm gut and silk in that order of preference. He recommended a wound dressing composed of six parts of pine tar to one part turpentine on the incision. The aftercare involved "daily application of iodoform to the operation site; removal of the end sutures on the seventh or eighth day if all is well, and the middle [sutures] on the tenth day." For those who were worried about wound infection, Dr. Reynolds recommended dusting the edges of the incision with boric acid powder or a combination of boric and salicylic acid powder before suturing.

Other Minnesota veterinarians who published papers in the American Veterinary Review included Dr. J. N. Gould of Worthington, Dr. Anton Youngberg of Lake Park, and Dr. J. S. Butler of Willmar.

A particularly important part of early veterinary practice involved dental work on horses. A common problem was the development of sharp corners on teeth which interfered with mastication. In severe cases, the animal would be unable to consume the food necessary to work properly. Sharp corners were treated by floating or filing the teeth. This procedure was often performed without the aid of a speculum to hold the mouth open. Consequently, it took great dexteri-

---

[5] Mineral lint is naphthalene rubbed into loose oakum.

[6] *An instrument which controls hemorrhage by looping a cord or chain around the tissue to be removed and gradually tightening to sever.*

SET OF INSTRUMENTS FOR HORSE DENTISTRY.

I have used this make of instruments for over fifteen years, and find them to be the very best made in the United States. Any kind of instrument can be had by addressing Haussmann & Dunn, Chicago, Ill.

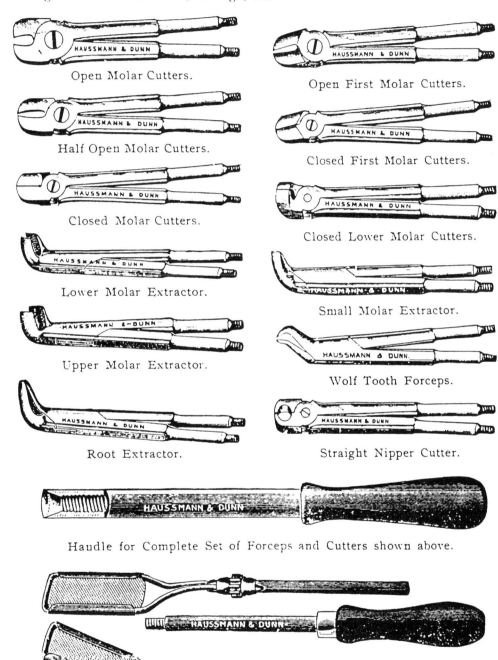

Open Molar Cutters.

Open First Molar Cutters.

Half Open Molar Cutters.

Closed First Molar Cutters.

Closed Molar Cutters.

Closed Lower Molar Cutters.

Lower Molar Extractor.

Small Molar Extractor.

Upper Molar Extractor.

Wolf Tooth Forceps.

Root Extractor.

Straight Nipper Cutter.

Handle for Complete Set of Forceps and Cutters shown above.

Haussmann & Dunn's Improved Float.

From Twentieth Century Horse Book by David Margan, 1902.

Plate XXIII.

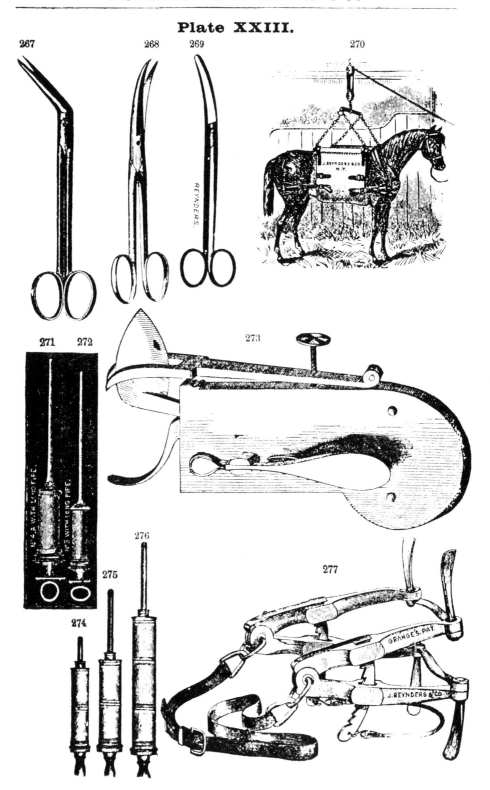

Items in 1881 catalouge of John Reynders & Co., various scissors, 267, 268, 269; horse sling, 270; fleam (used for blood letting), 273; dose syringes, 271, 272, 274, 275, 276: mouth speculum (used to hold a horse's mouth open), 277..

Plate XII.

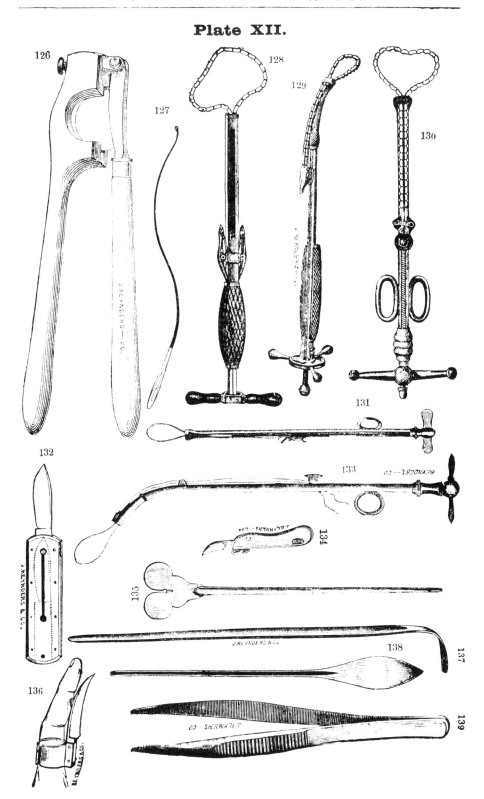

Items in 1881 catalouge of John Reynders & Co., horse tail docker, 126; seton needle, 127; chain ecraseurs (used in castration), 128, 129, 130; tumor snares, 131, 133; knives with concealed blades, 132, 134, 136; groove director, 135; tissue retractors, 137, 138; thumb forceps, 139.

ty on the part of the veterinarian to perform this procedure without having his fingers bitten. In farming areas and at a number of logging camps, there was a general practice to have the horses' teeth floated prior to the heavy work season so as to prevent mastication problems.

Other dental problems common at that time included abscesses at the roots of the teeth, and fractures of teeth that would result in non-fractured teeth becoming elongated and interfering with chewing movements.

CHANGES IN VETERINARY MEDICINE

There have been many changes in veterinary medicine since the first college trained veterinarian came to Minnesota in 1872. Until approximately 1930, veterinarians were for the most part large animal doctors and treated few pets. They primarily treated ailing animals, and little emphasis was placed on preventative medicine. Preventative medicine consisted mainly of trying to protect the other animals on the premises from the disease affecting the sick animal. The use of quarantine in cases of glanders, testing for tuberculosis, and vaccination for anthrax was the extent of preventative medicine at the time.

The development of the automobile enabled veterinarians to travel to farms more quickly and thus increased the number of calls made by veterinarians. As a result of World War

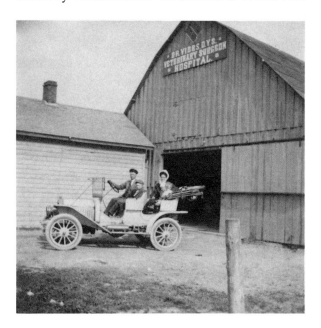

Dr. Carl Viers with his first automobile, in front of his veterinary hospital.

II, there was a shortage of veterinarians. In order to take care of all of the calls, the few remaining veterinarians would race their cars from farm to farm treating individual animals. Veterinarians became known as fast and reckless drivers. Many had large and heavy cars which were easier to handle at high speeds. They were known to travel down dirt roads at 90 miles an hour to treat a bloated cow. They were like a fire department going to a fire. Consequently, this was called "fire engine practice."

Over time, veterinarians began to have offices that were more professional in appearance and better suited to perform laboratory work. In the meantime, more bacterins and vaccines had been developed to aid in the control and prevention of diseases. As time passed, more small animal clinics were built, and the veterinarians began to specialize. Multiveterinarian practices began to be formed that allowed for specialization. This was true with both large and small animal practices. In the early days, laypersons would help in the office to answer the telephone, clean equipment, and perhaps restock drugs in the veterinarian's automobile. Today, specially trained personnel are required and institutions have begun to train veterinary technicians.

In the early days, veterinarians would compound their own medications if they did not have a working relationship with a pharmacist. Drug companies were subsequently formed and supplied prepared medications as well as drugs. The early veterinarians could purchase and use narcotics with no questions asked. Cocaine was readily purchased as a popular local anesthetic for mucous membranes in the mouth and larynx. Opium was often an ingredient in mixtures to control diarrhea. However, as drug addiction grew in humans, restrictions were placed on the purchase and use of narcotics and other drugs.

In the 1980s, dramatic changes occurred in both large animal and small animal practices. Small animal hospitals installed modern X-ray equipment, clinical laboratories, and modern surgical suites. The staffs have come to include veterinary technicians, receptionists, and laypersons. Staff veterinarians specialize and preventative medicine has become a central part of the practice. Specialized clinics have been developed in surgery, ophthalmology, and dermatology. Animal behavior experts now correct problems in the behavior of a pet. And, with the exception of emergencies, small animal hospitals see patients by appointment only.

In large animal practices, multiveterinary practices are common with specialization, either by system, such as reproductive, or by species, such as equine. Economics has caused changes in the size of farms. The smaller farms have merged into larger farms. Food producing animals are concentrated on these larger farms, leading to more problems in disease control. Practitioners travel from farm to farm in specialized trucks carrying their mediations, instruments, lab supplies, and even a source of hot water. They are in contact with their home office or with other vehicles via two-way or cellular telephones. Herd health has become the by-word in dealing with the larger farms and farm animal populations. Veterinarians have entered into contracts to oversee or consult in the management of a herd. This work has involved nutrition, vaccinations, ventilation, genetics, pregnancy testing, and treating problems associated with pregnancy. It has also involved monitoring weight gains in beef cattle, swine and sheep, and milk production in dairy herds.

The computer has became a very important part in the management side of a practice. In a survey conducted in 1990, 46 percent of Minnesota's veterinarians had computers. In small animal practices, patient and client records are all computerized. Programs became available for managing the practice and for assistance in making a diagnosis. In large animal practices, there may be a computer link with the farm to assist in monitoring herd health and maintaining records. In some cases, the veterinarian need not visit the herd but can instead monitor health matters by computer.

There has been a substantial increase in the number of women veterinarians in Minnesota. The first woman veterinarian, Dr. Joan Parent, Foley, Minnesota, began to practice in Minnesota in 1946. In 1990, it was estimated that one third of the veterinarians in Minnesota were women. The number will only increase as the majority of the students enrolled at the College of Veterinary Medicine at the University of Minnesota in 1990 were women.

If the pioneer veterinarians could see veterinary medicine as it is practiced today, they would be amazed at the changes and advancements. Indeed, they may even have great difficulty in realizing that veterinary medicine is the same profession they helped bring to Minnesota more than 100 years ago.

CHAPTER II

Board of Veterinary Medicine and Licensing of Veterinarians

The primary purpose of licensing persons in a profession is to protect the public from unqualified and often unscrupulous persons. Veterinarians looked upon licensing as a method to elevate the profession by limiting membership to qualified persons. Supporters of this view worked to achieve legislation to license and regulate veterinarians who practiced in Minnesota.

EARLY EFFORTS TO OBTAIN A PRACTICE ACT

In the 1880s, graduate veterinarians became concerned with the activities of persons with little knowledge or training who were posing as veterinarians. "Quacks," as these individuals were known, were victimizing the public and generating an unfavorable perception of the veterinary profession. Graduate veterinarians therefore set out to persuade the Minnesota legislature to create a board to prescribe the qualifications required to obtain a license and provide penalties for those who violate applicable regulations.

No record is available showing who was responsible for initially proposing the enactment of a veterinary practice act. However, this legislation could very well have been inspired at a meeting of the short-lived Northwestern Veterinary Medical Association. This association had its beginning at a banquet and smoker held at the first graduation exercise of the Northwestern Veterinary College in 1887. Representative E. J. Davenport of Hennepin County agreed to author and introduce a bill in the 1889 legislative session to create a board of veterinary examiners. When introduced, House File 113 was referred to the Judiciary Committee which, in due time, recommended the bill for passage. However, the bill was subsequently referred to the Agriculture Committee. The Agriculture Committee recommended that the bill be indefinitely postponed. This recommendation was adopted, and the first attempt at legislation died in committee.

The defeat of the practice act during the 1889 legislative session was caused by the objections of rural legislators. Thus, sponsors decided that graduate veterinarians would have to enlist the aid of reputable nongraduate veterinarians in the next attempt. A general meeting of all veterinarians in Minnesota was convened at the Astoria Hotel in St. Paul, Minnesota on December 26, 1890. After lengthy debate and failure to agree on a bill, a nine person committee was selected to draft proposed legislation. The Executive and Legislative Committee was given "power to act." The graduate veterinarians on the committee were C. C. Lyford, Minneapolis; Richard Price, St. Paul; and Olaf Schwartzkoff, St. Anthony Park. The nongraduates on the committee included Messrs. A. L. Button, St. Paul; William Dickson, Litchfield; J. Hinman, St. Paul; C. H. Parker, Minneapolis; E. Rowell, Minneapolis; and A. Scott, Owatonna. These men were chosen for their moral character and ability to provide credible veterinary services. Schwartzkoff was chosen chairman, Hinman, secretary and Lyford, treasurer of the committee.

The committee drafted a practice act that provided for the certification of graduates who had matriculated from legally authorized veterinary colleges and nongraduates who had both several years of experience and developed reputations for competence and integrity. Applicants would have 60 days from the date of passage of the act in which to apply for certification.

Representative R. M. McReeve, Hennepin County, agreed to introduce the bill. However, House File 31 was referred to the Agriculture Committee where it met with the same fate as the previous bill. It was passed out of committee with a recommendation of indefinite postponement. The recommendation was adopted.

THE ENACTMENT OF THE PRACTICE ACT

Following the unsuccessful coalition of "grads" and "nongrads," the "grads" decided to "go it alone" on the next attempt. However, it was the consensus of those who worked on the 1889 and 1891 proposals that to succeed they would have to offer a bill that officially recognized nongraduate veterinary practitioners who could meet certain specified qualifications. Accordingly, in 1893, Representative E. A. Fleming, a lawyer from Crow Wing County, introduced House File 201. This time the legislation passed in the House of Representatives, but was defeated by a 19 to 15 vote in the Senate on March 25. On that same date, Senator Jay La Due, a farmer from Rock County, moved that the bill be "laid on the table." This motion succeeded and kept the bill alive. On April 14, 1893, the bill passed in the Senate on a 35 to 7 vote, and

Governor Knute Nelson signed the proposal into law on April 18, 1893.

The Practice Act required the governor to appoint a Board of Veterinary Medicine that included both veterinarians and nonveterinarians. Governor Nelson promptly appointed Drs. J. J. Findlay of Duluth, B. W. Kirby of St. Paul, and W. H. Standish of Mankato, and Messrs. C. H. Pierce of Minneapolis, and W. H. Scruby of St. Cloud as members of the first Board of Veterinary Medicine. The Board was later renamed the Board of Veterinary Medicine.

The Board was authorized to execute and enforce the provisions of the act. Under the act, an individual could be certified and obtain a license to practice in two ways: (1) presentation of a diploma from a legally recognized veterinary college or (2) presentation of a sworn affidavit attesting to the fact that the applicant has practiced veterinary medicine in Minnesota for three years immediately preceding the passage of the act and letters of recommendation from freeholders and stock owners in his locality. The applications by nongraduates had to be made within six months of the passage of the Practice Act and were to be accompanied by a fee of $5.00. After the initial six month period expired, only graduate veterinarians could qualify for certification and license to practice veterinary medicine.[1]

Following the initial filing period, the Board granted licenses to 34 graduate veterinarians and 144 nongraduates. Only half of the eligible graduates applied for a license in 1893. The remaining graduates applied over the next several years.

The act further provided that persons practicing veterinary medicine for compensation without complying with the act would be guilty of a misdemeanor punishable by a fine or imprisonment. However, dehorning, castration, or giving assistance to an afflicted animal when a licensed veterinarian was not available were not regarded as violations of the Practice Act.

AMENDMENTS TO THE PRACTICE ACT

In 1901, the Board resolved to heighten the licensing standards beyond the mere possession of a diploma from a veterinary college. Consequently, the Practice Act was amended to require all applicants to submit to a written examination prescribed by the Board. Furthermore, a reciprocity amendment was added that provided

that a person licensed to practice in another state could, after establishing a residence in Minnesota and passing a written examination given by the Board, receive a license to practice veterinary medicine in the State of Minnesota.[2]

Amendments to the Practice Act in 1903 further defined the eligibility requirements of the applicants. The veterinary curriculum for which they received a diploma must have covered a minimum period of three and one-half years. Additionally, the fee that accompanied the license application was raised to $25.00.

In that same 1903 session, much to the surprise of the members of the Board of Veterinary Medicine and the Minnesota Veterinary Medical Association, the Practice Act of 1893 was amended to permit nongraduates to apply for a license without the payment of fees.[3] Eleven "quacks" subsequently took advantage of the amendment passed in 1903, and three more nongraduates followed their lead in 1906. This was the first, but by no means the last, bad experience in "opening up" the Practice Act.

THE "OPENING UP" OF THE PRACTICE ACT

There was an animated discussion about the amendments to the Practice Act at the Annual Meeting of the Minnesota Veterinary Medical Association in 1906. Some members expressed the opinion that the laws governing the practice of veterinary medicine in 1906 were no better than those in the original Practice Act of 1893.

In response to the criticism, members of the Board of Veterinary Medicine and the Association's Legislative Committee expressed their sincere regrets that the controversial amendment had been passed. They blamed the failure of the services that they had relied upon to alert them to legislative efforts that could weaken the Practice Act.

The members of the Association agreed that the Practice Act should be amended. However, there was a disagreement as to the timing of a proposed amendment. Drs. J. N. Gould and S. H. Ward believed that the time was not appropriate to seek a change. They counselled to delay amendment for five to ten years. They argued that to press for amendments now, and thus to again "open up" the Practice Act, could result in additional amendments favoring nongraduates. Drs. C. C. Lyford, Richard Price, and

[1]   Chapter 31, Laws of Minnesota, 1893.

[2]   Chapter 291, Laws of Minnesota, 1901.
[3]   Chapter 149, Laws of Minnesota, 1903.

G. Ed. Leech opposed this view, advocating immediate pressure on the legislature to adopt the proposed amendments. The Association's members became deadlocked on the question, the matter was tabled, and the veterinarians returned to their homes believing that no changes in the Practice Act would be sought during the coming legislative session.

Early in the following January, when the legislature was in session, Dr. M. H. Reynolds received a telephone call from a St. Paul attorney informing him that Senator Albert Schaller would be introducing a bill to license empirics. Schaller's proposed bill provided for the certification of persons who had filed their applications with the clerk of the District Court instead of with the secretary of the Board of Veterinary Medicine. The bill further provided that those who had failed to file applications during previous grace periods because of illness could be certified if they met the previous qualifications. Dr. Reynolds alerted the members of the MVMA Legislative Committee and members of the Board of Veterinary Medicine, and arranged a conference with Senator Schaller.

The conferees urged Senator Schaller to withhold the bill. Schaller declined to do so, and pledged "that if necessary he would fight to the finish for the enactment of" his proposal. Convinced that the senator would not yield, the veterinarians proposed that Schaller include the amendments discussed at the 1906 Annual Meeting of the MVMA. Schaller agreed to do so and the modified bill was subsequently introduced in the Senate where it was then referred to the Agriculture Committee.

Dr. Reynolds testified at a hearing before the committee that much had changed over the 14 years since the legislation had originally been proposed, and that it had become unreasonable to certify persons without formal education as qualified veterinary practitioners. He pointed out that the number of graduate veterinarians practicing in this state was increasing every year, and that the qualifications required for graduate degrees were becoming increasingly more stringent. However, at the conclusion of Dr. Reynolds' remarks, one of the committeemen declared that he would not consent to passing the bill out of committee unless the eligibility clause of the Practice Act of 1893 was retained.

Faced with this threat, Dr. Reynolds contacted key members of the Association through-out the state and urged them to inform their legislators that the pending legislation would permit empirics to apply for certification. The response was so prompt and effective that Senator Schaller came to Dr. Reynolds and requested that he prepare an amendment that would take cognizance of Schaller's commitment to interested empirics. Dr. Reynolds agreed to do so and drafted an amendment in which he included the proposals that were made at the Annual Meeting of the MVMA.

Dr. Reynolds' amendment provided, in part, that "any person who has practiced the profession of veterinary medicine, surgery and dentistry as a livelihood in this state for three years immediately preceding April 18, 1893, and who in the meantime shall not have been guilty of violating the provisions of the act . . . shall be deemed eligible to registration as a licensed veterinarians in this state (upon passing a practical and non-technical examination) and upon the payment of a fee of twenty-five dollars. . . . Providing that application for registration be made within ten days after the passage of this act."

The proposed legislation, as drafted by Dr. Reynolds, also provided that "penalties for violations of the practice act may be recovered in a civil suit instituted by the Board in the name of the state, or by a criminal prosecution upon complaint being made. In case the county attorney shall omit or refuse to conduct such proceeding, the board may employ another attorney for the purpose."

Finally, the amendment authorized the Board to revoke or deny renewal of a license, subject to review by the courts, where the license was obtained by fraud or when the licensee was guilty of gross moral or professional misconduct. The annual renewal fee was set at one dollar, payable on or before May 1.

The bill passed and was signed by the Governor.[4] The passage of this bill was regarded as a great triumph for the veterinarians. While the act allowed for the licensing of nongraduates, they were given only a brief ten-day period after passage in which to apply.[5] At the Semi-Annual

[4]   Chapter 419, Laws of Minnesota, 1907.

[5]   Seven nongraduates took advantage of the provision in the act to apply for a license in 1907. One of these men was Myron H. Higbee, Albert Lea, Minnesota. He later enrolled in the McKillip Veterinary College and received his veterinary degree in 1911. He then requested that he be allowed to take the examinations required of graduate veterinarians so
(continued...)

Veterinary Meeting in 1907, Dr. Reynolds declared that he did not know where he would change a single word in the act. Dr. C. E. Cotton, speaking on behalf of the Legislative Committee, stated that Minnesota veterinarians had the best practice act of any state in the union.

UNLICENSED PERSONS PRACTICING VETERINARY MEDICINE

The Board occasionally joined forces with licensed veterinarians to stop the ever present threat of unlicensed veterinarians. While some would heed a letter of warning from the Board, many unlicensed veterinarians ignored the warning and persisted in their illegal activities. The Board attempted to prosecute these violations. However, it was often difficult to obtain a conviction. To obtain a conviction, it was necessary to prove that the unlicensed person requested and received a fee for services. Many animal owners who had paid for such services were reluctant to testify because they believed the unlicensed veterinarians rendered valuable services. Moreover, these owners were reluctant to testify against a neighbor or a member of their community.

Prevailing in these cases was made even more difficult because the unlicensed person did not always expressly request payment of a fee. Recipients of these services were told that they could donate something of value to cover expenses. The value of this donation was invariably equal to or near the usual dollar amount donated for that particular service. Finally, elected officials were reluctant to prosecute unlicensed practitioners. The residents of the rural communities believed that the empiric was rendering valuable services. Thus, it was politically unwise for an elected official to prosecute such persons. Judges would also bow to political pressure and, when presented with a petition signed by numerous voters in support of a indicted empiric, they often dismissed the case or would impose only lenient sentences.

To prevail in the prosecution of unlicensed veterinarians, the evidence had to be "water tight" and proof of the violations had to be

5/(continued...)
that he might be classified as a graduate veterinarian. Higbee joined the Minnesota Veterinary Medical Association and was elected president of the organization in 1913 and 1914. He is the only person honored with two terms as president of the Association. His son, John Higbee, served a term as Head of the Diagnostic Laboratory at the College of Veterinary Medicine from 1961 to 1980.

supported by more than one witness. Of course, the best evidence was a confession by the wrongdoer. However, juries were also quite responsive to the testimony of livestock owners who had suffered losses as a result of treatments given by the indicted empirics.

Support for empirics was so strong that, if the local veterinarian filed a complaint against the unlicensed person, the community was likely to turn against the veterinarian and side with the empiric. Thus, it was better for the complaint to be filed by an outside agency such as the Board of Veterinary Medicine. However, the Board's ability to prosecute these matters was handicapped by the severe lack of funds. The Board's only source of funds was derived from the license and examination fees.

In 1925, the Minnesota Veterinary Medical Association agreed to underwrite the expenses of their Committee on Practice and Ethics to make an "all out" effort to convict persons who were practicing veterinary medicine unlawfully. It was felt that the number of persons practicing illegally was comparatively few and that the problem could be quickly resolved. The committee employed an investigator to gather evidence and build a case proving that an empiric rendered veterinary service for hire. The investigator lost no time in getting to work. In a report by the chairman of the committee, Dr. Ralph West stated that 21 empirics had been investigated and brought to trial. Fifteen of these individuals were eventually convicted. Dr. West further reported that many other empirics had ceased offering their services after they received official notice that they were under investigation and subject to prosecution.

During the depression of the 1930s and early 1940s, when farm income and the value of livestock were low, there was a great resurgence in the number of empirics and "neighborhood handymen." Unlicensed practitioners continued to flourish during World War II and for a time thereafter due to the shortage of licensed veterinarians. These empirics became rather bold and brash in areas where there were few veterinarians. Some of these empirics stated that they had a license to practice veterinary medicine and would threaten to prosecute any other persons who sought to treat animals in or around their communities. One man in Blackduck, Minnesota, set up a counterfeit licensing agency. He would grant a license to practice veterinary medicine for a fee and he threatened to prosecute anyone in the community who sought to treat animals who did not obtain one of his licenses. Another empiric in Pine City, Minnesota, claimed that he was trained in veterinary medicine at the University of Minnesota where he was allegedly taught to use a vaccine that would protect against 16 different diseases, including protein deficiency. In fact, his entire "training" consisted of holding pigs for vaccination while employed as an assistant at the University.

One of the complaints where the Board gathered sufficient evidence to bring a lawsuit for unlawful practice involved W. Strike from Cambridge, Minnesota. On September 8, 1940, Dr. R. J. Coffeen, Executive Secretary of the Board, was summoned to Cambridge to testify in Mr. Strike's trial. Strike was found guilty and the judge sentenced him to one year in jail. However, the sentence was suspended, and Strike was ordered to report to the judge every 30 days and to desist from further practice until he became qualified.

In another case, involving A. Bartlin of Hackensack, Minnesota, the Board did not have to prosecute the offender for illegal practice. The Board instead referred the complaint to the Cass County Attorney in early 1970. The Board subsequently received a letter from Mr. Bartlin's attorney stating that he would no longer practice in the future.

An example of prosecution for illegal practice that did not have satisfactory results in the eyes of the Board of Veterinary Medicine involved A. T. Leuck, a farmer in McLeod County. He was apprehended, brought before the District Court of McLeod County, and charged with unlawful practice of veterinary medicine. Drs. E. H. Gloss of Gaylord and A. C. Spannaus of Waconia, both members of the Board, and Knute Stalland of St. Paul, the Board's attorney, testified that Leuck had demanded money for performing veterinary services and represented himself as being competent to practice veterinary medicine. The court observed that a license to practice a skilled profession is a property right, and held that one or more members of the profession holding licenses have standing to bring suit on behalf of all members of the profession. The court further noted that licensed veterinarians could protect their property right through injunctive relief that would restrain unlicensed practitioners. Thus, the court enjoined Leuck from engaging in

further practice of veterinary medicine. However, Leuck refused to honor the court's order and continued to render veterinary services for hire. The Board petitioned the court to issue an order requiring Leuck to show cause why he should not be punished for contempt for failing to comply with the injunction. Leuck's attorney moved to dismiss the petition on the grounds that "the judge had no jurisdiction of [sic] the subject and that the proceeding now before the court was one in effect of punishing the defendant for alleged violations in a manner not in accord with the provisions of a law enacted in 1927 that prescribed the sole and only way of proceeding against persons who violate the practice acts." The court accepted counsel's argument and denied the Board's petition.

The Board of Veterinary Medicine appealed, but the District Court decision was later later affirmed by the Minnesota Supreme Court. The Court held that the Board, while having standing to sue for injunctive relief, had no right to seek an order for criminal contempt. Thus, the Board of Veterinary Medicine lost the case on a technicality.

ATTEMPT TO LICENSE AN EMPIRIC

In 1962, the Board of Veterinary Medicine made a seemingly innocent request to amend the Practice Act. The proposed amendment would penalize a licensee who failed to remit the annual renewal fee within 60 days of May 1. The Legislative Committee approved the amendment and arranged for its introduction during the 1963 legislative session. Although this amendment again "opened up" the Practice Act, the Legislative Committee relaxed their vigilance because they were unaware of any other pending amendments. However, a few days later, the members of the Legislative Committee learned that a second amendment had been proposed that provided that persons who had been actively engaged in the practice of veterinary medicine in Minnesota for 35 years should receive a bona fide license. Committee hearings had already been held in the House of Representatives by the time the Legislative Committee learned of this proposed amendment. Because there had been no opposition to the amendment by the veterinary profession, the committee passed it with the recommendation that it be adopted. The amendment was presented and passed in the House as a non-controversial matter.

The MVMA Legislative Committee lost no time in making contact with members of the Senate Committee on General Legislation. Upon informing the committee as to how the amendment was passed in the House, the veterinarians received a chiding that only added to their embarrassment. The author of the amendment in the Senate, Senator Harveydale Maruska, was contacted and urged to withdraw his proposal. While he refused to withdraw the amendment, Maruska did give the veterinarians the impression that he would keep an open mind on the matter.

The following Monday morning he summoned several of the veterinarians to his office where he showed them 60 or more letters, postcards, and telegrams he had received over the weekend from constituents in his district insisting that he make every effort to have the bill adopted as amended. The legislation was apparently aimed at licensing a particular empiric who actively provided services in Maruska's district. Based on these communications, Maruska told the veterinarians that he felt obliged to support the bill. He nonetheless agreed to a conference with members of the Board of Veterinary Medicine and others who opposed the legislation with the hope that the question could be resolved in a way that was satisfactory to both sides.

Senator Maruska, members of the Board of Veterinary Medicine and members of the Legislative Committee, together with Mr. T. Ryan, assistant attorney general, subsequently met to resolve the problem. After much discussion, Mr. Ryan stated that it was his opinion that the bill, as written, would not permit the licensing of persons who were not graduates of an acceptable veterinary college. Ryan also felt that the particular individual intended to benefit from this bill could not pass the prescribed examination. Based on Ryan's opinions, the parties agreed that Senator Maruska could return to his seat in the Senate and offer the bill for a vote. The legislation subsequently passed by a 49 to 6 vote and became law in Minnesota.

The true purpose of the amendment was to grant a license to one person, Conrad Berglund of Bagley, Minnesota, who had been illegally practicing veterinary medicine for approximately 35 years. He and his supporters had sought licensure in the face of mounting pressure to stop his "veterinary" activities. Complaints against him were discussed at the January 21, 1958, meeting of the Board of Veterinary Medicine. At this meeting, the Board instructed the secretary to write a letter to Berglund to request that he cease and desist his illegal activities. If he failed to do so, the secretary was to drive to Bagley and interview Berglund personally. Apparently this attempt to stop Berglund's illegal practice was unsuccessful. However, the county attorney refused to take action and the Board again addressed the problem at its July 10 and 11, 1962, meeting. At that time, Attorney Joseph H. Dingle of Rochester was engaged to prosecute Conrad Berglund for illegal practice. However, the amendment to license Berglund was introduced during the immediately following legislative session.

Upon passage of the amended Practice Act, the Board took action based on the assistant attorney general's opinion that the amendment would not allow the licensing of a nongraduate. The Board petitioned the District Court of Clearwater County to issue an injunction prohibiting Berglund from practicing veterinary medicine. The court granted the petition. It is ironic that shortly thereafter Conrad Berglund died and the matter became moot. However, the law used to license Berglund nonetheless remained on the books until 1976.

VIOLATIONS OF THE PRACTICE ACT BY VETERINARIANS

Complaints against licensed veterinarians in Minnesota have been variously handled by the Board of Veterinary Medicine, the Board of Animal Health, and the Practice and Ethics Committee of the Minnesota Veterinary Association. While each of these agencies has specific jurisdictions, they operate cooperatively. The Board of Veterinary Medicine is the only agency that can issue, suspend, or revoke a license to practice. The Board of Animal Health had the authority to suspend the accreditation of a veterinarian until the federal government took over that function through the Animal and Plant Health Inspection Service (APHIS). The Practice and Ethics Committee of the MVMA has no real power and must depend on persuasion and reason to resolve the complaints that fall under their jurisdiction.

The majority of the violations of the Practice Act have been resolved by bringing them to the attention of the veterinarian. However, serious violations have required more extensive action. One such case involved the license revocation of Dr. E. P. Walker of Willmar, Minnesota. His license was revoked for improperly operating a branch office at Melrose, Minnesota. The branch office was actually operated by a layman, C. A. Johnson, who rendered veterinary services for hire and split the fees with Dr. Walker. After it was revoked on July 31, 1940, Dr. Walker sought legal restitution to recover his license.

Dr. Walker had been formally charged as having "maintained a professional connection with, and lent his name to, a Mr. C. A. Johnson of Melrose, who was not a licensed veterinarian." The parties stipulated that Walker displayed advertisements in a local newspaper announcing that he was maintaining an office in Melrose under Johnson's management. The evidence demonstrated that Johnson collected a fee for the oral and intramuscular administration of medicaments to a horse he had diagnosed as afflicted with "spinal septicemia." Johnson shared the fee with Dr. Walker. The Board contended that this was an act of gross moral and professional misconduct that violated the Practice Act.

Dr. Walker and his counsel argued that the charge was "void and uncertain." The judge ruled in favor of the Board, stating "that the use of broad flexible terms in fixing such standards is inescapable and that the activities of Dr. Walker were in fact professional misconduct since the lending of a professional name to another is professional misconduct." The attorney for Dr. Walker appealed the decision to the Minnesota Supreme Court where, on May 23, 1941, the District Court's decision to revoke Dr. Walker's license was affirmed.

However, this did not end Dr. Walker's attempt to regain his license. On June 5, 1941, his attorney filed a petition for re-argument of his case before the Minnesota Supreme Court. On July 6, 1941, the Supreme Court stayed the revocation of Dr. Walker's license pending a rehearing. On Nov. 7, 1941, the Supreme Court again upheld the Board's revocation of Dr. Walker's license. Dr. Walker subsequently left Minnesota.

CORPORATE VETERINARY PRACTICE

The first reference to corporate veterinary practice in Minnesota occurred in 1934. A suit was filed in Dakota County District Court to enjoin the St. Paul Union Stockyards Company from collecting payment for conducting tuberculin tests on cattle that were to be transported to farms for milking and/or feeding. The suit was

filed by a group of veterinarians known as "The Associated Veterinarians" who had been providing veterinary service at the stockyards for many years.

The veterinarians based their lawsuit on the law that allowed only graduates of accredited veterinary colleges and duly licensed veterinarians to practice veterinary medicine for hire.

The defendants argued that:

1.   Both the animals tested and the Stockyards Company itself were part of the stream of interstate commerce.

2.   The state licensing law did not control the situation.

3.   The Packers and Stockyards Act contemplated the testing of cattle for infectious and contagious diseases, which were services stockyard companies were authorized to perform.

4.   The testing was actually performed by a veterinarian.

The veterinarians countered with the following arguments:

1.   The licensing law came into existence by virtue of the inherent police power of the respective states.

2.   Each state has the power to protect the public and morals of its people.

3.   This power never had been granted by the states to the federal government.

In considering the parties' arguments, the District Court observed that the laws of many states prohibited corporations from engaging in the practice of skilled professions such as medicine, dentistry, and law. Drawing an analogy to veterinary medicine, the court issued an injunction restraining the corporation at the St. Paul Union Stockyards Company from continued testing. The District Court's decision was affirmed by the Minnesota Supreme Court.

Although the Court had stopped corporate veterinary practice in this instance, the case nonetheless caused great concern among the members of the Minnesota Veterinary Medical Association. They concluded that, in order to prevent further attempts at corporate practice, the Practice Act had to be amended to specifically prohibit corporate veterinary practice. Dr. D. B. Palmer, chairman of the legislative committee, and Knute B. Stalland, legal counsel of the Association, were assigned the task of drafting a suitable bill and arranging for its introduction during the 1937 legislative session.

Palmer and Stalland drafted a bill and the Legislative Committee arranged for Dr. Lawrence McLeod, a physician and state senator from Itasca County, to introduce the bill in the Senate. The Senate passed the bill with little opposition. However, the bill received different treatment in the House of Representatives. Dr. R. H. Forsythe, a veterinarian from Dakota County and a member of the House of Representatives, introduced the bill. However, on the day that the legislature was due to adjourn, the bill still lay on the table of the committee to which it had been referred. On the final day of the session, Dr. Forsythe convinced the committee to put the bill on "special orders" so that it would come on the floor for a vote. The initial consideration of the bill fell a few votes short of passing. However, shortly after the vote was counted, four of the staunchest opponents of the bill retired to the anteroom. At approximately the same time, another legislator who had voted against the bill only a few minutes earlier made a motion to "reconsider." The motion to "reconsider" passed, and the bill then passed the House with a sufficient affirmative vote.

Although the bill was passed, Dr. D. B. Palmer, Knute Stalland, and the Legislative Committee were fearful of a "pocket veto" by Governor Elmer Benson. They contacted Dr. C. J. Anderson, of Luverne, who was a close personal friend of Governor Benson to arrange a personal visit. Dr. Anderson met with the governor and explained to his friend the importance of this legislation. Governor Benson agreed to sign the bill and the proposed legislation became law.

The bill provided that "it shall be unlawful in the State of Minnesota for any corporation to practice veterinary medicine." It also raised the annual renewal of license fee to $2.00 and provided that the fees collected by the Board were to be turned over to the state treasurer where they would be credited to the Board's account.[6]

As time passed, groups in other professions obtained legislation that allowed them to incorporate. Veterinarians soon became aware of the many business advantages of incorporation and eventually sought legislative action that would allow them to incorporate. Finally, a bill was passed during the 1971 legislative session that permitted the formation of corporations by veterinarians. The legislation stated, "One or more persons licensed as veterinarians may form a corporation only for the purpose of practicing veterinary medicine and services ancillary thereto . . . and not to engage in any other business." In order to incorporate, veterinarians were required to obtain the approval of the Board of Veterinary Medicine. At the January 4, 1972, meeting, the Board approved the following initial applications: North St. Paul Veterinary Hospital, Ltd., dated 12-23-71; Faribault Veterinary Hospital, P.A., dated 12-29-71; and Park Pet Hospital, Ltd., dated 12-31-71. Since that time, many veterinary practices have taken advantage of the privilege to incorporate.

BOARD AUTHORIZED TO ACT IN MORAL AND ETHICAL MISCONDUCT

In 1965, a revision of the Practice Act gave the Board the power to revoke or suspend a license to practice for chronic inebriety, addiction to habit-forming drugs, violation of the Harrison Narcotics Act, fraud in testing and reporting biological tests, lending one's name to an illegal practitioner of veterinary medicine, license revocation in another state, conviction of a felony, or adjudication of insanity or mental illness. New applicants for license examination were required to present affidavits from at least two veterinarians and three adults regarding their habits and general reputation. The Board also was given the power to inspect the premises of a veterinarian upon receiving a written complaint.[7]

Previously, the actions of a few had affected the overall quality of the veterinary medicine offered to the public and reflected unfavorably upon the profession. This amendment allowed the Board to address this situation. Since this amendment of the Practice Act went into effect, only a few veterinarians have been suspended because of alcoholism or drug addiction. However, their licenses have been restored only after they have undergone treatment and satisfied the Board that they were no longer chemically dependent.

---

[6] Chapter 199, Laws of Minnesota, 1937.

[7] Chapter 204, Laws of Minnesota, 1965.

REORGANIZATION OF LICENSING BOARDS

In 1969, a movement began to reorganize many branches of the state government. The various proposals included the creation of a Super Board directed by a commissioner appointed by the governor. The Super Board was to be placed in the Department of Commerce and Consumer Services. The veterinary profession vigorously opposed this reorganization and it was defeated. However, some changes were nonetheless made in that all 10 of the health related boards were required to be housed in the Minnesota Department of Health Building in Minneapolis near the University of Minnesota Medical School. There were some advantages in this arrangement in that the various boards could easily confer with each other on common problems. They also were able to use the Department of Health computer system and have their accounting done at a centralized location. At the same time, this arrangement greatly increased the expenses of the Board of Veterinary Medicine. Until this time the executive secretary of the Board conducted the business and stored the records of the Board in his home. Under the new arrangement, the Board of Veterinary Medicine had to pay for the cost of the services provided by the Department of Health, including rent, utilities, and computer services. In 1985, the Department of Health determined that it needed the space that was rented to the 10 health-related boards and asked them to vacate the premises. On January 3, 1986, the Board moved its office to a vacated insurance building at 2700 University Avenue W., St. Paul, Minnesota. The new quarters, while more costly than the previous location, have provided a larger space and greater accessibility.

In 1973, laypersons were added to the examining boards so as to provide the general public with greater input on the control of licensure in the professional fields. The first public members of the Board of Veterinary Medicine, Robert Stegmaier of Farmington and Shirley Wilcox of Minneapolis, were appointed in 1974. Stegmaier and Wilcox, as well as their successors, proved to be very capable members of the Board. The public members have brought concerns of the public to the Board and have helped increase public respect for veterinary medicine.

FUNDING FOR THE BOARD OF VETERINARY MEDICINE

The Board is required by law to be a self-supporting entity. The funds for its expenses are raised through the fees that it collects. The Board, in addition to rent and utilities, must pay for items such as attorney fees, salaries, mileage, examination costs, and office supplies. The budget is set by the legislature. Each biennium, the secretary of the Board appears before the Appropriations Committee to present the Board's budget request. The amount that the legislature approves must then be raised through examination and renewal fees.

The increase in the cost of operating the Board and carrying out its functions is reflected in fees charged for examinations and license renewals. The fee for license renewal is controlled by the legislature and has increased over the years from $1.00 to $10.00, and the examination fees have increased from $25.00 to $50.00. Additionally, since 1955, the Board has contracted with the Professional Examination Service for use of its written examination as part of the process of granting licenses to practice veterinary medicine in Minnesota.

To allow the Board of Veterinary Medicine to keep more current with rising costs, the 1976 legislature amended the Practice Act to allow the Board to set examination and license renewal fees.[8] Presently, the renewal fee is $40.00 and the examination fee is $250.00. No doubt these will be raised in the near future.

BOARD ESTABLISHES COMPLAINT REVIEW PANEL

The establishment of a Complaint Review Panel in 1974 was an innovative step and streamlined the handling of complaints. The panel is composed of four members: a veterinarian; a layperson from the Board; the executive secretary of the Board; and an attorney who is assigned to the Board. The presence of two nonveterinarians on the panel has given it more credence with the public. Other states have become interested in the Complaint Review Panel and have requested information on its operation.

Under the new system, complaints must be made in writing. Copies of the complaints are sent to members of the panel for study prior to conducting a conference to evaluate the complaints. The panel may vote to dismiss the complaint, pursue further investigation, conduct a hearing, or decide that the complaint does not fall

[8]   Chapter 285, Laws of Minnesota, 1976.

under the jurisdiction of the Board. The panel makes recommendations to the full Board which, in turn, decides what action is to be taken. Many of the complaints are resolved by the panel without requiring the involvement of the entire Board. Under the provisions of the Privacy Act, complaints, investigations, findings, panel deliberations, and records of the informal hearings are confidential and not available to the public. The records become public information only after a veterinarian has been formally disciplined by the Board.

BOARD OF VETERINARY MEDICINE HAS NATIONAL REPUTATION

Over the years, the Minnesota Board of Veterinary Medicine has gained the reputation of being one of the better veterinary licensing boards in the nation. The Board has been able to operate as an independent body free of political influence to protect the interests of the public and members of the veterinary profession. One of the reasons for the excellence of the Board is the quality of the persons appointed by the Governor to serve. The MVMA has forwarded recommendations to the governor as to whom they considered qualified to serve. These recommendations have usually been followed.

During the 1937 legislative session, an amendment was added to the Practice Act stating that, when the occasion arises to appoint a member of the Board of Veterinary Medicine, the MVMA shall recommend three veterinarians qualified to serve on the board and the governor "may appoint one of these persons."[9] In 1973, the words "may appoint" were deleted, leaving the governor free to appoint whom he pleases. However, the MVMA still sends recommendations to the governor and these recommendations are usually given serious consideration.

Another reason for the excellence of the Board is the orderly manner in which the members are appointed. The terms are staggered, fostering continuity. There has also been great continuity in the offices of secretary and executive secretary.[10] The first secretary of record was Dr. Leopold Hay of Faribault who served for several years. He was followed by Dr. M. H. Reynolds

and others whose names are not available. Dr. Robert Coffeen of Stillwater served as secretary from 1938 until 1943 when he resigned. Dr. D. B. Palmer of Wayzata was secretary from 1943 until 1956 when he failed reappointment to the Board. Dr. A. C. Spannaus of Waconia succeeded Dr. Palmer and continued until 1958 when he too failed reappointment. The Board, however, then appointed Dr. Spannaus as its first executive secretary. He served until 1965 and was succeeded by Dr. Glen Nelson of St. Paul, who retired in 1987 after 22 years of service. Mary Nelson, wife of Dr. Nelson, served as administrative secretary and then office manager for the Board, serving her initial ten years with the Board as a volunteer. Mrs. Nelson retired in 1989 after 24 years of service. The Board presented plaques and passed resolutions honoring both Dr. Nelson and Mary Nelson for their many years of faithful service.

Dr. Roland Olson was appointed Executive Secretary of the Board of Veterinary Medicine effective July 1, 1987, and Donna Carolus replaced Mary Nelson as office manager in 1989. Dr. Susan Poirot has been appointed to the Board of Veterinary Medicine to replace Dr. Milton Crenshaw and Dr. Ron D. Kuecker has been appointed to replace Dr. William F. Maher. Both Dr. Poirot and Dr. Kuecker's terms will expire in 1995.

---

[9]   Chapter 119, Laws of Minnesota, 1937.
[10]   Unfortunately, minutes of Board meetings prior to 1938 have been lost and in various reports the secretary's name is not stated. Thus, it is not possible to list all of the early secretaries.

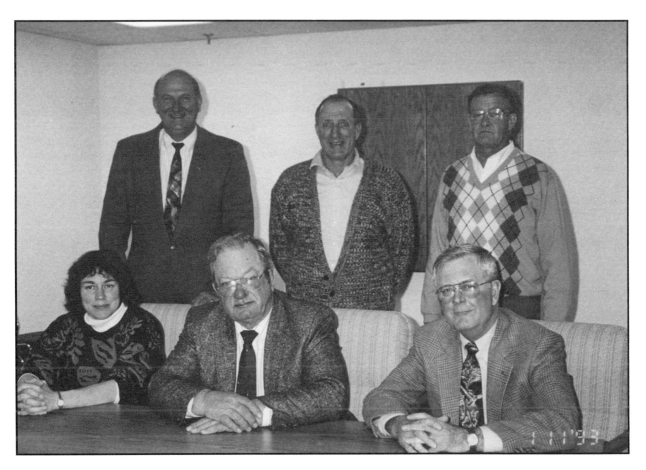

Board of Veterinary Medicine, 1993, left to right. seated, Dr. Susan Periot, Dr. A.J. Eckstein, president, Dr. Roland Olson, executive secretary, standing, Dr. Ronald Kuecker, vice president, Mr. Greg C. Abnet. Not in photograph, Mr. Marion Fogarty, and Dr. Joseph Glenn. Courtesy Dr. Roland Olson.

CHAPTER III

Control of Animal Diseases

The outbreak of disease or plagues would occur when groups or herds of animals were assembled together in villages or on the plains. In the early days, when the food for a village depended on these animals, a plague that destroyed the animal population could result in starvation of the local population. This situation inspired people to coordinate their efforts to control these diseases. These efforts took on particular significance with the development of the germ theory for infectious and contagious diseases. The most logical method to coordinate efforts to control a disease was through government supervision and regulation. Minnesota's state agencies, in cooperation with the United States Department of Agriculture, have effectively coordinated the control of animal diseases in the state.

The control of animal and poultry diseases in Minnesota has required the concerted effort of all persons connected with those industries. Primary responsibility to carry out the disease control programs has resided with owners and veterinarians. However, a governmental agency has been created to control animal and poultry diseases on a statewide basis.

In 1903, the Minnesota legislature created the Live Stock Sanitary Board (LSSB) in recognition of the need for a statewide agency to deal with animal diseases. The LSSB operated under this name until August 1, 1980, when the agency was renamed the Board of Animal Health to more accurately reflect its functions.[1]

ANIMAL DISEASE CONTROL PRIOR TO 1903

The earliest investigations into the control of animal diseases in Minnesota were made by the Minnesota State Board of Health (now the Minnesota Department of Health). The Board of Health was established in 1872 by the legislature to investigate and control human diseases and it did not become involved in animal diseases that were communicable to humans until 1883. At that time, the Board of Health was uncertain of its role, the scope of its authority, and the appropriate procedures it should follow.

On August 9, 1883, Dr. C. R. Bacon, a physician in St. James, Minnesota, wrote to Dr. C. N. Hewitt, a physician in Red Wing, who was the Board of Health's secretary and executive officer, that the local health officer had informed him two horses stabled in the village had glanders. Dr. Bacon requested guidance as to the appropriate actions to take under these circumstances.

Dr. Hewitt wired back a simple message: "Quarantine." On the same day, Dr. Hewitt asked the Minnesota attorney general for an opinion on whether local health Boards were authorized to control glanders in horses. The attorney general eventually answered in the affirmative: "Yes, as a nuisance, cause of sickness or disease."

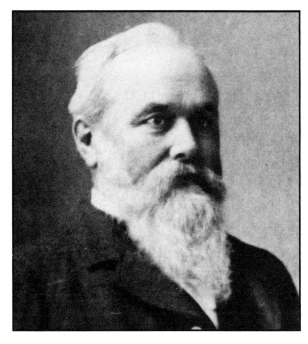

Dr. Charles N. Hewitt, executive secretary Minnesota State Board of Health. Courtesy Minnesota Historical Society

Following the St. James incident, the Board of Health regularly dealt with glanders as a disease communicable to humans. In its 1883 annual report, the Board of Health stated that

1/ In this chapter, the agency originally known as the LSSB and later renamed the Board of Animal Health or simply the "Board." The achievements in the control of animal and poultry diseases in Minnesota would not have been possible without the assistance of the agencies of the U.S. Department of Agriculture. Therefore, references will also be made to the valuable cooperation and assistance received from the U.S. Department of Agriculture, through the Bureau of Animal Industry (BAI) and the Animal and Plant Health Inspection Service (A.P.H.I.S.).

glanders was prevalent in many localities throughout Minnesota, and announced that it had hired a veterinarian to inspect two or three localities where glanders was suspected.

In the same report, Dr. Hewitt made the following uncomplimentary comments concerning the veterinary profession and the manner in which it had dealt with glanders:

The first difficulty which local Boards have met in regard to dealing with glanders is the unorganized condition of veterinary surgery in the state. The majority of those calling themselves veterinary surgeons have had no systematic professional education. A few are graduates of eastern veterinary colleges. There has been a conflict of veterinary testimony, making legal measures difficult and uncertain.

At the time Dr. Hewitt made this statement, there were less than a dozen graduate veterinarians in Minnesota.

In 1883, the legislature enacted a law requiring "Town Boards . . . to pay the expenses of preventing local outbreaks of disease." The Board of Health also ruled that local health boards were responsible for controlling animals suffering with diseases communicable to humans. However, local health boards often were either unwilling or unable to take on these substantial responsibilities. Some local health boards had only one member, and many local boards had no members with medical training. Some communities did not even have health boards. Local boards generally had inadequate funds, and the costs of enforcing the regulations sometimes threatened the local town or village with bankruptcy. Moreover, local board members were hesitant to burden friends and neighbors with financial hardships. Finally, the authority of the local boards of health was frequently questioned and often ignored. As a result, little or nothing was done on the local level to control animal diseases.

During this period, the Board of Health issued the first forms to local health boards and veterinarians for use in ordering quarantines and destruction of diseased animals.

The earliest reference in the state Board of Health's annual reports of diseases in cattle was recorded when Mr. J. D. McBroom of Butterfield, Minnesota, wrote Governor L. F. Hubbard of his sick cattle who "cough badly." McBroom was afraid to tell his neighbors that he suspected the cattle suffered from pleuropneumonia for fear of causing panic. The governor referred the letter to Dr. Hewitt who, in turn, informed Mr. McBroom that the Board would not get involved unless the cattle had a disease that posed a danger to humans. Dr. Hewitt then advised McBroom to treat the disease as dangerous until he was sure that it was not pleuropneumonia, and provided him with sources to obtain additional information.

However, Governor Hubbard did not let the matter rest and issued the following order to Dr. Hewitt:

In view of epidemic disease among cattle in some of the States and Territories of the West and danger of contagion to cattle of our own state I desire that you take steps at once to investigate the diseases referred to and the possible danger of spread to herds in Minnesota. If you deem it necessary, you are authorized to visit other states and also appoint a competent veterinary surgeon to aid you.

Dr. Hewitt subsequently traveled to Memphis, Tennessee, to obtain further information. Upon his return, he reported that "neither in Kansas, Missouri, Iowa or Illinois or in any Territory has there been a case of foot and mouth disease this winter." Strangely, Dr. Hewitt made no reference in his report to pleuropneumonia, which was the cause of the governor's initial concern. However, he did opine that the disease present in the suspected herds "is due chiefly to insanitary conditions of the animals, due to carelessness or neglect by the owners." As it turned out, McBroom's cattle did not have pleuropneumonia and the trouble eventually subsided.

Following the McBroom incident, the Board retained a veterinarian, Dr. Richard Price, to investigate several outbreaks of disease in cattle. Reports of losses had been delayed in reaching the Board of Health. Investigations were further delayed by slow and arduous travel. Dr. Price traveled by train to the town with a railroad station nearest to his ultimate destination, and then hired a horse-drawn vehicle to travel the remaining distance to the farm. By the time he finally arrived, most of the dead animals were too badly decomposed for adequate examination. On those few occasions when Dr. Price could express an opinion, he usually diagnosed the cause of death as anthrax.

During 1884, Dr. Price was sent to Marshall County to investigate reports of glanders. He subsequently wrote two reports confirming the diagnosis of glanders. Dr. Hewitt was not satisfied and requested an additional report. Dr. Price, irked by the request, did not know what more information he could provide Dr. Hewitt. He pointed out to Dr. Hewitt that he had already taken considerable time away from his business with no remuneration to prepare these reports and a detailed history of the disease. Expenditure to control glanders in Minnesota was only $47.75 in 1884. Dr. Price noted that veterinarians in other states who had been appointed to perform such duties had received regular annual salaries of $2,500, as well as $10 per day for expenses. "From this fact you can perceive that it is a great loss to me to have to give many hours from my business in preparing reports, and that the fees are so small that they do not begin to recompense a qualified man for his services."

Dr. Price's "attitude" only enhanced Dr. Hewitt's poor opinion and disrespect for the veterinary profession. Dr. Hewitt responded to Dr. Price:

> County Boards are finding it difficult securing the services of competent veterinary surgeons, and some of the fees demanded are extortionate. Pay before services rendered is one form. The state's 91 Board of Health has no difficulty in securing the services of competent physicians as Health Officers in charge of small pox at $10.00 per day and expenses. There is no reason competent veterinarians should charge more.

Despite this disagreement, Dr. Price continued to perform investigations for the Board.

The state Board of Health subsequently enlisted the support of livestock breeders and other supporters to obtain legislation to control animal diseases. These efforts resulted in legislation passed by the 1885 legislature "to prevent the spread of contagious or infectious diseases among cattle, horses and other domestic animals." The law clarified procedures for quarantining animals and indemnifying owners whose animals were destroyed, and uniformly authorized all local boards to act in their district, regardless of the size, to control animal diseases. The Board of Health was authorized to coordinate and assist these local boards.

In 1895, Dr. M. H. Reynolds, professor and chief of the University of Minnesota's Division of Veterinary Science in the College of Agriculture and Experiment Station, was appointed to the Board of Health. However, before Dr. Reynolds could assume the post, Dr. Hewitt successfully prevailed upon the governor to rescind the appointment.[2]

In 1897, Governor Clough declined to reappoint Dr. Hewitt. He was not notified of his nonreappointment by the governor or any of his staff; he was instead informed by a fellow Board member. Removal in this manner was a great blow to Dr. Hewitt. The situation was only made worse by the fact that the governor had appointed Dr. Reynolds to replace him on the Board. Dr. Hewitt had spent nearly 25 years of his professional life as the Board's secretary and executive officer, and he had guided it through some very trying and difficult times. There were some who believed that Dr. Hewitt had become too autocratic and arrogant, and that the time had come for him to step down. Dr. Hewitt nonetheless received widespread sympathy due to the manner in which his removal was handled.

The members of the state Board of Health elected Dr. H. M. Bracken to succeed Dr. Hewitt as secretary and executive officer. Dr. Bracken immediately focused on the fact that the Board's duties concerning animal disease problems were substantially intertwined with its responsibility to prevent human diseases.

The state Board of Health soon established a veterinary department and appointed Dr. Reynolds its director. He organized the department, promulgated its rules and regulations, and used his office at the University of Minnesota as its base of operations. Unfortunately, Dr. Reynolds was given little enforcement authority. While he was authorized to quarantine animals, Dr. Reynolds was otherwise limited to offering suggestions and hoping that the livestock owners would abide by the rules and regulations. Dr. S. D. Brimhall was subsequently appointed to assist Dr. Reynolds in the control of animal diseases as field veterinarian.

In 1900, Governor John Lind objected to the Board of Health's practice of appointing one

2/ Information of these events is sparse and the name of the governor who was asked to rescind the appointment is left to speculation. Knute Nelson was governor until January 31, 1895, when he resigned to become U.S. Senator from Minnesota. He was succeeded by David Marston Clough who, as governor, later appointed Dr. Reynolds to the Board.

of its members as director of the veterinary department. Consequently, Governor Lind reappointed Dr. Reynolds to the Board with the express understanding that Reynolds would not direct the veterinary department. Consequently, Dr. Reynolds resigned as director in August 1900, and Dr. Brimhall was appointed to take his place in April 1901. Dr. J. G. Annand was appointed field veterinarian, W. J. Pomplun was appointed the department's inspector, and the department's base of operations was moved to the Board of Health's offices in St. Paul.

BOARD OF ANIMAL HEALTH

Problems with animal disease grew proportionally with the increase in the livestock population of Minnesota. (See Table III-I.) More people were convinced that a separate Board or commission should be established to control domestic animal diseases. In 1901, a bill was introduced in the legislature to separate the veterinary department from the Board of Health. However, the sponsors were unable to agree on the terms of this bill and the proposal was subsequently defeated. In 1903, a revision of the original bill passed with the support of the Livestock Breeders Association, the Minnesota Veterinary Medical Association, the stockyard companies, and the Board of Health.

The new law created the Live Stock Sanitary Board, made up of five members appointed by the governor for staggered terms of five years. Three members were to be financially interested in the breeding and maintenance of livestock, and the two remaining members were to be qualified veterinary surgeons who were graduates of regularly organized and recognized veterinary colleges who practiced in Minnesota.

> To protect the health of domestic animals of the state, to determine and employ the most efficient and practical means of prevention, suppression, control and eradication of dangerous, contagious and infectious diseases among domestic animals of the State of Minnesota, and for these purposes it is hereby authorized and empowered to make all such rules and regulations for the conduct of business of said Live Stock Sanitary Board as it may deem necessary.

The legislation also required the local boards of health to cooperate with the Live Stock Sanitary Board (Board of Animal Health) to carry out its functions.

TABLE III-I

LIVESTOCK POPULATION OF MINNESOTA FROM U.S. CENSUS

	1860 Census	1900 Census
Horses	93,011	782,129
Mules, asses, and burros	2,350	9,382
Working oxen	43,176	—
Dairy cows	121,467	789,683
Other cattle, including dairy bulls and heifers	145,736	972,762
Swine	148,473	1,458,651
Sheep	132,343	594,006

	1860 Census	1900 Census
Goats	—	663
Chickens	4,448,331*	7,730,940
Ducks and geese	—	411,753
Turkeys	—	159,561

* 1880 census.

The governor traditionally appointed the chief of the Veterinary Division of the University of Minnesota as one of the members of the Board of Animal Health. This practice continued until Dr. W. T. S. Thorp determined that it was unwise for the head of the Veterinary Division to serve as a full member of the Board, and proposed that that individual should instead serve as a consulting nonmember of the Board. Thereafter, the Minnesota Veterinary Medical Association would submit a list of veterinarians as candidates for appointment, and livestock groups were asked to do likewise for proposed livestock representatives on the Board. The governor has usually selected Board members from these proposals. However, on occasion these lists have been ignored, and appointments have been made before the lists were even submitted.

Board members have always selected nonmember veterinarians licensed to practice in Minnesota to serve as the Board's secretary and executive office. The secretary and executive office serves at the pleasure of the Board on a year-to-year basis.

Because the position of secretary and executive office (state veterinarian) has been less political than Board positions, only six men have

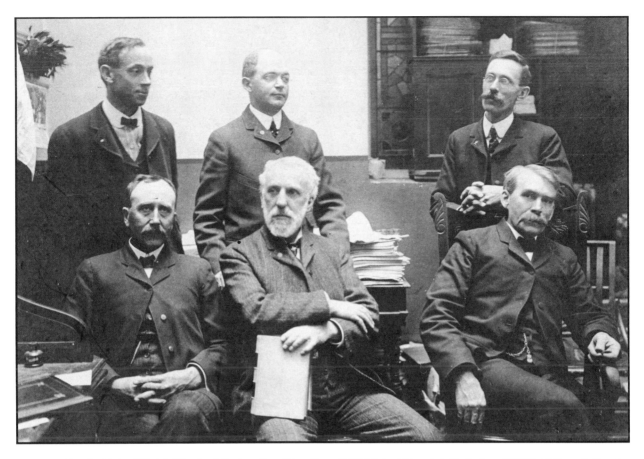

Board of Animal Health (Live Stock Sanitary Board) in office c. 1905; left to right, seated, J.J. Furlong, W.W.P. McConnell, Forest Henry (?), standing, Drs. Myron H. Reynolds, Charles E. Cotton, S.H. Ward. Courtesy Board of Animal Health.

served in this position: Dr. S. H. Ward, 1903-1907 and 1908-1918; Dr. M. S. Whitcomb, 1907-1908; Dr. C. E. Cotton, 1918-1942; Dr. R. L. West, 1942-1959; Dr. J. G. Flint, 1960-1984; and Dr. T. J. Hagerty, 1985 through the present time. In many states, a new state veterinarian is appointed each time a new governor is elected.

Governor Samuel R. Van Sant appointed Messrs. J. J. Furlong of Austin, Forest Henry of Dover, W. W. P. McConnel of Mankato, Dr. C. E. Cotton of Minneapolis, and Dr. M. H. Reynolds of the University of Minnesota to the first Board of Animal Health. The members of the Board held their organizational meeting on May 1, 1903, at the Merchant's Hotel in St. Paul. Furlong was elected as president, Henry as vice president, and Cotton as secretary pro-tem.

The Board eventually selected Dr. S. H. Ward, a veterinarian from St. Cloud, Minnesota, as its secretary and executive officer. Dr. Ward had served as an early resident secretary for the American Veterinary Medical Association and, in that capacity, he had given disease reports at the organization's annual meeting.

The Board selected Dr. S. D. Brimhall to serve as field veterinarian. This represented a demotion for Dr. Brimhall, who had been director of the Veterinary Department in the Board of Health. However, Dr. Bracken, the Board of Health's secretary and executive officer, had complimented Dr. Brimhall very highly in his report on the Veterinary Department, observing that, before Dr. Brimhall had become director, very little laboratory work had been done in the investigation of animal diseases. This had changed under the direction of Dr. Brimhall and had yielded "very useful results."

Six months after Dr. Brimhall accepted the appointment, a committee from the Board of Animal Health questioned Dr. Brimhall's "work and loyalty." Although the matter was later dropped, Dr. Brimhall's year-long appointment was not renewed. Dr. M. S. Whitcomb of Austin was hired to replace Dr. Brimhall as field veterinarian.

The secretary and executive officer's annual salary was $2,400 and the field veterinarian received $2,100 per year. The Board of Health was originally supposed to receive a general appropriation of $19,000, and an additional special appropriation of $2,500 to operate the Veterinary Department during the 1902-1903 fiscal year. However, the budget that was subsequently approved by the legislature did not authorize the special appropriation of $2,500, and $4,002.77 was actually provided to the Board of Animal Health to operate from May through August 1902.

At the same time, the legislature also passed the Krostue Act to establish procedures for reimbursement for animals destroyed to control disease. Horses with glanders and cows with tuberculosis could be appraised for up to $75.00 and $35.00, respectively. The state would pay three-fourths of the appraised value less any salvage. The remaining cost of the appraised value was assumed by the owner. This expansion of indemnity to include horses with glanders and the increased level of the appraised value of cattle placed even greater strain on the Board's budget. Conversely, the Krostue Act benefitted local boards by repealing existing requirements that these boards indemnify animal owners. As a result, local boards were more likely to take action to control animal disease in their communities.

The Board of Animal Health held its second meeting on May 21, 1903, at which time the staffing was completed and the initial rules and regulations were issued. Miss Nellie Carroll was elected assistant secretary with a salary of $1,000 per year. Miss Carroll had begun working in the Veterinary Department of the Board of Health under Dr. Reynolds in 1897. In the Board's 1901-1903 report, she was referred to as registering clerk and stenographer. She worked for the Board of Animal Health until June 30, 1946, when she retired after 49 years of faithful and dedicated service to the control of animal and poultry diseases in Minnesota.[3]

At the same meeting, the Board approved the hiring of Mr. William Pomplum as field investigator with the understanding that he would furnish his own horse. He too had worked in a similar capacity for the State Board of Health under Dr. Reynolds.

Finally, Mr. John Day Smith, of Minneapolis, was retained as consulting attorney at a salary not to exceed $500 per year. When Mr.

---

[3] Nellie Carroll, who never married, was a tall stately woman. She retained her youthful appearance and good health until the day she retired. Miss Carroll always adhered to the medical advice of her brother, Dr. Bill Carroll, a well-known St. Paul surgeon who performed so many gallbladder operations that he was nicknamed "gallbladder Bill." Nellie enjoyed a long retirement, and was well in her nineties when she died.

Smith resigned his position in January of 1905 to become a judge, the Board selected Mr. Robert Jamison as the Board's counsel. Shortly thereafter, on May 19, 1905, the Board was informed that the law required the attorney general to act on its behalf. Since that time, the attorney general's office has acted on the Board's behalf in all legal matters.

Upon completing the staff, the Board lost no time identifying glanders, tuberculosis of cattle, hog cholera, and sheep scabies as priority diseases for control. The Board issued rules and regulations relating to these diseases. The Board regulated the importation of range horses, dairy or breeding cattle, and breeding hogs and sheep. The regulations prohibited importation without a proper health certificate and required all inspections and related tests to be conducted by a qualified veterinarian.

The standard health certificates used at that time required the following statement by the owner:

I do hereby certify that the above _____ mentioned animals have been in my possession for _____ and they have not to my knowledge been exposed to any contagious or infectious disease the past three months.

Local officials were authorized to seize and quarantine all animals imported to the state without the proper health certificate.

To make the regulation more effective, the Board notified all of the railroads doing business in Minnesota of their legal right to refuse shipments of livestock without proper health certificates.

DIAGNOSTIC INVESTIGATIONS

The Board of Health continued to assist the Board of Animal Health through the early years. For example, Dr. F. F. Wesbrook of the Board of Health performed the bacteriological work for the new Board of Animal Health. However, the substantial amount of time and cost of supplies involved soon became too much, and the Board of Health notified the Board of Animal Health that it could no longer cover the cost of this service. After several meetings in 1904, the State Board of Health submitted their estimate of the cost of this service, which included the $2,500 salary for a bacteriologist and $500 for expenses.

The members of the Board of Animal Health decided that this was more than their budget could support and rejected the proposal to perform these services under these terms.

In setting the Board's policy in regard to bacteriological work, Dr. Reynolds proposed "that it shall be the purpose of this Board to confine its bacteriological work essentially between the lines of police control of infectious diseases of domestic animals and in the main avoid expensive, elaborate research work as not being within the scope of our legitimate work." Dr. Cotton seconded the motion, and the proposal was adopted by the Board.

In June of 1904, the Board accepted the offer to use the University of Minnesota's Experiment Station's laboratory equipment and animal housing facilities for use in performing the Board's laboratory and research work. Thereafter, within six weeks after rejecting the Board of Health's proposal, the Board hired Dr. W. L. Beebe as its bacteriologist.

In 1905, Dr. Beebe sent a letter to veterinarians throughout Minnesota directing them to send specimens for diagnosis to the Experiment Station in St. Anthony Park, in care of Ballard's Express. A laboratory was later equipped for Dr. Beebe in the basement of the Old Capitol Building. Dr. Beebe's numerous field investigations are reflected in the Board's reports. Dr. Beebe remained with the Board until April 1912, when he resigned to establish the Beebe Laboratories, which produced veterinary vaccines, bacterins, and anti-serum for sale to the general public.

Following Dr. Beebe's resignation, the Board asked Dr. Willard L. Boyd of the Veterinary Division of the University of Minnesota to become its bacteriologist at a salary of $1,600 per year. Although this salary was approximately $200 more than Dr. Beebe had received, Dr. Boyd nonetheless refused the offer. Thereafter, the Board of Animal Health proposed to move its laboratory to the College of Agriculture, and entered into negotiations with Dean W. F. Woods of the University of Minnesota's College of Agriculture. On July 12, 1912, the parties agreed to move the laboratory from the Old Capitol Building to the St. Paul campus of the University of Minnesota where all of the equipment would be under the Board's control. The Board would employ a laboratory assistant for six months of the year. The University of Minnesota would furnish the sup-

plies needed, and Dr. Boyd would conduct the laboratory diagnostic work for the Board of Animal Health.

EFFORTS TO GAIN PUBLIC ACCEPTANCE

Initially, the Board of Animal Health enjoyed little public support or respect. To gain acceptance as the authority on animal disease control, the Board issued regulations that contained positions generally supported by the public. One example of these efforts involved the Board's regulation of public watering troughs.

For years, villages and cities provided public watering troughs for horses as a convenience for persons coming to town to shop or to engage in other business. Some of the watering troughs were supplied by running water from a fountain or spring while others, especially in small villages, received their water from a well. These public watering troughs provided a perfect medium for the spread of respiratory diseases and glanders in horses. More observant horse owners recognized the correlation between drinking from a public watering trough and respiratory infection in their horses, and avoided watering their horses at these troughs.

In 1905, the Board took note of growing public opposition to public watering troughs. However, the Board proceeded cautiously and requested an opinion from the attorney general as to whether the Board had the authority to close public watering troughs throughout Minnesota. The attorney general opined that the Board had the necessary authority to make any regulation it deemed necessary for the suppression and control of contagious diseases. While the Board realized that it would be fiscally impossible for them to enforce the closing of all the public watering troughs, the Board nonetheless adopted a measure closing all public watering troughs and condemning these troughs as dangers to livestock health.

In 1906, the Board stepped up its efforts to regulate cattle brought into the state for breeding purposes. Great numbers of these animals entered via the South St. Paul Stockyards and were then transported throughout the state without being tested for tuberculosis. Veterinary inspector Dr. R. J. Coffeen, of Albert Lea, was hired and stationed at the South St. Paul Stockyards by the Board to inspect and test all breeding cattle brought into the state. The Board's action received the public support necessary to stop the importation of diseased breeding cattle.

BOARD REPRIMAND OF VETERINARIANS

As early as 1905, cattle owners complained that veterinarians were improperly conducting the tuberculosis test.[4] The owners variously charged some veterinarians failed to take the required number of temperatures, temperatures were falsified on the report, temperatures were not recorded, and veterinarians did not personally conduct the test. In 1908, the Board instructed the secretary and executive officer "to refuse to accept the inspection work of any veterinarian when there is good reason to believe that the work was not carried out in a competent way or [was] dishonest."

While the Board of Animal Health did not have the authority to revoke or suspend the veterinarian's license to practice, it could revoke or suspend their accreditation and thus deprive veterinarians the authority to issue health certificates.[5] The first veterinarian called before the Board was charged with failure to properly conduct the testing of a herd of cattle. The veterinarian, who was represented by counsel, was found guilty and his authority to issue health certificates was suspended. To gain reinstatement, the veterinarian was required to convince the secretary and executive officer that he would carry out the tests correctly in the future. This hearing set the format for future hearings in cases where veterinarians failed to adhere to the rules and regulations promulgated by the Board.

In 1911, the Board heard the first case involving veterinarians who falsified information on the health certificate to import cattle. Three shipments of cattle from Illinois tested for tuberculosis after their arrival were found to have four reactors. The Board obtained affidavits from the original owners stating that the cattle had not "been looked at" for tuberculosis. The Board subsequently decided to bar importation of cattle from Illinois that were not accompanied by a certificate of tuberculosis test signed by a veterinari-

an of the U.S. Bureau of Animal Industry. After a few days, the Board placed the same restrictions on cattle imported from New York to deal with a similar problem.

CHANGES IN EXECUTIVE OFFICER AND SECRETARY

In May of 1907, Dr. Ward submitted his resignation as executive officer and secretary of the Board to accept the position of Chief of the Meat Inspection Bureau for the Dominion of Canada. Dr. M. Whitcomb was elected to succeed Dr. Ward. There were other shifts in personnel as Dr. McDonald advanced to Dr. Whitcomb's former position, Dr. Coffeen was placed in the field, Dr. Lyons of Hutchinson was hired as field veterinarian, and Dr. Edmund Mackey of Janesville was hired as inspector for the South St. Paul Stockyards. In addition to his salary, Dr. Mackey received an allowance of $15 per month for the expense of keeping a horse used in his work for the Board. Dr. Mackey was the uncle of Dr. Walter Mackey of St. Paul. Dr. Ward remained only a short period of time in the position in Canada. In April 1908, Dr. Ward returned and was rehired as secretary and executive officer.

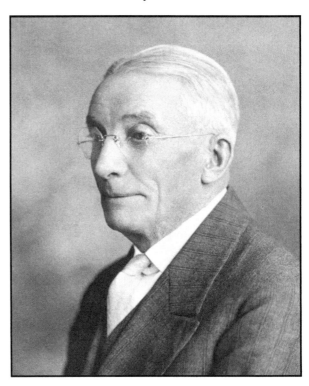

Dr. M.S. Whitcomb, secretary and executive officer, June 15, 1907-May 1, 1908. Courtesy Board of Animal Health

[4] The temperature test was used in testing for tuberculosis since this was before the development of the intradermal test.
[5] The procedure was changed in 1983 so that suspension of accreditation may now only be ordered by the U.S. Animal and Plant Health Inspection Service. The Board investigates the charges and, if a hearing is held, the Board's chief officer is "allowed" to be present and "may" give his opinion.

At approximately the same time it took action to curb falsified health certificates, the Board also formulated regulations to bar the importation of animals with infectious or contagious diseases. The Board sent these regulations to the attorney general for review. An assistant attorney general issued the opinion that "such regulations are a discrimination against the citizens of that state to which the regulation is operative." The Board apparently received the same legal opinion when it considered asking the legislature to pass a law prohibiting the importation of diseased animals as in October of 1912: "The state cannot prohibit the bringing into the state of animals from another state irrespective of whether they are infected with a contagious or dangerous disease."

In 1913, the Board tried another approach to the problem by asking the attorney general if it could prevent the importation of hog cholera virus into the state. Assistant Attorney General C. Louis Weeks informed the Board that the "Legislature of this state has no authority to prohibit the importation into this state . . . in due course of interstate shipment of hog cholera virus."

The refusal of the attorney general to approve the Board's regulations in regard to the importation of diseased animals is strange in light of the wording of the 1903 statue creating the Board. The following is from General Laws of Minnesota for 1903, Chapter 350, Section 3:

> Authority is hereby given to the state live stock sanitary board and the several local boards of health of towns, villages and cities, to take all steps they deem necessary to control, suppress and eradicate all contagious infections and diseases among any of the domestic animals in this state, . . . ; and said live stock sanitary board is hereby expressly given authority to regulate or prohibit the shipment into this state any domestic animal which is in judgment of said board may injure the health of live stock in this state; . . .

In 1914 foot and mouth disease broke out in the state of Illinois. This was a crisis situation and the Board issued a regulation prohibiting the shipment of cattle, sheep, and swine from the state of Illinois into Minnesota. The attorney gen-

eral apparently approved this regulation as there is no recording of any question about it.

The Board over the following years kept getting more power by issuing regulations to stop the importation of certain diseased animals such as dogs with rabies. Finally the Board received unquestionable authority according to the following, taken from Mason's Minnesota Statutes of 1927, Chapter 30, Section 5399:

> ". . . the state board may regulate or prohibit the bringing of domestic animals in the state, which in its opinion, for any reason, may injure the health of live stock therein."

DEATH OF DR. WARD

On December 14, 1918, Dr. Ward died of influenza. He became ill while attending a meeting of the Livestock Sanitary Association in Chicago. After being confined to his hotel room, Dr. Ward's condition eventually improved enough to return to his home in St. Paul where he died a few days later.

The sudden death of Dr. Ward was a great loss to the control of animal diseases in Minnesota. He was a patient and even tempered man who enjoyed great respect from all who

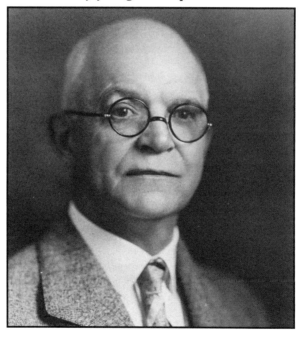

Dr. Charles E. Cotton, secretary and executive officer. Jan. 1919-Feb. 15, 1942. Courtesy Board of Animal Health.

knew him. He guided the Board from a time when there was a widespread tendency to ignore rules and regulations in regard to livestock diseases to a period when the public had begun to accept the Board's authority to control animal health issues. During his tenure in office, Dr. Ward established the foundation for the control of several diseases such as glanders, scabies, and tuberculosis. Dr. Ward was the right person for these challenging times.

At the Board's meeting following Dr. Ward's death, Dr. Charles E. Cotton announced his resignation from the Board. Dr. Cotton's resignation made him eligible to become the Board's executive officer and secretary. The Board subsequently elected Dr. Cotton to succeed Dr. Ward.

TROUBLE WITH THE GOVERNOR

In October of 1926, the College of Agriculture of the University of Minnesota notified the Board the university could not continue to furnish the laboratory services unless its funding was increased. The university requested appropriations of $7,500 for the first year and $6,000 for the second year to cover the costs of these laboratory services.

The Board of Animal Health included these amounts in its 1927 legislative request for appropriations. However, Governor Theodore Christianson refused to include these funds in his budget request. The governor felt he could persuade the university's Board of Regents to appropriate the funds necessary to perform the laboratory services for the Board.

At approximately the same time, the Board established the new position of quarantine officer. The governor recommended Sever Nelson for the position. The Board interviewed Nelson and found that he had no farm or animal experience. The Board determined that Lester Tate was better qualified and offered him the job.

Governor Christianson insisted that the Board rescind its decision and hire Mr. Nelson for the position. He further stated that, if the Board did not comply, he would order the Commission of Administration and Finance to change the employment classification so as to eliminate the position of quarantine officer. Despite the Board's attempts to explain the reason Mr. Tate was selected over Mr. Nelson for the position, Governor Christianson insisted that he had the right to have his "recommendation" accepted by the Board. The Board records reveal a series of very strong letters about this matter between Dr. Cotton and Governor Christianson.

The Board refused to rescind the appointment of Mr. Tate, and Governor Christianson proceeded to carry out his threat. The Board hired outside attorneys to defend their position. The case was delayed because Governor Christianson entered the Mayo Clinic for major surgery. Although the details of the case are unclear, Lester Tate eventually went to work for the Board and the Board's attorney's fees were forwarded to the attorney general for payment.

To relieve the financial burden of maintaining the laboratory services at the university, the Board was allowed to contribute $2,000 toward the salary of a laboratory specialist in the Division of Veterinary Medicine at the university. The Board of Regents supplied the remainder of the funds needed to pay for these services for that year. Both boards also agreed to work on a request to the legislature for approval of a supplementary budget for the laboratory. In 1929, the legislature appropriated $7,500 for maintaining the laboratory, and agreed to pay the salary of a technician for pullorum testing.

DROUGHT AND STARVING ANIMALS

In the 1930s, there was a severe drought in North and South Dakota, western Iowa, and Minnesota. Starving animals were brought by truck or railroad into the nondrought areas of northern Minnesota to graze or be fed. Some animals were even driven on foot across the Minnesota border.

Some of the animals went to grazing land where previous arrangements had been made with the owner. Other animals were taken to the northern part of Minnesota and turned loose on state and federal land. The owners planned to return in the late fall or winter to "round up" the animals. However, subsequent attempts to catch these animals were not very successful because they had become very wild during the interim. As a result, many of the animals who were not caught fell prey to wild animals and hunters.

The majority of the animals that were imported during this time entered the state without health certificates. To avoid detection, many of these animals were taken across the state line at night and on little traveled roads. In addition to their threat as possible carriers of disease, these animals also had less resistance to disease because of their debilitated condition.

With the importation of thousands of these animals, great concern arose as to whether there would be sufficient grazing land in the non-drought area for starving Minnesota animals. This concern increased with the leasing of grazing land by speculators for imported animals. These concerns prompted a group to meet with Governor Floyd B. Olson on May 31, 1934.

Dr. C. E. Cotton was called to the governor's office where a conference involving representatives of the federal and state drought officials was in session. Among those present were Dean W. C. Coffey, University of Minnesota; Dr. M.I.V. Shears; Colonel M. T. Morgan; Mr. R. E. Miller; Mr. F. M. Rarig, Jr.; Mr. L. T. Zimmerman; Mr. H. T. Forsburg, the Commissioner of Agriculture; R. A. Trovatten; Mr. E. L. Aamodt; and Adjutant General E. E. Walsh.

The governor explained to Dr. Cotton that he was going to issue an executive order preventing the movement of livestock from drought counties into nondrought counties. However, the governor noted that from a legal standpoint the only authority he had to issue such an embargo was derived from the Board of Animal Health's power to protect the health of the livestock and to inspect livestock prior to importation. The governor observed that a larger number of livestock would be imported for feeding and grazing, and it would be impossible for the Board to ensure that all of these animals would be properly inspected and certified free of disease.

The governor asked Dr. Cotton to work with the attorney general to prepare an executive order. The executive order was prepared and signed by the governor on that same afternoon. The hastily prepared executive order was subsequently modified later that same day to allow livestock to enter the state for immediate slaughter at an establishment that provided for a federal government inspection. The order was further amended to allow importation of feeder cattle for finishing in a dry lot feedlot under special permit.

Adjutant General Walsh, who was directed to assist in carrying out the embargo, insisted that he would not attempt to police the borders unless he was able to do it properly. To provide the necessary manpower, Governor Floyd Olson ordered out the National Guard effective Saturday, June 2, 1934. On that date, troops were stationed along the western border of Minnesota. On the following Monday, June 4, 1934, troops were also placed on the western half of the southern Minnesota border.

On Thursday, June 14, 1934, the Governor withdrew the National Guard from the borders and ordered the Minnesota Highway Patrol to police the highways to maintain the embargo. The State Patrol was ordered to stop all trucks with livestock and check for the proper health certificate. This arrangement failed, and on June 21, 1934, the governor dissolved the embargo explaining that a change in climatic conditions had reduced the need for an embargo. The Board of Animal Health subsequently rescinded the rules and regulations it had adopted as the result of the governor's executive order. Livestock could again enter Minnesota freely if accompanied by an official health certificate.

SALES BARNS AND COMMUNITY SALES

Another method of marketing livestock made its appearance during the drought era of the 1930s. Owners of livestock would assemble their animals at a central point for sale at auction. These sales were eventually held at regular intervals in converted barns or sheds, giving rise to the name "sales barn." Most of these sales were later held in a building specifically designed for that purpose. Livestock auctions were also held by breed associations to sell breeding stock.

At the same time, a new type of livestock auction made its appearance as part of trade promotion for a village or city. These auctions were often held annually, and were referred to as community auctions.

In 1934, three sales barns were in operation in Minnesota. By the end of 1935, there were sixteen sales barns operating in Minnesota. Sales barns sold cattle imported from the drought areas of Iowa, North Dakota, and South Dakota, as well as animals raised in Minnesota. The animals imported from out of state that went directly to slaughter did not pose a threat of disease. However, many of these imported animals, because they were very thin in flesh, were transported to Minnesota farms to improve their physical condition. Most of these animals eventually went to market as soon as their physical condition warranted, but some were used as breeding stock. Of course, when animals from these sources were assembled, the likelihood of exposure to an infectious disease greatly increased. The problems associated with animals being disseminated from auction sales prompted the Board to issue regulations in 1935 pertaining to the operation of sales barns and community sales.

The Board's regulations required the operators of the auction sales to obtain a permit to conduct livestock auction sales. Operators were required to hire a veterinarian who had been approved by the Board and would represent the Board at auction sales. The veterinarian would inspect the premises and the animals being offered for sale, supervise the dipping of sheep, administer antihog cholera serum, issue quarantines, and administer other disease control measures deemed necessary. The Board further required all animals imported from out of state to have an official health certificate.

For the most part, there were and are many fine and honorable persons associated with the operation of sales barns, and there were and are many highly regarded and respected veterinarians who act as agents of the Board of Animal Health at the sales. However, the regulations have been violated frequently since they were promulgated in 1935. Most of the violations are such that a warning is sufficient to correct the problem. However, there have been other violations of a more serious nature where the Board has suspended the operations of sales barns for a period of time and even required changes in management. The Board has also suspended veterinarians from acting as Board agents at the sales.

Sales barns attracted livestock dealers, or "jockeys," who buy and sell animals. These persons made their living by outwitting other participants in the sales, and to be successful they had to be "sharp." The jockeys merely regarded the regulations to control diseases as another challenge. They were quick to identify and take advantage of loopholes in the regulations. They would interpret the regulations in a way that would circumvent the Board's intent, and they always raised situations that they claimed were exceptions to the rules. To deal with those dealers who tried to obtain unfair advantages, veterinarians at the sales barns had to be on their constant guard and remain thoroughly familiar with the regulations. If they learned or sensed that the veterinarian was a little vague or uncertain on a rule, these dealers would exploit the situation to the fullest extent. The dealers sought to put the veterinarians in a position where they could exert pressure on the veterinarian to make a decision in a gray area that would be favorable to them or, alternatively, convince the veterinarian to overlook violations of the regulations.

Examples of some of the ploys that the dealers would use involved brucellosis testing at the sales barns. They would typically arrive with a load of cattle just as the sale was starting or otherwise wait until the sale had started before they would unload their cattle. The dealers hoped the veterinarian would be too rushed to complete the proper test and inspection before the animals were due to enter the sales ring. They knew that the veterinarian had to draw a blood sample, wait for the sample to clot, and then draw off serum to run the plate test. In this rushed situation, the dealer would have one or more clinical brucellosis reactors in the load. This was to test the veterinarian as to whether he would take short cuts to have the animals sold that day. If the animals passed the test and were allowed to be sold as free from brucellosis, the next load would have more clinical reactors in it.

Another ploy used by these unscrupulous dealers involved the presentation of an outdated brucellosis test chart with manure conveniently soiling the effective date. The dealers would, of course, claim the test occurred on a date that made the chart acceptable under the regulations. A variation of this same trick involved the claim that the veterinarian who conducted the test had been confused and had written the wrong test date.

Other examples of these ploys occurred in vaccination certificates of swine when hog cholera was prevalent. The veterinarian would record the date of vaccination, the number of pigs, and their size on the certificate. Some dealers would substitute "stunted" pigs for those animals referred to on the certificate and, unless he was alert, the veterinarian would not notice that the pigs were older than stated on the certificate. In cases where the pigs were not sold and were not accompanied by a vaccination certificate, the dealers would claim that they had been vaccinated and the certificate would be supplied later. This ploy was used to avoid payment for the administration of hog cholera antiserum to the pigs. In the event any of these actions were detected, the dealers would invariably blame someone else, usually the veterinarian.

There were many cases in which the dealers clearly violated the regulations and were simply betting they would not be caught. Frequently, dealers imported animals without an official health certificate. The animals would sometimes go directly to the sales barn and at other times be unloaded at a farm in the state where they would then be transported to the sales barn. If animals had ear tags that would indicate their place of origin, the tags would be removed and perhaps replaced by counterfeit ear tags. Some sales barn operators were involved in the illegal importation of animals for the purpose of increasing the volume of their barn in a manner that would avoid the expense and delay in obtaining an official health certificate.

Generally, sales barns had the reputation of being dirty and unethical places where unhealthy or nonproductive animals were sold. The number of sales barns owned and managed by responsible persons gradually increased until, with a very few exceptions, sales barns became known as healthy and responsible operations. The second generation of owners and managers had better business training and were more interested in long-term returns than in a "quick buck" from questionable dealings. They improved the facilities and made conditions more sanitary. Sales have come to be known as livestock auction markets. Swine auction markets have also been developed.

Today, if a person purchases an animal at a livestock auction market that is not honestly represented, or nonproductive, or introduces disease into the herd, the likelihood of a lawsuit is high. Thus, the managers of the auction markets do the best to comply with all of the rules and regulations. This lessens the possibility of a lawsuit but increases the amount of work for the managers. They must keep more complete records in regard to testing, vaccinations, and the origin of animals. In 1990, there were 63 livestock auction and swine auction markets operating in Minnesota.

DR. COTTON RETIRES, REPLACED BY DR. WEST

Dr. C. E. Cotton retired as secretary and executive officer of the Board of Animal Health on February 15, 1942, after 24 years of service. Dr. Cotton had begun his career as a practitioner in Minneapolis and had done considerable tuberculosis testing of cattle. Dr. Cotton also was employed by the railroads as an expert witness. In the early days, railroad right-of-ways in many areas were not fenced. Livestock would often wander onto the railroad tracks and be struck by a train. The livestock owners would occasionally sue the railroad for the loss of their animals. In many of these cases, Dr. Cotton appeared as a wit-

ness for the railroad. This litigation experience helped prepare him for subsequent court cases that involved the Board of Animal Health.

Dr. Cotton was never known to back away from a fight. This was a quality that the Board needed during his tenure in office to keep the disease control programs moving forward. Dr. Cotton always gave veterinarians in the state his unqualified support when he believed that they were in the right. On the other hand, if he believed that a veterinarian had made a mistake or committed some transgression, he would not hesitate to call the veterinarian on the telephone and air his opinion in no uncertain terms. In these instances, there would be no opportunity for rebuttal or explanation because, when he had finished talking, Dr. Cotton would slam down the receiver and end the conversation.

During Dr. Cotton's term as chief officer of the Board of Animal Health, glanders was eradicated, Minnesota became a modified accredited tuberculosis-free state, and a firm foundation was established for the control of brucellosis and several other diseases.

Dr. Ralph L. West was selected by the Board to succeed Dr. Cotton as secretary and executive officer. Prior to his appointment, Dr. West had been a practitioner in the Waseca area for 22 years. To prepare himself for the position of sec-

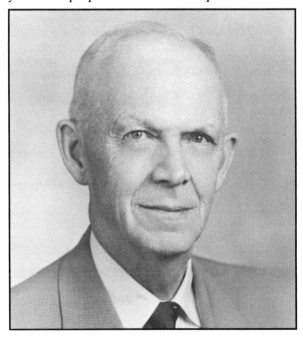

Dr. Ralph L. West, secretary and executive officer, Feb. 16, 1942-Dec. 31, 1969. Courtesy Board of Animal Health.

retary and executive officer, Dr. West began working as a field veterinarian for the Board on June 30, 1941.

REORGANIZATION OF STAFF AND BOARD

On July, 1, 1947, laws modifying civil service classification and salary schedules for state employees went into effect. This resulted in the implementation of civil service examinations, and staff reorganization as follows: Dr. W. C. Bromaghim became assistant secretary; Dr. George E. Keller was placed in charge of Bang's disease (brucellosis); and Dr. L. E. Jenkins became responsible for diseases of poultry.

GARBAGE FEEDING

For many years, some swine producers collected garbage that contained food wastes from restaurants and butcher shops to feed their hogs. Over time, this practice raised objections because of public health hazards such as trichinosis in persons eating insufficiently cooked pork, and the unsanitary conditions in which much of the garbage was collected. Several states experienced hog cholera outbreaks as a result of the feeding of uncooked garbage. Many of the collecting vehicles were uncovered, had objectionable odors, and attracted flies in warm weather.

In 1953, the Board issued regulations for the collection and cooking of garbage that was fed to hogs. The cooking guidelines were intended to prevent the spread of trichinosis that might result from consuming pork and to reduce the spread of hog cholera. The Board required garbage to be heated throughout for 30 minutes at 212 degrees Fahrenheit. The cost of the equipment necessary to comply with the regulation caused many garbage feeders to cease operation. There has been a decline from a high of 42 garbage feeding permits issued in the 1966-1967 fiscal year to 3; the number remained at 5 or below until 1991-1992, when it increased to 10. (See Table III-2.) This was due to eating places having trouble disposing of their garbage.

TABLE III-2

GARBAGE FEEDING PERMITS
ISSUED BY BOARD OF ANIMAL HEALTH

Fiscal Year	Number
1966-67	42
1967-68	37
1968-69	35
1969-70	26
1970-71	19
1971-72	19
1972-73	13
1973-74	9
1974-75	10
1975-76	5
1976-77	5
1977-78	4
1978-79	4
1979-80	4
1980-90	3
1990-91	5
1991-92	10
1992-93	13
1993-94	14

Source: Courtesy of Dr. Robert Pyle, Board of Animal Health.

KEEPING FOOT AND MOUTH DISEASE OUT OF MINNESOTA

In 1914, animals in Illinois were diagnosed with aphthous fever, also known as foot and mouth disease. On November 7, 1914, the Board issued a regulation prohibiting importation of cattle, sheep, swine, hides, skins, or hoofs of cattle, sheep, or other ruminants, hay, straw, similar fodder, or manure from Illinois. The regulation provided exceptions for those animals consigned for immediate slaughter in a plant where there was government inspection, and carcasses could be imported if the hides, horns, and hoofs had been removed. On February 26, 1915, the scope of this regulation was expanded to include other states, including Iowa and Wisconsin.

In the spring of 1915, a shipment of cattle destined for sale to farmers in Minnesota arrived in South St. Paul from Chicago, an area under quarantine for foot and mouth disease. The Board ordered the shipment promptly returned to Chicago. There were no further attempts to evade the quarantine by shipping cattle to Minnesota.

On August 11, 1915, the Bureau of Animal Industry's inspector in Chicago advised the Board that "hog cholera serum" suspected of being contaminated with foot and mouth disease had been shipped to West Concord, Minnesota. Dr. S. H. Ward, chief officer of the Board, and Dr. D. B. Palmer, field veterinarian and father of Dr. Richard Palmer, immediately went to West Concord where they were met by a Bureau of Animal Industry veterinarian. Once they learned that the serum had been administered four days previous to their arrival, the veterinarians assumed the cattle were infected. For purposes of preventing a possible outbreak of the disease all of the cattle on the premises were appraised, killed, and buried.

A quarantine, effective August 14, 1915, was established in Kenyon, Cherry Grove, and Roscoe Townships of Goodhue County, and in Ellington, Concord, Milton, Claremont, Wasioja, and Mantorville Townships of Dodge County. On September 2, the quarantine was scaled back to include only the territory in Goodhue and Dodge Counties within a three-mile radius of the premises of A. H. Evarts, Section 12, Concord Township, Dodge County. Eventually, the entire quarantine was lifted after authorities could find no evidence of the disease.

Foot and mouth disease appeared in Texas in 1925, and later in California in 1929. These were the last instances of foot and mouth disease diagnosed in the United States. At both times, the Board issued a regulation similar to the one issued when foot and mouth disease broke out in Illinois. The Bureau of Animal Industry quarantined the infected areas and enforced the quarantine.

In 1952, there was an outbreak of foot and mouth disease in the Province of Saskatchewan, Canada. The Board ordered the northern borders of the state closely watched to prevent the entrance of Canadian cattle. The outbreak, which proved to be minor, was quickly contained and eradicated. From 1946 to 1953, there was a serious outbreak of foot and mouth disease in Mexico.

In 1949, Dr. W. G. Andberg, Anoka, Minnesota, reported mouth lesions in two herds of cattle. The Board sent Dr. W. L. Boyd to investigate. In July 1949, Dr. Boyd reported that the disease was vesicular stomatitis. By September, the disease had spread into northeastern Minnesota. However, during the following winter, the incidence of vesicular stomatitis decreased markedly.

In 1952, another disease appeared in Minnesota that had lesions similar to foot and mouth disease. The disease primarily affected swine, but also affected cattle. Fearing that the disease might be foot and mouth disease, the Board banned the importation of swine except for immediate slaughter. The Board also banned the exhibition of swine at fairs and other shows and the sale of swine in the state except under special permit given for feeding purposes. The disease was eventually diagnosed as vesicular exanthema.

DR. WEST RETIRES AND IS SUCCEEDED BY DR. FLINT

Dr. R. L. West retired as the Board's secretary and executive officer at the age of 71 on December 31, 1959, after 17 years of service. Dr. West introduced the Board to many ideas that the veterinarians in the field had conceived to control disease. He was an extremely hard worker who was always the last one to leave the office on regular working days. He opened the office on Saturday forenoons in case there was an emergency, and he always came to the office on Saturdays to work with those on duty except when he went out to investigate a possible disease outbreak. While Dr. West would carefully consider alternative programs, he did not veer from a course of action once he had made up his mind.

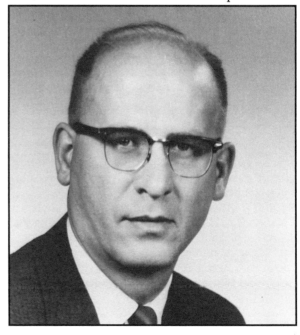

Dr. Jack G. Flint, secretary and executive officer, Board of Animal Health, Jan. 1, 1960-Dec. 31, 1984. Courtesy Board of Animal Health.

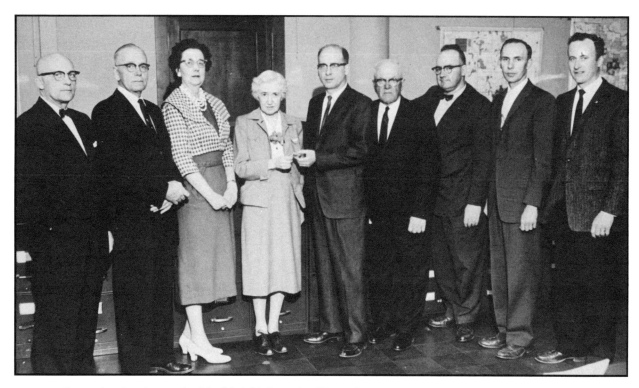

Presenation of service award to Miss Marie McGee, early 1850s; staff and members of the board, left to right, Dr. Ralph Bergman, Lester Tate, Miss Evelyn Rolfing, Miss Marie McGee. Dr. Jack Flint, E.H. Knodt, Clem Chase, Dr. Henry Ruebke, Dr. James Flanary.

He was so involved in carrying out the programs that, at times, it was difficult for him to delegate responsibility to others on the staff.

When he took office, Dr. West faced many challenges in maintaining existing disease control programs. One of his most perplexing problems was caused by the shortage of veterinarians during World War II. He also was challenged by the low salary that he could offer to veterinarians to work for the Board. As a result of these two problems, the Board's testing programs fell behind schedule. But Dr. West did manage to bring the test programs back on schedule after the war. During his tenure, programs to eradicate tuberculosis continued and great strides were made in the control of brucellosis.

Dr. Jack Flint, Faribault, Minnesota, was elected to succeed Dr. West effective January 1, 1960. Dr. Flint spent seven of his twelve years of practice in Faribault. Dr. Flint began employment with the Board on April 1, 1956, and became the Board's assistant secretary in July 1958. In addition to his state duties, Dr. West was also very active on the national level. He served on several AVMA committees and, in 1952, he was the president of the U.S. Animal Health Association.

INDEPENDENT STATUS OF BOARD IN DANGER

The Board of Animal Health is an independent body that is appointed by the governor and is therefore responsible to him for matters of policy. The Board members are appointed to staggered terms and the Board itself selects its executive secretary. These features enable the Board to carry out unpopular policies without undue political pressures.

There have been several attempts over the years to place the Board under the authority of the commissioner of agriculture who is a political appointee that serves at the pleasure of the governor. The commissioner is therefore sensitive to political pressure from members of the agricultural industry. If it was placed under the commissioner of agriculture, the Board's budget requests would be subject to the commissioner's approval before being submitted to the governor. The commissioner could lower the budget request so as to hinder the enforcement of particular rules or regulations. The commissioner also could put pressure on the Board to modify programs for disease control so they would be less effective.

Most of the attempts to place the Board of Animal Health under the commissioner of agriculture took place "behind the scenes" outside the view of the public.

The most serious attempt to place the Board under the Commissioner of Agriculture occurred in 1968. Governor Harold LeVander created the Governor's Council on Executive Reorganization. Although the council was made up of an impressive panel of fifty-three persons,

Governor's Reorganization Plans Are Under Attack

ST. PAUL (AP) — Administration proposals to streamline state government operations came in for a tug-of-war at a meeting of some 300 interested parties in the state office building auditorium Monday night.

Gov. Freeman and Arthur Naftalin, administration commissioner, presided at the session designed to sample reaction to the program which lost out both in the 1955 and 1957 legislatures.

Main feature of the reorganization plan, expected to be introduced as one bill this session centers around regrouping some 105 functions within 10 departments, three of them new ones.

Naftalin said the ideal situation would be to have 10 appointed commissioners, plus their deputies, with everyone else in state government under civil service.

Would Reduce, Appointees

He said this would greatly reduce the number of appointees and assure a continuity in government experience in the lower ranks.

Loudest objections came over proposals to incorporate the Iron Range Resources and Rehabilitation Commission within the framework of a newly - created commerce department, put the Livestock Sanitary Board and Soil Conservation Department under the Agriculture Department, and have the labor conciliator under a new department of labor.

The third new department would involve state colleges.

Reps. Jack Fena of Hibbing and Peter Fugina of Virginia and Sen. Elmer Peterson of Hibbing argued against revamping the current set-up of the Iron Range Resources and Rehabilitation Commission.

Veterinarians Give Support

Backing up the Livestock Sanitary Board in opposition to the proposed change were representatives of the Veterinary Medical Assn., South St. Paul Union Stockyards and the Turkey Growers Assn.

Otto Christenson, vice president of the Minnesota Employers Assn. said he was expressing the sentiment of practically every industry in voicing objection to the labor conciliation change.

Freeman's proposal to combine the Youth Conservation Commission Parole Board and penal institutions under a division of corrections within the Welfare Department also drew fire.

Judge Theodore Knutson, of Hennepin County District Court, spoke against the suggested change on behalf of the State Assn. of District Judges. He said the association feels corrections should be a separate department, not part of a division, and equal to the other 10.

From Albert Lea Tribune, Feb. 3, 1959

only one of them, Mr. Norris Carnes, had any meaningful contact with the livestock industry. The council, among other things, recommended that the Live Stock Sanitary Board (Board of Animal Health) be transferred to the Department of Agriculture. Governor LeVander eventually endorsed legislation that contained this recommendation. However, the veterinary profession, led by the Minnesota Veterinary Medical Association and with the help of livestock organizations, rallied their forces to successfully defeat the proposed legislation.

To date, all attempts to transfer the Board of Animal Health have been similarly defeated. However, future attempts are inevitable. In times of budget shortfalls, there is a tendency to search for ways to make state government more efficient. Unfortunately, because those persons who are appointed to consider these issues know little of animal disease problems, transfer of the Board of Animal Health to another department appears to make sense to cut administrative costs. However, this narrow approach is unwise and should be guarded against in the future.

DISEASES THAT HAVE DEFIED ERADICATION

There are some diseases that, because of their very nature, have defied eradication efforts in Minnesota. Some of these diseases have been a problem since the 1800s and early 1900s, while other diseases are of more recent origin.

ANAPLASMOSIS

Anaplasmosis is a disease that has appeared relative recently in Minnesota. The first outbreak worthy of note occurred near Worthington in 1949. State Senator Davis of Worthington imported a group of cattle that, upon arrival, became sick and were placed under quarantine. After laboratory tests diagnosed sweet clover poisoning, the quarantine was dissolved and Senator Davis disposed of the cattle at auction. After the cattle were sold and dispersed, further laboratory tests revealed that the cattle had anaplasmosis. The Board immediately located all of the cattle that had been sold at the auction, and quarantined those which had not yet been sent to slaughter, or castrated, or dehorned on the farms. In all, 287 cattle on 15 farms were quarantined, all of which were sent to slaughter.

Cases of anaplasmosis continued to increase. In 1970, the Board found it necessary to modify its approach from quarantine and slaugh-ter of the exposed animals toward programs where owners could choose treatment. While the herd was quarantined as before when reactors were disclosed, owners of nondairy herds could elect to treat the animals at their expense or to slaughter reactors without indemnity. Owners of dairy herds had the option to slaughter the reactors with indemnity or retain the reactors and treat them when not lactating.

Because of the importation of cattle from southern states, anaplasmosis has become more widespread in Minnesota, and is now also found in herds with no history of imported cattle. Anaplasmosis titers have recently been found in deer. Thus, it appears that the disease has become endemic in Minnesota.

ANTHRAX

The first reference to anthrax in Minnesota was made in 1884. In 1908, the Board of Animal Health reported a case of anthrax in Dakota County. By 1911, the Board declared the Mississippi River flats in Dakota County were the most widely infected area in the state. The Board issued regulations for handling and disposing of animals that had died of anthrax. The regulations provided that the remains of anthrax infected animals must be either cremated or buried no less than six feet deep.

During the summer of 1919, an outbreak of anthrax near Montevideo involved animals in Lac qui Parle, Yellow Medicine, and Chippewa Counties. The area was placed under quarantine and a vaccination program was instituted. Forty-six farms were infected before the outbreak was brought under control. By fall, the quarantine had been lifted with the exception of a few infected farms. However, the difficulty of eliminating the disease is reflected by the fact that at least 15 outbreaks occurred in the Montevideo area from 1919 to 1952.

Anthrax is characterized by long-term survival of the organism in soil. Under favorable conditions in warm and damp alkaline soil, the anthrax organism has been reported to survive for 37 and 60 years. In 1949, reports stated that anthrax had appeared on 147 Minnesota farms over the preceding forty years.

The current measures employed to control anthrax involve quarantine and mandatory vaccination in areas where anthrax has appeared within the past 10 years. While the incidence of the disease has decreased, anthrax has been diagnosed in Pope County as recently as 1984.

EQUINE ENCEPHALOMYELITIS

In the midst of the problems created in the 1930s by the drought, equine encephalomyelitis, or sleeping sickness, appeared

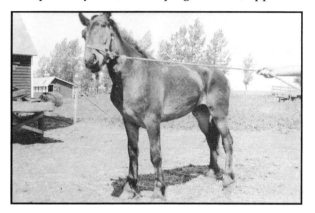

Equine Encephalomyelitis (sleeping sickness)

in Minnesota. The first case of sleeping sickness was diagnosed by Dr. C. H. Wetter of Princeton, Minnesota, from clinical signs in 1933. During the 1934-1935 fiscal year, sleeping sickness was again diagnosed in Nobles, Cottonwood, and Murray Counties. Quarantines that were placed on the premises to prevent spread were unsuccessful. The erratic incidence of the disease is shown in Table III.

TABLE III-3

INCIDENCE OF EQUINE ENCEPHALOMYELITIS

Year	Cases	Deaths
1934	330	110
1935	3,337	1,244
1936	112	31
1937	45,275	10,120
1938	23,368	4,979
1939	691	176
1940	409	101
1941	6,777	1,320
1942	319	49
1943	423	109
1944	1,470	307
1945	182	45

Source: Board of Animal Health records.

When equine encephalomyelitis first appeared in Minnesota, no effective treatment or method of prevention was available. With the exception of nursing care, treatment varied from veterinarian to veterinarian. Almost every imaginable type of drug treatment was used to combat the disease. Once it became established in a community, sleeping sickness spread rapidly. Veterinarians worked long hours with little sleep. Many veterinarians hired people to drive their cars and would take naps between farms. Because veterinarians were so busy and because there was no effective treatment, "quacks" began to offer treatments for sleeping sickness. The quacks revived bloodletting and other treatments that had previously been discarded as worthless. The quacks were helped by the fact that an occasional case would make a satisfactory recovery regardless of the treatment.

Many drugs and procedures were developed to treat the disease. An anti-encephalitis serum became available and appeared to have some benefit if given early in the disease. However, the serum was in limited supply and quite expensive. Later, a vaccine prepared from horse brain was used on an experimental basis. The potency of this vaccine varied and some horses experienced a severe local reaction. In 1938, a chick embryo vaccine was introduced by Lederle Laboratories that proved much more effective in preventing the disease than the horse brain product. The vaccine was given subcutaneously and intramuscularly in about three different sites in the cervical region. Two 10-milliliter doses of the vaccine were given to the animals 7 to 10 days apart. Some horses had a local reaction to the vaccine. In 1941, a refined vaccine became available. This vaccine was given intradermally in two 1 milliliter doses. This product, which was also developed by Lederle Laboratories, was in short supply until other laboratories began to produce it under a royalty agreement.

The severity of the equine encephalomyelitis outbreak speeded the replacement of draft horses by tractors as the source of power for farm work. After the outbreak of the disease was brought under control, the majority of the farmers who still did use horses as work animals continued to practice vaccination. In later years, when pleasure or light horses have become popular, the owners have, as a rule, maintained their horses on a vaccination program to prevent equine encephalomyelitis. Consequently, there have been only sporadic cases of the disease in horses in recent years. However, because of the reservoir of infection in wild life, a large percent of the horses must continue to be vaccinated each year to prevent another outbreak of the disease.

EQUINE INFECTIOUS ANEMIA (EIA)

Equine infectious anemia was an important disease in the early days of the Board of Animal Health. The disease was called "swamp fever" because it was more common in horses located near low lands. In 1907, the Board began supporting a swamp fever research project through the University of Minnesota. The Bureau of Animal Industry later cooperated in the project, which continued until 1917.

The disease was difficult to diagnose because it resembled other diseases at certain phases. The initial diagnosis on a farm was often made in an advanced case where the anemia was severe.

With the replacement of the draft horse by the tractor and the accompanying drop in the horse population, equine infectious anemia became less of a concern. However, the disease became a problem again when the light horse became popular. The spread of equine infectious anemia was also aided by the transportation of horses through sales, horse shows, and racing. Diagnosis was hampered by the lack of a reliable laboratory test that could be easily performed. The development of the Coggins test[6] enabled earlier diagnosis with a higher degree of confidence. Since 1974, imported horses were required to test negative to the Coggins test.

PSEUDORABIES

Pseudorabies, or PRV, variously known as Aujeszky's disease, "mad itch," and infectious bulbar paralysis, has occurred as a sporadic disease of cattle in the United States since the early 1800s. In the 1970s, a more virulent form of the pseudorabies virus appeared in swine herds throughout the country. The disease caused losses as high as 100 percent in very young pigs.

In the United States the more virulent form of the virus appeared first in Indiana, and then in Ohio, Illinois, and Iowa. The disease spread rapidly in all of these states. In 1975, two cases of pseudorabies were the first ever diagnosed in Minnesota. The disease spread rapidly in Minnesota. See Table III-4. In 1980, 69 herds were infected. By 1982, the number of infected herds had increased to 132. The losses in many

[6] Agar gel immunodiffusion test (AGID).

swine herds were very severe and caused great financial hardships for the producers. Much of the early spread of PRV was due to the movement of untested breeding swine and feeder pigs. Many herd infections were traced to Iowa herds.

TABLE III-4

INCIDENCE OF PSEUDORABIES IN MINNESOTA AS REPORTED TO BOARD OF ANIMAL HEALTH

Year	Positive Herds
1975	2
1976	13
1977	26
1978	21
1979	53
1980	69
1981	132
1982	101
1983	82
1984	72
1985	145
1986	77
1987	109
1988	172
1989	253
1990	294
1991	396

Note: Due to the reluctance of owners to have their herds quarantined, it is believed that only part of the infected herds were reported during 1982, 1983, and 1984. To avoid being quarantined, owners would refuse to call a veterinarian when they suspected pseudorabies or would insist that none of their animals be tested and that no specimens be sent to a laboratory for diagnosis.

The increase in cases reported for 1985 is believed to be due to required testing of breeding swine sold and the new pseudorabies control rules.

Source: Courtesy of Dr. Walter J. Mackey, Board of Animal Health.

Animal health officials in Iowa had allowed the wide use of vaccines. When pseudorabies began to spread in Minnesota, swine producers and veterinarians pressured the Board of Animal Health for the same freedom to use vaccines. There was no agreement among the authorities as to the best method to control pseudorabies, and there was no uniform program for its control in the states where it was present. Thus, the Board decided to allow the use of pseudorabies vaccines with few restrictions.

In late 1978, the Board decided that further measures were needed to control the spread of pseudorabies and issued rules for its control, effective 1979. The rules provided for quarantine of the herd if a reactor was diagnosed by official pseudorabies test, clinical diagnosis, or laboratory diagnosis. The rules also outlined the procedure for establishing a qualified pseudorabies negative herd. The rules also required that vaccinations were to be performed by an accredited veterinarian, and that the vaccinated animals must be identified with a numbered pink ear tag. Finally, vaccinations had to be promptly reported to the Board.

The seemingly unchecked spread of pseudorabies caused heavy losses. A study by the Board of Animal Health in 1983 indicated that the livestock industry in Minnesota lost approximately $1,000,000 per month due to pseudorabies. Among veterinarians and swine producers, there was much disagreement on how to deal with the disease and many proposals on how to control pseudorabies, including learning to live with the disease; uncontrolled vaccinating; testing herds for pseudorabies and slaughtering the reactors; and eliminating the disease by depopulation.

Vaccination programs received popular support for the control of pseudorabies because vaccinations are relatively inexpensive, reduce the severity of the outbreak, reduce the death loss in infected herds, and are less disruptive for swine operation. Moreover, the other methods proposed to treat infected herds were difficult for the individual swine producers to apply.

Opponents of vaccination based their opinion on the fact that vaccination does not produce a solid immunity against the disease. A vaccinated animal, when exposed to pseudorabies, could develop a latent infection. An animal which contracted an infection following vaccination would not exhibit any of the clinical signs of an unvaccinated animal with pseudorabies, but would nonetheless be a carrier of the virus with the ability to spread the disease. Thus, while it could lessen the severity of an outbreak, vaccination could not eradicate pseudorabies because of the "carrier status" of exposed swine.

Some of the leaders of the swine industry were hesitant to admit that the disease was a serious problem. As late as 1982, swine organizations in Minnesota sought to remove all pseudorabies regulations, including quarantines, and let the swine producers control the disease through vaccination. These suggestions were rejected by the Board of Animal Health.

In 1982, the Board of Animal Health set up the Pseudorabies Advisory Committee in an effort to obtain input and support from the swine industry on the problem of pseudorabies. The committee was composed of representatives from the swine producers, auction markets, packing industry, South St. Paul Stockyards, practicing veterinarians, and the College of Veterinary Medicine. See Exhibit III-1. Dr. Flint, the Board's secretary and executive officer, was also a member of the committee. Dr. Robert A. Martens of Nicollet, Minnesota was chairman of the Committee.

EXHIBIT III- 1

PSEUDORABIES ADVISORY COMMITTEE MEMBERSHIP LIST

Minnesota Pork Producers Association appointees:
> Mr. George Coy, West Concord
> Mr. Jim Girard, Lynd
> Mr. Merlin Mackenthun, Brownton
> Mr. Ron Westrich, Bertrum
> Mr. Todd Resler, Owatonna
> Mr. Jim Lewis, Welcome

Minnesota Purebred Producers Association appointees:
> Mr. Arno Moenning, Dodge Center
> Mr. Ben Bartusek, New Prague
> Mr. Allen Routh, Owatonna

Minnesota Livestock Breeders Association appointees:
> Mr. Keith Thurston, Madelia
> Mr. Paul Pierson, Lake City
> Mr. Mike Casky, Holland

Minnesota Veterinary Medical Association appointees:
> Dr. Conrad Schmidt, Worthington
> Dr. Bob Martens, Nicollet
> Dr. Milton Stensland, Austin

(Exhibit II-1 continued)

Other appointees:

Mr. Frank Schiefelbein, Kimball, Minnesota Cattlemens Association

Dr. Jack Flint, St. Paul, Board of Animal Health

Mr. Dale Melin, Sauk Center, Feeder Pig Dealer

Mr. Don Kampmeier, South St. Paul, Central Livestock Association

Dr. Jerry Hawton, St. Paul, Animal Science, University of Minnesota

Dr. David Thawley, St. Paul, Veterinary College, University of Minnesota

Other nonvoting resource members:

Mr. Neal Black, St. Paul, Livestock Conservation Institute

Dr. Page Eppele, St. Paul, U.S. Department of Agriculture

Dr. Martin Bergeland, St. Paul, Diagnostic Lab, University of Minnesota

Dr. Bob Morrison, St. Paul, Veterinary College, University of Minnesota

Dr. Kent Kislingbury, Fairmont, Fairmont Veterinary Clinic

Dr. Rodney Johnson, Morris, American Swine Practitioners

Mr. Jim Lieske, Henderson, Lieske Genetics

Mr. Vern Ingvalson, St. Paul, Farm Bureau

Mr. Willis Eken, St. Paul, Farmers Union

The conscientious and hard working group met for five full day sessions over an 18 month period. The committee eventually came to the conclusion that the swine industry in Minnesota was not prepared to support an eradication program. The committee developed a program designed to control the spread of pseudorabies that was accepted by the Board of Animal Health.

In the meantime, the 1983 Minnesota legislature passed a law requiring the Board of Animal Health to adopt a program to control pseudorabies in swine, including pseudorabies testing of breeding swine sold in Minnesota, and control of the movement of feeder pigs to prevent the spread of the disease.

To carry out the mandate of the legislature, the Board adopted the program that had been developed by the Pseudorabies Advisory Committee. Committee members helped get the proposed rules through the public hearings required by law, and the Board's rules were formally adopted by the rule promulgation process on July 23, 1984.

These new rules strengthened those regulations adopted in 1979. When a herd of swine was quarantined, all livestock owners within a radius of one mile were to be notified by the Board. If swine had been purchased within 12 months of the diagnosis of infection, the new regulations required attempts to locate the source of the infection by testing 10 percent of the herd from which the purchased swine originated. Another provision of the rules required that, when an animal of another species should die on a farm of signs that could be pseudorabies, 10 percent of the swine herd would be tested for that disease. This procedure is supported by the rationale that other species are more severely affected by pseudorabies, and are thus more likely to die and provide an earlier diagnosis of the disease on the farm.

The new regulations also clarified the establishment of a qualified pseudorabies negative herd. Owners whose herds achieve this herd status can sell breeding swine without testing each animal sold. These herds must have been free from pseudorabies for the past 12 months. To retain that classification, at least 25 percent of the breeding herd must be tested every 80 to 90 days, and the entire herd has to be tested every year. A positive test at any time disqualifies the herd as a qualified pseudorabies negative herd.

The new rules also established the pseudorabies-controlled vaccinated herd. As the title suggests, vaccination of a negative breeding herd is an important part of this program. The progeny do not need to be vaccinated until they enter the breeding herd, and 25 percent of the progeny between four and five months of age must have a negative pseudorabies test every 90 days to maintain this classification.

The extent of pseudorabies in the state was shown by a study conducted by the Animal and Plant Health Inspection Service of the Department of Agriculture from March 1983 to February 1984. Serum of 1,025 samples taken from pigs being slaughtered were tested for pseudorabies. Out of those samples, 10.17 percent tested positive, placing Minnesota second in the nation only to Iowa, which had 15.3 percent positive samples, in the incidence of pseudorabies.

From 1982 to 1985, 17 percent of the pure-bred herds in Minnesota were lost because of pseudorabies. The purebred herds are the source of seed stock to improve the quality of market hogs. Thus, this herd infection represented a major loss to the state.

On the national level PRV infection markedly increased in the United States during the late 1970s and early 1980s. The prevalence of PRV seropositive market hogs in the United States steadily increased from 0.56 percent in 1974 to 8.18 percent in 1984. Due to much concern over the rapid spread of PRV, the USDA initiated five pilot studies to examine the feasibility of eliminating PRV from infected herds and regions. These studies began in 1983 and included 119 herds in five states. Successful elimination of the infection was achieved in 116, or 97.5 percent, of the herds.

After much discussion by all segments of the livestock industry, a National PRV Eradication Program was begun on January 1, 1989. The program is proceeding well. As of March of 1993, 12 states were declared free of PRV. The goal of the program is to have the nation free of PRV by the year 2000. History will record whether that goal is realized.

Minnesota reached its peak of 903 PRV infected herds in September of 1992. As of the summer of 1993, Dr. John Landman reported the total infected herds in Minnesota was down to 813 herds.

RABIES

The Board of Health first identified rabies as a problem in the 1890s. By 1904, the Board of Animal Health's initial report stated that 45 cases of rabies had occurred in that past fiscal year. In 1907, the Board ordered the quarantine or muzzling of all dogs in the vicinity where a dog with rabies had been found. Public cooperation with law enforcement officials was poor in enforcing the regulation. In 1916, there was an outbreak of rabies among dogs in Minneapolis. The Board was obliged to send a letter to the mayor and call his attention to the lax observance of the order to quarantine or muzzle dogs.

During another outbreak of rabies in Minneapolis, when the order to quarantine or muzzle dogs was still effect, Dr. Cotton was stopped by a patrolman for speeding. As the patrolman began to write out a ticket for speeding, Dr. Cotton, who was the chief officer of the Board, noticed unmuzzled dogs on the street and he asked the patrolman if this area was his regular beat or territory. When he replied that it was,

Dr. Cotton identified himself as a health officer and asked why he was not enforcing the order to quarantine or muzzle the dogs. Suffice it to say, Dr. Cotton did not receive a speeding ticket.

No cases of rabies were reported in the state from December of 1920 to December of 1925. However, rabies reappeared in a small area in Sibley County, and, by May 26, 1926, the disease had spread to McLeod County. On December 28, 1925, a case of rabies was found near Wheaton in Traverse County. The source of this infection was believed to be a dog with rabies that had wandered across the border from South Dakota. Although the dogs in all of the townships in Traverse County were ordered quarantined or muzzled, rabies spread to the northern part of Big Stone County and to nearby Morris in Stevens County. The outbreak was eventually brought under control by the action of the Board.

The Board's regulations now require a six month quarantine for dogs that have been exposed to rabies unless the animal has been vaccinated. If a vaccinated dog is revaccinated immediately, the period of quarantine is markedly reduced. If the exposed animals are food animals, they are quarantined for six months, but can be released by a veterinarian when he inspects the premises 90 days or more after the quarantine is established.

The incidence of rabies has remained low because of the large scale vaccination of dogs and the control measures of the Board. Killed and modified live virus vaccines are effective and available for vaccination against rabies. However, rabies has remained a sporadic disease. The reason that the disease has not been eliminated is the reservoir of infection in wild animals such as skunks.

SWINE ERYSIPELAS

Swine erysipelas appeared in southwestern and western Minnesota in the late 1930s. In 1943, Dr. Kernkamp received permission from the Board to obtain a live culture vaccine for experimental purposes.

The Board ordered the quarantine of farms where swine erysipelas had been diagnosed and would not allow the use of live culture vaccines. In 1948, a number of veterinarians from the southwestern part of the state complained to the Board about its refusal to authorize the use of live culture vaccines. The Board felt there were insufficient cases of swine erysipelas reported to justify the use of a live vaccine. The veterinarians noted that the swine owners did not like the inconvenience of being quarantined. If the veterinarian reported the diagnosis of swine erysipelas on a farm, and the farm was quarantined, the swine producer would no longer employ him as a veterinarian. Thus, veterinarians were not reporting many of the cases and the number of infected farms was much greater than the Board realized.

The Board later voted to discontinue the quarantine for swine erysipelas infection and allowed the use of live culture vaccine by permit on premises where infection was high. The restrictions on the use of the vaccine were finally removed and swine erysipelas is no longer a reportable disease.

DISEASES ERADICATED IN MINNESOTA

Glanders, scabies in sheep, hog cholera, tuberculosis and brucellosis have been eradicated from the State of Minnesota.

ERADICATION OF GLANDERS IN HORSES

Glanders, or farcy, is a highly contagious and fatal disease of horses that is transmissible to humans. Infection with glanders is usually fatal. Glanders was the first economically important livestock disease that was eliminated in Minnesota through the efforts and guidance of the Board of Animal Health.

EARLY ATTEMPTS TO CONTROL GLANDERS: MALLEIN TEST

In 1879, the legislature passed a law establishing as a criminal misdemeanor for an owner of a horse affected with glanders to drive it on a public highway or permit it to run at large. The state Board of Health became concerned with glanders in 1883. The diagnosis of glanders was very difficult in the early stages of the disease when it resembled other diseases of the horse. This created many disputes between the owners and health officials. There was a scarcity of graduate veterinarians to make a diagnosis. When no qualified veterinarians were available, the diagnosis was made by local health officials.

Because indemnity was not paid on horses ordered destroyed, there was no incentive to report the disease. However, a few local boards would pay $3.00 to $5.00 to the owner to cover the cost to kill and bury the animal. Horses suspected of glanders were often sold to unscrupulous dealers who, in turn, would sell the diseased animals at very low prices to unsuspecting farmers with little money who were struggling to make a living. The losses that eventually followed the purchase of these horses caused even greater financial hardships among the already poor farmers.

In 1900, in an effort to locate horses affected with glanders, the City of Minneapolis offered to pay veterinarians $3.00 for each horse with glanders reported to the Department of Health. However, this program enjoyed little overall success.

The development of the mallein test for glanders was a great step forward that eventually led to the elimination of glanders. The test made earlier diagnosis possible and provided a reliable tool for separating glanders from other horse diseases. During the 1893-1894 fiscal year, an ample supply of mallein became available in Minnesota. However, there were few qualified persons to administer the test in some of the outlying sections of the state.

The state Board of Health issued regulations for the control of glanders that called for the destruction of reactors to the mallein test that also showed clinical signs. The Board did permit the destruction to be delayed until the work season was over, or until the disease had progressed to the point that the animal was unable to work. Reactors with no clinical signs would be quarantined. But quarantines were difficult to enforce and were often ignored. Moreover, under these conditions, a horse with glanders could continue to expose other horses after it had been diagnosed as having glanders.

INDEMNITY PAYMENTS AID CONTROL

The Board of Animal Health was originally authorized to pay indemnity for horses destroyed because of glanders. However, the legislature failed to appropriate funds for indemnification. During the following session, in 1905, the legislature appropriated sufficient funds to pay the claims on file and indemnification for the next biennium. These appropriations did much to encourage reporting glanders.

The Board of Animal Health soon issued a regulation that required immediate destruction of all clinical cases of glanders. The Board's regulation further required all horses in contact with a glanders-infected horse not be placed with other horses until they tested negative for glanders.

During the 1911-1912 fiscal year, glanders was eliminated in Minneapolis and St. Paul due to the closing of the public watering troughs and the extensive use of the mallein testing. The only cases reported after this date were in horses that had originated outside of the Twin Cities.

The number of horses destroyed each year because of glanders peaked at 606 during the 1905-1906 fiscal year. The disease subsequently declined dramatically and, in the 1911-1912 fiscal year report, the Board announced that glanders was well on its way of being eliminated in Minnesota. This announcement proved to be premature. Horses imported from western states without testing for glanders provided a continuing source of infection. Dealers brought the horses into Minnesota and sold them at an auction or peddled them individually to farmers before quickly leaving town. In 1912, for example, a shipment of 40 horses from South Dakota contained 23 glanders reactors. The horses were sold and taken to farms before authorities learned many of the animals had glanders. The buyers of the horses suffered heavy losses because they were not eligible for indemnification. This unfortunate practice was eventually controlled by greater vigilance and public education of the danger of buying untested animals.

The logging camps of Northern Minnesota were another source of new infection. The logging companies would import horses for logging that would be sold within the state after the completion of the logging season. Some of the horses were purchased outright, and others would be leased for the season. However, it was customary for many companies to simply dispose of them after the logging season. Most, if not all, of these horses were imported without a glanders test. This practice resulted in substantial losses in horses and in days of work.

This source of infection was handled by convincing the logging companies that it was to their financial advantage to purchase or lease only those horses that were negative to the mallein test. The problem was again solved through awareness and education.

OPHTHALMIC TEST AND ERADICATION

The Board approved ophthalmic testing for glanders during the 1913-1914 fiscal year. This test was much easier to perform than the subcutaneous injection of the mallein. In the subcutaneous test, the horse was observed for a local reac-

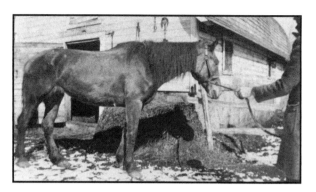

Glanders, glanders was found again in Minnesota in 1937 when Dr. A.O. Garlie diagnosed glanders in a horse on the Olaf Tviet farm in Pembina Twp., Mahnomen Co., Minnesota. Dr. C.A. Mack of the Board of Animal Health tested all of the horses on the farm for glanders. Six horses reacted and five were in serious condition. All of the horses were destroyed. The horses came from South Dakota in 1929, Courtesy Dr. A.O. Garlie.

tion at the injection site and for a rise in body temperature over a period of as long as 18 hours. The number of horses diagnosed as having glanders during this period fluctuated below 100 per year, and was usually below 50. The adoption of the ophthalmic test greatly speeded the testing process. During the 1929-1930 fiscal year, no cases of glanders were reported and the Board of Animal Health declared glanders eliminated from Minnesota.

ERADICATION OF SHEEP SCABIES

Sheep scabies or sheep scab, known by the scientific community as psoroptic mange, was already a problem when the Board of Animal Health was created in 1903. One of the Board's first actions was to issue regulations for the control of sheep scabies. In the control program, sheep scabies was diagnosed on a flock basis. If one animal was found to be infected, the whole flock was considered infected and quarantined until it was declared negative. While the death loss due to sheep scabies was low, it did cause sheep to lose wool, weight, and fertility. The causative agent for the disease was a mite. The prevention and treatment involved dipping the sheep in solutions of tobacco and sulphur or lime and sulphur. Although there were some problems in inclement weather, generally, the sheep owners cooperated in dipping their sheep.

The disease proved difficult to eradicate because of the importation of infected sheep, usually feeder lambs, from western states. Flocks of sheep with scabies can be easily identified

Scabies Inspection

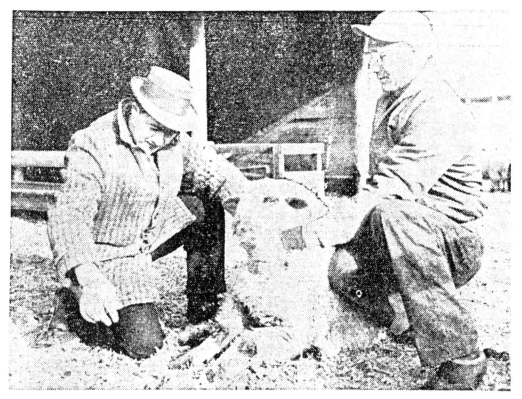

SCABIES INSPECTION. Pictured are County Agent Russ Bjorhus and Paul Warga as they take a close look at one member of a herd of sheep on the Guy Flint farm, east of Elbow Lake. The inspection, which is being conducted in the county by the county agent, is part of a state-wide drive to eliminate scabies in Minnesota. Herald Photo.

★　　★　　★　　★

A state wide drive to eradicate sheep scabies in Minnesota started December 17 and will be completed by January 18. By that date every sheep flock in Minnesota will be inspected.

County Agricultural Agents in each county have been given the job of doing the inspection. This will result in the State saving some $200,000 by not having to use State Veterinarians.

The results of this inspection will be for Minnesota to be declared Scabies-Free and sheep men in this state will not be faced with continued embargoes and shipping restrictions from states now scabies free. Nearly all western states, including North and South Dakota have eradicated the disease.

Any sheep flock owner in Grant County, who does not have his flock inspected by Friday, January 4, should call the County Agent's Office in Elbow Lake. Some flocks may have been over-looked and all flocks, regardless of size must be inspected.

From Elbow Lake, Herald, January 3, 1963.

Official Hog Cholera quarantine signs were posted when hog cholera was diagnosed on the premises.

because the wool falls off in patches. The difficulty in the complete eradication of sheep scabies arose from the problem of disclosing all of the mite-infested herds. Finally, in 1962, a cooperative scabies reporting effort was organized between the Board of Animal Health and the State Agricultural Extension Division. In each county, each county agent would inspect each flock of sheep in the county. He would report to the Board which flocks had "falling wool," and that flock would be "dipped." Finally, in June 1963, sixty years after the initial effort by the Board of Animal Health and those connected with the sheep industry, sheep scabies was declared eradicated in Minnesota.

ERADICATION OF HOG CHOLERA

The State Board of Health's first official reference to hog cholera in Minnesota occurred in 1894. During the previous fall and winter, there had been "a wide-spread and fatal epidemic [in hogs] of a combination of diseases imported into Minnesota, it is believed, chiefly from Iowa and perhaps some other Western States."

EARLY ATTEMPTS TO CONTROL

A circular entitled "So-Called Hog Cholera and Swine Plague" was prepared in 1894 and distributed to local boards where the disease was known to exist. The circular included instructions on how to dispose of the dead swine and methods to disinfect the premises.

There was great indifference on the part of local health boards and farmers to reporting and trying to control the disease. Dr. J. G. Annand, a veterinarian from Minneapolis, was employed by the State Health Department from May to November 1898 to do special hog cholera field work. During the same year, A. K. Bush was hired as a special agent to aid in the campaign to educate farmers and local boards on hog cholera.

When the Board of Animal Health was established in 1903, one of the first items on its agenda was the control of hog cholera. This was before the discovery of the etiological agent and the development of hog cholera antiserum. The only means at the Board's disposal to combat the disease involved the restriction of the movement of swine through the use of quarantines. The Board also required that hogs shipped for breeding or exhibition purposes had to be transported

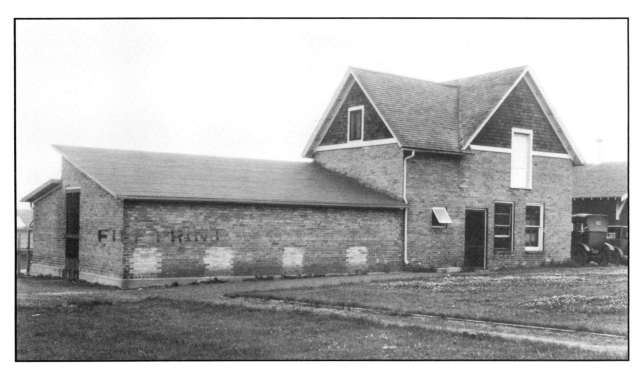

Virus Building, where hog cholera virus producing hogs were housed. biult in c. 1915. Courtesy of University of Minnesota Archives.

in crates. The hogs also had to be accompanied by a certificate stating they were free of hog cholera and the disease had not occurred on the premises or in the neighborhood from which they originated for at least six months prior to shipment.

There were 119 reported outbreaks of hog cholera during the 1903-1904 fiscal year. A severe epidemic occurred in Yellow Medicine County that began on farms occupied by farmers who had recently moved to Minnesota from Iowa. The Board minutes concluded, "beyond question," the disease was imported from Iowa. During the following year, 206 outbreaks of hog cholera were reported. As the etiological agent was unknown, the efforts to control hog cholera were not effective.

DISCOVERY OF ETIOLOGICAL AGENT

In the meantime, researchers at the U.S. Bureau of Animal Industry were trying to find the specific cause of hog cholera. In 1903, the Bureau reported that hog cholera was due to a filterable virus. This report led to the development of an effective antiserum by Dorset, McBryde, and Niles at the Bureau of Animal Industry field station at Ames, Iowa. A small amount of available funds were to be used by the Bureau to produce as much antiserum as possible for use in the expected fall outbreak of hog cholera. These researchers eventually learned the most efficient way to obtain hog cholera virus and to produce

antiserum. They subsequently staged a conference in Ames, Iowa, to announce their findings. During the conference, they demonstrated the procedures to produce and use hog cholera virus and antiserum to control hog cholera. The conference, held in June 1908, extended over a period of six days. The heads of the veterinary departments in the agricultural experiment stations located in the corn belt were invited. The Bureau of Animal Industry hoped these men would convince the administration of their respective stations that it was necessary to provide the facilities and equipment to immediately produce hog cholera antiserum.

STATE SERUM PLANT

Dr. M. H. Reynolds, who represented the University of Minnesota at the conference, convinced Minnesota authorities of the need to produce hog cholera antiserum. The university authorities approved the proposal. The Board of Animal Health used a portion of its funds to help start the project in 1908. Twenty-four pigs weighing from 240 to 260 pounds were used to produce the serum. Some of the pigs were housed in horse stalls on the adjacent Minnesota State Fair Grounds. And, in 1909, legislature appropriated funds to erect, equip and operate a "serum plant."

The serum plant was constructed on the College of Agriculture campus that is now occupied by the College of Veterinary Medicine. The plant was located approximately 100 feet south of the Old Anatomy building. A small amount of antiserum was produced in 1909. By February 1910, a sufficient amount was produced to have a conference where its use was described to practicing veterinarians. The demand for antiserum increased, and the plant was operating at capacity by 1913.[7]

At the end of the fiscal year in 1914, the Board reported the state serum plant was unable to "fill all" of its orders. Although the demand for serum was high, the serum was being sold at a loss. In appropriating $10,000 to manufacture the serum, the legislature had also required sale of the serum for 1/3 cent per c.c. The cost of production was 1-1/3 cents per c.c. This caused a deficit in the operation. The Board requested funds from the 1915 legislature to enlarge the "serum plant." The Board proposed an increase in the $10,000 level of operating funds in order to increase production and take care of the deficit. The legislature appropriated $10,000 to enlarge the facilities and an additional $20,000 to defray the cost of production and erase the deficiency.

As the demand for hog cholera antiserum increased, the Board of Animal Health and the College of Agriculture, who operated the plant jointly, found it necessary to issue the following regulations in regard to its sale and use:

Serum to be sent express C.O.D. or for cash.

Must have satisfactory evidence that cholera exists in the herd or vicinity

Serum sent only in quantities needed.

Serum sent only to persons who have attended a course of instruction and obtained a certificate from the Board.

The recipient must report the number of hogs treated and the dosage within 10 days and notify the town supervisor or local health officer of herds in which diseased animals have been given serum.

Commercial plants eventually began producing hog cholera virus and antiserum. These commercial operations took customers away from the state serum plant. They could produce the products at nominal cost, and thereafter sell them at lower prices. By 1926, only five individuals purchased serum and virus from the state serum plant. Early in 1927, the Board agreed to simply purchase serum and virus from the St. Paul Serum Company rather than produce its own. However, the Board was prevented from going out of the serum and virus business entirely by the legislature, which felt that, in case of an epidemic of hog cholera, there must be a sufficient source of serum and virus available to prevent any potential disaster in the swine industry. The St. Paul Serum Company thus continued to produce and store hog cholera serum and virus. This contract has subsequently been terminated.

SERUM AND VIRUS VACCINATION FOR IMMUNITY

The simultaneous administration of hog cholera virus and hog cholera antiserum in different location on the hogs produced an immunity to the disease. However, the Board of Animal Health was cautious in using this method for fear of spreading the disease. The Board started by allowing limited use of vaccination by their field veterinarians.

Early in 1914, Drs. J. N. Gould, A. F. Lees, L. Hay and K. J. McKenzie — all highly respected veterinarians — appeared at a Board meeting to urge wider use of the anti-hog cholera serum and virus method of vaccination. Following this meeting, the Board voted to permit the use of the anti-hog cholera serum and virus method in and near infected areas.[8] This method could also be used under other exceptional conditions on written permission from the Board. Only graduate and licensed veterinarians were authorized to use hog cholera virus.

HOG CHOLERA "CURES"

During the early days when hog cholera was spreading rapidly there was a proliferation of hog cholera "cures." Some of the agents that were sold to livestock owners were billed as medicinal concoctions and often marketed by vendors going from farm to farm. Advertisements in farm magazines offered products, as well as directions, to eradicate the disease. Some of the "cures" were ridiculous. But pigs were dying and there was no

[7] When Dr. H. C. H. Kernkamp was a veterinary student, he worked at the serum plant during the summers and, after graduation in 1914, he was hired to work full time.

[8] An infected area was defined as an area within a radius of four miles of a premise where hog cholera had existed within the past six months.

MINNESOTA STATE LIVESTOCK SANITARY BOARD
NOTICE
HOGS QUARANTINED

Hogs on these Premises Have Been Vaccinated With Hog Cholera Serum-Virus [Double Treatment] And Are Under Quarantine

THE MINNESOTA STATE LIVE STOCK SANITARY BOARD RULES AND REGULATIONS WHICH HAVE THE FORCE OF LAW AND VIOLATION OF WHICH IS A MISDEMEANOR PROVIDE AS FOLLOWS:

The owner or person in charge of any domestic animal affected with or which shows symptoms of, or has been exposed to a contagious or infectious disease shall, upon discovery of the existence of such disease, or symptoms thereof, or exposure thereto, cause each of such animals to be isolated from all well or unexposed domestic animals and to so keep them until the State Live Stock Sanitary Board, its Executive Officer or its duly authorized agent or officer, shall certify in writing that such animal is free from any such disease or that there is no longer any reasonable necessity to keep it isolated from other domestic animals.

No person except the owner, attendants or medical advisers shall enter any enclosure where any animal so isolated is being kept and upon which a placard shall have been placed, during the time such placard is so displayed. No person shall remove, obliterate, mutilate or destroy this placard until the quarantine has been released.

SECTION 35.70 MINNESOTA STATUTES, 1949

Provides that every person violating any rule or regulation made by the Live Stock Sanitary Board shall be guilty of a misdemeanor, the minimum punishment whereof shall be a fine of $25.00 or imprisonment for 30 days. Said section also provides that any member of a local Board of Health who shall neglect or refuse to perform any duty imposed upon him by law or by the direction of the State Live Stock Sanitary Board or who refuses or neglects to enforce the regulations of said State Board shall be guilty of a misdemeanor, the minimum punishment whereof shall be a fine of $25.00; and each day's neglect or refusal to perform any duty imposed upon him under this chapter shall constitute a separate and distinct offense.

Official Hog Cholera vaccination quarantine signs were posted when pigs on the premises had been vaccinated with hog cholera serum and virus.

treatment recommended by veterinarians or health officials. The farmers had no alternative but to buy these "cures."

One example of these ridiculous "cures" could be obtained for one dollar from a magazine advertisement. The "cure" consisted of feeding salt to the sick pigs. To determine if the pig had taken a sufficient amount of salt, a straw was placed in the anus of the pig and the farmer was instructed to then suck on the straw. If the farmer could taste the salt, then the pig had taken enough of the "cure."

With the advent of antiserum and virus methods of prevention, the vendors of cures sensed the end of their profitable business. While some of the persons were honorable citizens who were sincere in their objections to the antiserum and virus method of vaccination, the majority of the objectors were unscrupulous and dishonest persons who took advantage of the misfortunes of others. They attacked vaccination by spreading rumors that it was ineffective, caused the disease, cost too much, and benefited no one except the veterinarians. They caused some swine raisers to consider all methods to control and prevent hog

cholera as a form of graft. The Board hired a temporary staff member to lecture and work with county agents to counter this propaganda.

QUARANTINE OF VACCINATED PIGS

In 1914, the Board required that swine vaccinated at the stockyards be quarantined for a period of fourteen days, in conformation with the Bureau of Animal Industry's regulations. In 1923, the Board required all hogs given antiserum and virus be quarantined for 21 days, and further required that a quarantine placard be placed both in a conspicuous place on the enclosure holding the hogs and by the public road. Some animal owners regarded the quarantine placard as a status symbol and were proud of it, while others were embarrassed by the sign and sought to have it put in an inconspicuous location. Those who did not like the placard generally lived in neighborhoods where antiserum and virus vaccination was an uncommon practice. They feared being ostracized by the neighbors who did not vaccinate.

Hog Cholera Vaccnation School At Blue Earth

At the request of farmers in Fari-bault and Martin County, the Minnesota Livestock Sanitary Board has authorized Hog Cholera vaccination school. This school will be held on March 9 and 10 in the Courtroom in the Blue Earth Courthouse. Dr. Raymond B. Solar, Extension Veterinarian, University of Minnesota, will conduct the school.

This school is open to hog producers so that they may become informed to take a test in securing a permit to vaccinate their own hogs. Blanks for enrolling in the school are available from Faribault County Agent James V. Johnson, or Martin County Agent, Floyd Bellin.

The school will begin at 10:00 a.m. March 9 and runs until 4.00 p.m. March 10th. Those enrolled must be present both days. Members enrolled must take a written exam on the second day. The names of all who pass are sent to the Minnesota Livestock Sanitary Board, who in turn issues the permits, which are good for one year and must be renewed.

Fourteen farmers have enrolled in Faribault County and a like number in Martin County.

From Bricelyn Sentinel, March 3, 1960

FARMER (LAY) VACCINATION

Graduate licensed veterinarians were the only persons authorized by the Board to vaccinate swine with the antiserum and virus method. This limitation angered some swine producers who believed that veterinarians charged too much for their services. They believed they were just as capable of vaccinating pigs. These owners became politically active and pressed for the passage of legislation that became known as the "Farmer's Vaccination Bill." The legislation was supported by the "Farm Block" in the legislature in 1919 and again in 1921 only to be defeated both times. However, much to the dismay of the Board of Animal Health and the veterinary profession, the legislation did pass in 1923.

The new law provided that a school of instruction would be convened upon presentation of a petition signed by seven or more owners of swine in an eligible county. An "eligible county" was defined as one that contained an area the Board of Animal Health had declared an "infected territory." A school could not be convened more than once a year. One of Dr. W. A. Billings' duties was to conduct these schools.

The school "term" covered a period of 6 to 7 hours. The morning session was devoted to lectures and demonstrations with the afternoon designated for examinations. Those students who passed the examinations could then apply for a permit that would allow them to purchase anti-serum and virus to vaccinate their own pigs. The permit was renewable after one year.

During the first two years, the vaccination schools were quite popular with attendance ranging from 30 to 70 persons at each school. Attendance subsequently dropped, and only 50 percent of those who passed the examinations eventually applied for a vaccination permit. These schools were actively promoted by serum companies that sold their product directly to laymen. In some counties, the serum companies were able to obtain the enthusiastic support of county agents to get the requisite number of signatures to start a school. During the 1926-1928 fiscal years, 925 new and renewal permits were issued.

In some localities, farmer vaccination had a significant effect on the local veterinarian's practice while in others it had a minimal effect because of the "breaks" that occurred in farmer vaccinated herds. "Break" was the term applied to an outbreak of hog cholera following vaccination with antiserum and virus. These "breaks" convinced many swine raisers that vaccination was an unsafe procedure. While there were several causes of the "breaks" in farmer-vaccinated herds, the main sources were due to ignorance of the appropriate vaccination process. Insufficient antiserum to control the virus would be given because the weight of the pig was misjudged or because the dosage was intentionally reduced in an effort to lower costs. Hog cholera virus would not be kept properly refrigerated or had low potence because it was outdated. "Breaks" also occurred from vaccinating unhealthy pigs.

FARMER VACCINATION PERMIT CHALLENGED IN COURT

Over time, the great majority of the laymen eligible to obtain a vaccination permit did not take advantage of the privilege. In hope of reviving the sale of its products, the American Serum Company of Sioux City, Iowa, challenged the constitutionality of the law that required laymen to take a special course for a permit to administer the hog cholera antiserum and virus in "infected territory." Vernon Anderson, a farmer in Renville County, consented to become plaintiff on behalf of the serum company. The Board of Animal Health was named as a defendant in the lawsuit.

In early 1943, Attorney Leo Lauermann obtained an injunction to prevent the county attorney, sheriff, and justice of peace from interfering with vaccination of Vernon Anderson's hogs. Anderson then purchased hog cholera antiserum and virus from the American Serum Company, without a permit, and proceeded to vaccinate his pigs. Anderson then proceeded to have himself arrested. In June of 1943, Anderson's case was presented to Judge Howard Baker in the District Court of Renville County without a jury. Lauermann represented Anderson and Tom Streisguth, a special assistant attorney general, defended the Board.

Dr. T. B. Huff, president of the American Serum Company; Dr. E. Stubbs, former state veterinarian of the State of Arkansas; a practicing veterinarian from Illinois; and several Renville County farmers were called to testify in the plaintiff's case. Dr. H. Evanson, a practicing veterinarian from Sacred Heart; Dr. C. C. Frank, state veterinarian of Iowa; Dr. R. L. West, secretary and executive officer of the Board of Animal Health; and Dr. H. C. H. Kernkamp, from the University of Minnesota, testified for the defense. The trial lasted nearly three weeks, and a decision was not rendered until more than a year later. Judge Baker found Vernon Anderson guilty of a misdemeanor.

NATIONAL PROGRAM TO ERADICATE HOG CHOLERA

Although properly performed vaccination with hog cholera antiserum and virus immu-nized pigs against hog cholera, the disease nonetheless continued to be a serious problem in the swine producing areas. Live virus capable of producing hog cholera was used in the vaccination program. Some swine raisers would vaccinate their animals only after the disease was reported in the neighborhood or their pigs began to sicken.

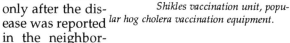

Over 5,000 Satisfied Users
SHIKLES BROS., VETERINARIANS
Sole Manufacturers of

Shikles vaccination unit, popular hog cholera vaccination equipment.

Continued outbreaks of hog cholera resulted in heavy losses. Many believed the disease could never be eliminated as long as live virus was used in producing immunity. These people began to urge a national program to eradicate hog cholera.

The breakthrough for eradication of hog cholera came in 1961-1962 when representatives of the swine industry, mindful of the eradication programs for bovine tuberculosis and brucellosis, requested Congress enact legislation for eradication of hog cholera throughout the United States. Legislation was eventually enacted to authorize the U.S. Department of Agriculture to take whatever steps deemed necessary to carry out the program. Minnesota Senate Senator Eugene McCarthy was one of the authors of the bill.[9]

The 1961 plan adopted for eradication of hog cholera was developed jointly by the National Hog Cholera Advisory Committee, the U.S. Animal Health Association, and the U.S. Department of Agriculture. It was to be carried out in stages or phases in cooperation with the livestock control agencies in each of the states:

Phase I: Informational approach to explain the program.

[9] These efforts were preceded by Congressman James McCleary, of the Second District in Minnesota, who in 1906 introduced a bill for federal appropriations and cooperation with the states in a nationwide hog cholera control program.

Phase II: Discontinuance of the use of hog cholera virus. Destruction of swine sick with hog cholera. Exposed swine given antiserum or marketed.

Phase III: Limited use of hog cholera vaccines. Destruction of swine sick with hog cholera and indemnity to owner, and all apparently healthy swine marketed for slaughter.

Phase IV: Discontinuance of the use of vaccines. Cholera-affected herd destroyed and hogs taken to rendering plant and indemnity to owner. Premises quarantined and general disinfection.

Minnesota adopted this program in 1962. In 1963, the "Farmers Vaccination Bill" was repealed. Minnesota achieved Phase II in 1964; Phase III in 1968; and Phase IV in 1969. On March 10, 1972, Minnesota was declared cholera-free.

It is almost unbelievable that hog cholera, a disease that caused sickness and death of thousands of swine since it was first recognized in 1833, is now a disease that has been eradicated in the United States. However, the Board must continue to remain vigilant to prevent hog cholera returning through other countries.

ERADICATION OF TUBERCULOSIS IN CATTLE

EARLY HISTORY

Tuberculosis of cattle in America was brought by the early settlers in foundation stock from Europe at the time tuberculosis was prevalent among the herds of cattle in Europe and before the development of the tuberculin test. Tuberculosis is very difficult to diagnose by physical examination except in advanced or chronic cases. As a result, many animals that appeared healthy but actually had tuberculosis were imported to Minnesota.

In the 1880s and 1890s, many veterinarians and physicians believed that tuberculosis in cattle could be transmitted to humans. They warned of the danger from the use of milk produced by tuberculous cows. Many of these individuals advocated the sterilization of milk from tuberculous cows.

In 1890, Robert Koch announced the development of tuberculin as a treatment rather than as a diagnostic test for tuberculosis. Russian veterinarian Dr. Gutmann and Danish veterinarian Dr. Bernhard Bang learned that tuberculin was a safe and highly accurate product for the diagnosis of tuberculosis in cattle. In the early part of 1892, Dr. Lester Pearson of the University of Pennsylvania visited Koch's laboratory and obtained a small quantity of tuberculin.

On March 2, 1892, Dr. Pearson, with the assistance of a veterinary student, Charles E. Cotton of Prescott, Wisconsin, performed the first test with tuberculin on a herd of cattle in the United States. The herd was composed of 79 purebred Jersey cattle owned by J. E. Gillingham of Villa Nova, Pennsylvania. Fifty-one cattle reacted to the test, and six of these cattle were taken to the veterinary college where they were killed and necropsied. All of these cattle showed lesions of tuberculosis.

EARLY TESTING FOR TUBERCULOSIS IN MINNESOTA

In 1894, the executive officer and secretary of the state Board of Health, Dr. Hewitt, obtained a supply of tuberculin from the Bureau of Animal Industry and supervised the testing of 335 head of cattle. The thermal test that was used at that time was made by the subcutaneous injection of tuberculin. Diagnosis was based on the temperature reaction. Forty-one of the reactors were slaughtered, and the tuberculosis lesions found in the carcasses proved the effectiveness of the test. Citing these results, Dr. Hewitt began to promote the tuberculin test to control tuberculosis in cattle. He also contended there was proof beyond a doubt that tuberculosis had been communicated to humans by milk from infected cattle.

Dr. Charles E. Cotton was employed by the Minneapolis City Health Department to test cattle for tuberculosis from July through August of 1895. From 1895 to 1901, Dr. Cotton was city veterinarian of Minneapolis. In that capacity, he convinced the Minneapolis councilmen to adopt an ordinance to require all raw milk marketed in Minneapolis to come from cattle that had passed the tuberculin test. Minneapolis was the first city in the United States to adopt such an ordinance.

The enforcement of this ordinance caused some cattle owners to challenge the validity of the test. They became powerful enough to convince the legislature to pass legislation in 1897 "that cattle in this state should not be adjudged infected with tuberculosis or condemned as being infected, except and until, they are subjected to at least two separate tuberculosis tests and such tests shall not be nearer than two months or further than three months. Tests to be made by a duly licensed veterinarian." This law had the effect of allowing reactors to remain in the herd for a time after being diagnosed, and caused further exposure to other animals in the herd. Fortunately, this law was subsequently repealed.

Early in its existence, the Board of Animal Health promoted the "test and slaughter" program as the most effective way to suppress and control tuberculosis in Minnesota. The Board began by encouraging the use of the program in purebred herds because these herds were the main source of new animals brought into a farmer's herds.[10]

OPPOSITION TO TUBERCULOSIS TEST

In the meantime, those who opposed the tuberculosis test had not been idle. In its 1905 and 1909 annual reports, the Board made reference to rumors the Board was forcing farmers to test their cattle for tuberculosis. Newspapers had printed some of the same rumors. These rumors had arisen from objections that were made when the cities of Albert Lea, Mankato Willmar and Winona had passed ordinances similar to the ordinance passed by Minneapolis that required milk being marketed in those cities to be from cows free of tuberculosis.

In 1909, opposition to the tuberculin test had reached the point where the legislature considered placing prohibitions on the condemnation and slaughter of cattle reacting to the test. The sponsor of the bill, Senator L. E. Swanson of Hennepin County, was out to devalue the test and discredit the Board of Animal Health. He also introduced a resolution accusing the Board of making expenditures and incurring debts greatly in excess of appropriated funds. The resolution further directed the Board to immediately submit a detailed report of all claims, and placed a moratorium on any new obligations except as directed by a legislative committee. The Board was also directed to aid and cooperate with the Senate Committee on Dairy Products and Livestock in

---

[10] For example, owners of grade herds would purchase a purebred bull to upgrade their herd. A purebred breeder would purchase or trade bulls from another purebred breeder to avoid too much inbreeding.

conducting a tuberculosis test on a group of cattle in the usual manner. Senator Swanson was convinced that conducting the test under the direction of the committee would prove the incompetence of the test and discredit the Board of Animal Health.

As the bill and resolution of Senator Swanson had not been voted on by the Senate, the Board of Animal Health arranged for a supervised demonstration of the tuberculin test and subsequent postmortem examinations. Swift and Company allowed 25 head cattle that were "fed out" in their feedlots in South St. Paul to be tested and slaughtered. The postmortem examinations were performed by veterinarians in the federal meat inspection service at Swift's meatpacking plant. None of the cattle reacted to the test and none showed lesions of tuberculosis at the postmortem examinations.

Some of the committeemen from the legislature who were disappointed by the test results asserted that the demonstration was not conclusive. Senator B. E. Sunberg, a farmer in Kittson County, suggested that his herd be tested and agreed that any of the animals that reacted could be shipped to South St. Paul for postmortem examination. The committee accepted the offer and traveled to Sunberg's farm to witness the application of the test. Fourteen of the 19 animals that were tested reacted to the test. The 14 reactors were shipped to South St. Paul where they were slaughtered and necropsied. All of these specimens showed gross lesions of tuberculosis. In its report to the legislature, the committee concluded, "the results show that tuberculin is a reliable diagnostic agent." The report on the fiscal part of the resolution noted that the accumulated deficit was incurred only after the Board had conferred with the governor, the attorney general, the treasurer, and the auditor, and observed that each of these officers had agreed that the testing program should continue. The Senate sitting as a committee of the whole received the report and returned the bill to its author.

PROBLEMS WITH DISTRIBUTION OF TUBERCULIN

The Board also had trouble with unscrupulous persons injecting tuberculin into cattle before the scheduled "official test" to negate the reaction and the diagnosis of tuberculosis. In an infected animal a second injection of tuberculin within 30 days may result in no reaction. Thus the animal would be considered free of the disease.

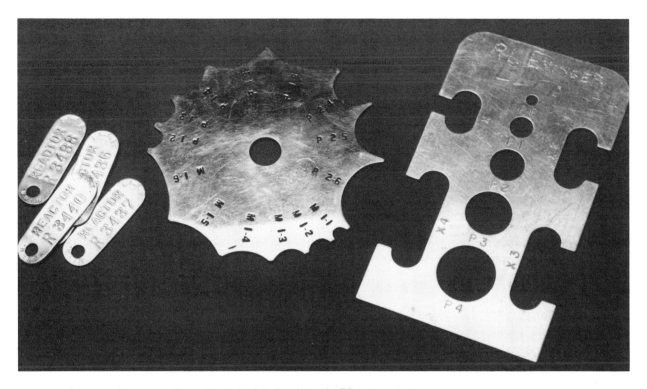

Guages used to measure the reaction in the intradermal test for T.B. and reactor tags.

The same was being done with mallein in horses. At the time there was no restriction on the sale of these two diagnostic agents. In an effort to identify one who had tuberculin and mallein, the legislature passed a bill in 1909 requiring every drug vendor to immediately report the name or names and address or addresses of the purchasers in every transaction in which they dispensed tuberculin or mallein.

Tuberculin and mallein had been supplied to the Board by the Bureau of Animal Industry of the Department of Agriculture with the understanding that the products would be distributed only to licensed graduate veterinarians and local health officers approved by the Board. In a significant event in the chronicles of bovine tuberculosis control, licensed nongraduate veterinarians persuaded the legislature to pass a law that prohibited the Board from distinguishing among licensed veterinarians in supplying them with mallein and tuberculin.

The Board asked the attorney general for an opinion on the new law. The attorney general stated that, as agents of the Bureau of Animal Industry, the Board would have to follow its directions and issue to licensed graduate veterinarians the tuberculin and mallein that they supplied. The state law provided, however, that these products be furnished to licensed veterinarians regardless of whether they were graduates or nongraduates. Therefore, the Board had the duty

to supply itself with tuberculin and mallein from other sources and distribute them to any qualified applicant. The Board complied with the attorney general's interpretation.

MINNESOTA "TEST AND SLAUGHTER" PROGRAM INCORPORATED IN NATIONAL PROGRAM

The early certification of many herds in the state made Minnesota a pioneer in the use of the "test and slaughter" program for the control and elimination of tuberculosis in cattle. As the result, the Minnesota plan was incorporated into the nationwide modified free herd tuberculosis plan of the Bureau of Animal Industry. In September of 1917, the Board of Animal Health signed a memorandum of agreement with the Bureau of Animal Industry for the purpose of eradicating tuberculosis from purebred herds and establishing tuberculosis free herds of grade cattle.

Under the cooperative agreement each was to detail veterinarians who would "spend their entire time in the eradication of tuberculosis." The number of veterinarians furnished by the state would determine the number furnished by the Bureau of Animal Industry. The Bureau furnished a competent veterinarian known as Inspector in Charge of Federal Tuberculosis Work. He supervised the federal veterinarians. The Board of Animal Health furnished a veterinarian to have similar responsibilities in regard to state employed veterinarians. To insure cooperation, the leaders of the state and federal programs met at least every two months. Both leaders were to receive copies of all charts and reports. In addition, the state enforced the regulations governing the handling and disposition of cattle that reacted to the tuberculin test.

Dr. W. J. Fretz, who later became Inspector in Charge, represented the B.A.I. and Dr. S. H. Ward, secretary and executive officer, represented the Board of Animal Health in signing the agreement. The agreement proved to be a model for subsequent programs to control animal diseases.

AREA TEST PLAN DEVELOPED

The success of the plan to control and eliminate tuberculosis in herds led to the development of a plan to do the same in all herds of an entire county through an area test program. Such an agreement was signed in 1922 with Dr. W. J. Fretz again representing the Bureau of Animal Industry and Dr. C. E. Cotton representing the Board of Animal Health.

The plan was called the modified accredited tuberculosis free area plan. Under this plan, all cattle of age six months and over were tested. According to the regulations in the plan, all reactors were to be promptly removed and sent to slaughter at a location where there was federal inspection and the premises used by the reactors cleaned and disinfected. The herds with reactors would be retested in 60 days and again in six months after the last negative test. The herd was considered free of tuberculosis after two consecutive negative tests. When the infection rate in a county declined to one-half of one percent, the county would be accredited as a modified tuberculosis free area.

After the adoption of the modified accredited tuberculosis free area plan, it was necessary to convince cattle owners and others, including county commissioners and legislators, that the plan was in the best interests of the livestock industry and the people of Minnesota. The Board appointed the Special Committee on Control of Tuberculosis to promote the plan. The committee was chaired by Thomas E. Cashman, and included J. E. Montgomery, C. E. Glotfelter, John B. Irwin, and D. D. Tenny. In January of 1923, Dr. W. J. Fretz reported that he had held meetings in 38 counties and "practically all" of the representatives of the counties in attendance were

Farm Bureau Weekly News' Service

TUBERCULOSIS ERADICATION POSSIBLE

State legislature permits two or three counties to have "area" testing that will clean up disease.

Meeker County is out to clean up the tuberculosis in the county. The first step necessary to do this is to secure the signature of 1200 farmers to a petition requesting the state to perform such service. After this has been secured the County Commissioners may make application to the live stock sanitary board and the first to make application will be accepted in this campaign. Two tests are necessary to clean up the county of the disease.

Meetings have been held and petitions are being circulated in every part of the county. The campaign is on and is going over big unless all signs fail. We believe that such a movement will be of great benefit to Meeker County, not only as a community where there is healthy livestock, but also in disposing of our butter.

At Ellsworth, a large meeting listened to the discussion on this question by County Agent Stitts and everyone signed the petition;also drives were secured for a house to house canvass. Darwin reports to the County Farm Bureau office that practically everyone is signing.

The same reports come from Watkins and Kingston. Swede Grove, Acton and Danielson are reported as being much interested in this and everyone is signing who is approached. In fact, it is entirely a matter of approaching the farmers in order to get the necessary signatures.

There are petitions in every creamery that may be signed. Lets go to it.

The County Farm Bureau is in charge of the work in lining up this work. Petitions will be returned to that office.

Petition to test signing in Meeker Co. From Litchfield Independant, May 2, 1923.

in favor of the program. They agreed to send committees to the legislature to lobby for larger appropriations for the area test.

The testing of cattle for tuberculosis in Minnesota became much easier and less time consuming with the adoption of the intradermal test. It was officially adopted on March 6, 1923, after Minnesota took a conservative approach on approving the test. The U.S. Sanitary Association and others had already adopted the test in 1921. Until the adoption of the intradermal test, the subcutaneous test was the official test in Minnesota.

The subcutaneous test was expensive because it required veterinarians to take several rectal temperatures over a 24 hour period. The test was performed by taking two pre-injection rectal temperatures not less than 4 hours apart to establish the normal temperature of the animal. Tuberculin was then injected subcutaneously, usually in the neck region. The amount varied between 2 c.c. and 4 c.c. according to the concentration of the tuberculin. Temperatures were taken beginning not later than 11 hours after the injection. They were taken not less than 2 hours and not more than 3 hours apart. This process was continued until at least 20 hours after the injection. A rise of 2 degrees Fahrenheit or a temperature above 103.8 degrees was regarded as positive for a tuberculosis reaction. Many reactors developed a temperature of 105 degrees and higher. Besides being time consuming and expensive, the test was not pleasant to conduct. This was especially true in the summertime when cattle were on green grass. Grass caused the cattle to have loose stools and cattle tended to defecate when disturbed or excited. With the veterinarian having to take several rectal temperatures, the cattle often seemed to anticipate when the veterinarian would be behind them. When they aimed at him, the veterinarian was not able to always dodge successfully.

In the intradermal test, tuberculin is injected within the skin in the caudal fold under the tail. Three days later the veterinarian returns to check the injection site for a reaction. This test is much easier and less time consuming to conduct than the subcutaneous test.

The program for the control and elimination of tuberculosis in cattle was greatly enhanced by the development and adoption of the intradermal test. The support of these committees helped the Board of Animal Health obtain the passage of a bill that gave the county commissioners the authority to appropriate a sum not to exceed 25 cents per head for each test of cattle for tuberculosis when presented with a petition signed by a majority of the cattle owners in the county. After voting the funds, the county commissioners were to sign an agreement with the Board of Animal Health to test the cattle in the county for tuberculosis. The agreement specified the rules and regulations that were to be observed if the test was to be undertaken and indemnity paid on the reactors.

After the bill was passed, the Board of Animal Health, the Special Committee on Control of Tuberculosis, veterinarians, county agents, livestock associations, and livestock owners along with others began trying to get the required number of signatures on petitions. The first county to sign the agreement for an area tuberculosis test was Meeker County on May 10, 1923.

HOW AREA TESTS FOR TUBERCULOSIS AND BRUCELLOSIS WERE CONDUCTED

The Board of Animal Health and the federal government officials would schedule a complete test of all the cattle in a county. This was known as an area test and was to be completed in two weeks. It applied to tests for tuberculosis, brucellosis, or a combination of the two. The agencies assigned veterinarians from their staff to perform the test. However, they did not have enough veterinarians to complete the test in two weeks. To obtain the requisite number of veterinarians, practicing veterinarians were hired on a per diem basis. Assistants for each veterinarian were also hired to help in the test. The county agricultural agent selected the assistants and tried to obtain farmers who were well respected and lived in the area assigned to the veterinarian.

Before an area test would begin, the veterinarians and assistants would gather at the county courthouse on Sunday afternoon. Dr. Cotton, the executive officer of the Board of Animal Health at that time, liked to arrange an elaborate organizational Sunday meeting. Whenever possible, he would arrange for local dignitaries to address the veterinary session. On one occasion, Senator Knute Rockne addressed such a gathering. Senator Rockne started his speech with great formality and recognized the group as "Dr. Cotton and members of the cow testing association." The veterinarians were not pleased with this salutation.

The veterinarians were given instructions

and cards with the names of owners of the herds of cattle that they were to test. They also received supplies such as tuberculin, cotton, alcohol, and ear tags. There was no official number of cattle set for a veterinarian to test during the two-week period. However, under favorable conditions, the proper assignment was approximately 1,000 head of cattle per week. The lists of owners of cattle herds were based on the county tax lists. In the northern counties, there were problems with out of date or incomplete herd lists.[11] Thus, the veterinarians occasionally had more herds of cattle to test than they originally expected, and might not be able to finish the testing during the standard two week period.

The assistants would start to line up the herds for testing on the same Sunday afternoon they would meet with the veterinarian. During the first three days of the week, they would inject tuberculin in the mornings and early afternoons. During the last three days of the week, they would observe the reactions of the animals, and brand and appraise the reactors. In area tests for brucellosis, cattle were bled every day of the week. In a combination test, cattle were usually bled and injected the first three days of the week.

In 1937, the veterinarians worked at a per diem rate starting at $10.00 plus $2.00 for "subsistence." The assistants received $4.00 per day. In 1942, the pay was raised to $11.00 per day due to the shortage of veterinarians during World War II. If the veterinarian furnished a car, he was paid an additional 5 cents per mile. The pay for assistants was raised to $5.00 per day if they furnished the car. During the war, veterinarians usually had better cars and it was easier for them to get extra gasoline ration stamps. In 1945, the federal government paid veterinarian assistants $6.00 per day. Minnesota began to have trouble hiring assistants and was forced to raise the pay to $6.00 per day. In 1947, the per diem pay for veterinarians rose to $13.00 with $4.00 for subsistence. The mileage was raised to 7-1/2 cents per mile. Later, the veterinarians were paid on a per head basis, primarily for testing for brucellosis.

Some veterinarians left their practice to follow the area tests from county to county. Other veterinarians would only help test in their county or in neighboring counties. They would test cattle

and answer calls in the late afternoon or evening.

A few of the veterinarians taking part in the tests are worthy of note for their individual characteristics. For example, Dr. C. G. Jennings of Morris would give his assistant a physical examination when they first met at the courthouse. He once rejected an assistant as unfit after such an examination. This caused consternation among the organizers of the test and shocked the assistant. After a time, another assistant was found who could pass Dr. Jenning's physical examination. Dr. Jennings also injected the caudal fold of cattle in a unique way. He would have his assistant and the farmer hold a door behind the cattle. He would stand behind the door and inject the cattle. In this way, the cattle kicked the door rather than him. However, this would cause a chain reaction with all of the other cattle kicking right down the line.

Dr. M. J. Jones of Milaca raised Red Poll cattle. He was very proud of his herd and took every opportunity to promote the breed. He became known as "Red Poll" Jones. Dr. Jones would take his assignment on Sunday afternoon and leave with his supplies to his assigned neighborhood. He would not be heard from during the two weeks unless he ran out of supplies. At the end of the second week, he would reappear at headquarters with all of his herds tested and all of his records up to date.

Dr. R. A. Hallquist of Brainerd was envied for his professional dress. Others would need a change of clothes and a shower to appear presentable after a day of testing. He would test cattle all day in a white shirt and tie and his clothes never got dirty!

In the early 1920s, state and federal authorities began to indemnify the owners of cattle that reacted to the tuberculosis test to assist the owners bear their financial loss. The reactors were appraised and sent to market for federal inspection. The net amount an owner received for the animal was subtracted from the appraised value of the animal. The difference of these amounts represented the farmer's loss. The state paid one-third, the federal government paid one-third, and the owner assumed the remaining one-third. The maximum indemnity that could be paid by the state and federal governments could not exceed $25.00 for grade females and $50.00 for purebred cattle with registration papers. The indemnity could not be paid until all the reactors had been shipped and the premises had been

---

[11] In sparsely settled counties, the assessor might not visit every farm if he had reason to believe that there was little to tax on the farm or if the farm was off the "beaten path" and the roads were poor.

cleaned and disinfected. Indemnity was calculated in the same way for reactors of cattle with tuberculosis, brucellosis, and paratuberculosis, and for horses with glanders.

OBJECTORS TO AREA TEST ACTIVE

The introduction of the area test stimulated objections because of the financial loss that they would suffer if they had to send many animals to slaughter. While animal owners received indemnity, it did not adequately cover the cost of replacing the animals and the expense of cleaning and disinfecting the premises.

Rumors were circulated to discredit the test. For example, it was rumored the test was unreliable on cows in late pregnancy and those that had recently calved; cows aborted after the test; and milk production would drop after the test was administered. Other rumors included that the test was not accurate on excited or overheated animals, and that some animals became ill and even died after the test. If an animal died after the tuberculin test, these rumors would be widely circulated regardless of whether the owner blamed the test for the animal's death.

Dr. John Arnold and his assistant conducted an area test in Aitkin County. They went to the home of Johannes Olson who lived on the edge of the small village of Redtop. When Dr. Arnold informed Mr. Olson that they had come to test his cattle, Mr. Olson replied that he had no cattle. Dr. Arnold's assistant, who lived about a mile away from Mr. Olson, knew his livestock and asked him what happened to individual cows. For the most part, Mr. Olson was able to tell to whom he had sold the cows. However, when he hesitated on one cow, the assistant said, "You still have her." Mr. Olson became enraged. He believed the tuberculin test would kill his cattle. When Dr. Arnold tried to explain that his cattle would be quarantined, Olson ordered them to "get off the place or I'll get my gun!" At his assistant's recommendation, Dr. Arnold decided to leave before Olson got his gun.

Mr. Olson's actions were reported to Dr. Andrew Walsh, the veterinarian in charge of the test. The following day, Dr. Walsh and three other veterinarians drove to Mr. Olson's place and parked their car in his driveway. Unnoticed by Mr. Olson, they walked directly to the barn where they found the cow in question, a yearling heifer, and a calf. They obtained a sample of blood from each and injected tuberculin in the cattle. When they had finished, they went to the house and told Mr. Olson what they had done. Dr. Arnold and his assistant returned three days later to read the reaction to the tuberculin. They also went directly to the barn to check the reaction. When they were done, they went to the house and informed Mr. Olson that his cattle did not have tuberculosis or brucellosis. Mr. Olson said, "They are all going to die. Testing for TB kills them."

The objectors were quick to invoke any statement, article, or publication that repudiated or cast doubt on the validity of the tuberculosis test. If the statements or writings suited their purpose, the objectors accepted them as authentic with no consideration of the author's background. They gave special attention to any author who attached the title of doctor to his name. But they made no effort to learn how the degree had been "earned" or whether the degree was even in the field of medicine. At least two of these so-called experts published pamphlets solely for financial gain.

Stories were circulated about the veterinarians, or "cow testers," as they were called, who conducted the tuberculin test. When the temperature test was used, veterinarians were said to use dirty syringes and needles, and alleged to have injected infection into the animal to cause a rise in temperature. There were other rumors that the temperatures were not taken at proper times; records were falsified; and veterinarians had to fill a quota of reactors.

When the intradermal test replaced the temperature test, the rumors were that a dirty syringe or needle was used to inject the tuberculin and cause a swelling that would be called a tubercular reaction. The rumor that veterinarians had to fill a quota of reactors was commonly heard.

The arrogance of a few veterinarians caused resentment among the cattle owners. They would order the owners and their families around as if they were servants. Some did not seem to understand the problems of keeping animals confined without water during the hot summer months. In some cases, the resentment was so great that farmers refused to have their animals tested. Many farmers who had originally been in favor of the test or planned on having their cattle tested subsequently changed their minds because of the attitude of these veterinarians. One veterinarian would notify farmers to have their cattle in the barn for a test by driving into the farmyard and blowing the car horn until somebody came to the car. He would then say, "Have your cattle in tomorrow morning for test," spin the car wheels, and drive off. Another veterinarian would call a farmer on the telephone and say in a loud and gruff voice, "This is the government. Have your cattle in tomorrow morning for test." He would then hang up the receiver before the farmer could answer. Veterinarians would often arrive just after the cattle were turned out. Instead of waiting for the cattle to drink, the veterinarian would bawl out the farmer and his help. This often would result in the veterinarian being ordered off the place. Those who objected to the test were quick to spread these negative stories about the conduct of these few veterinarians.

Political pressure by the objectors to the tuberculin test had its effect on some county commissioners. As elected officials, they had the authority to vote funds to conduct the test for tuberculosis. Incumbents who voted for funding were threatened with being voted out of office in the next election. However, there were some county commissioners who voted against or dragged their feet on approving the petition to area test because they genuinely did not believe in the test.

Various methods or ploys were used to avoid the tuberculin test. The legality of the signers of the petition would be questioned, the petition could be tabled, and there were campaigns to encourage signers to withdraw their signatures. County commissioners claimed that the county did not have the funds to make the appropriation necessary for the test, or they would delay signing of the agreement by requesting changes in the regulations.

In spite of these efforts, counties signed the agreements at a rapid pace. In 1923, nine counties signed agreements. In 1924, four more counties signed agreements. By 1928, a total of 50 counties had signed agreements and 24 counties were officially approved as modified tuberculosis free counties.[12]

Even after the funds had been appropriated and the agreement had been signed, problems still remained in conducting the tuberculin test. Some objectors refused to confine their animals. Others would confine their animals but would refuse to assist in restraining them. Some would

move some or all of their herd to another pasture or across the line into another county. Where there were confrontations, the veterinarian and his helper would be ordered off the premises by the farmers or the farmers would block the driveway to prevent them from entering to test the cattle. In some instances, groups of farmers would escort veterinarians to the county line and tell them to stay out of the county. In at least one case, veterinarians were loaded into a truck and hauled to the county line and told to go home. These situations often made it necessary for the county sheriff or his deputies to accompany veterinarians to test the cattle.

In Iowa, objections to the TB test had been more violent. In 1931, a confrontation took place in Cedar County over TB testing. The authorities assembled 63 state agents, sheriffs and deputy sheriffs to test the cattle of the alleged ringleader, J. W. Lenker. These officials were met at the farm by approximately 150 angry farmers who forced the officers off the farm.

Shortly after the officials had left, the state veterinarian, Dr. Peter Malcolm, arrived from Des Moines. His car was surrounded by the farmers who hurled insults at him and took his suit and briefcases. The windows on his car were smashed, the tires slashed, the radiator filled with mud, and the gas line cut. Dr. Malcolm was lucky to have escaped with his life. As a result of this violence, Governor Dan Turner ordered three regiments of the Iowa National Guard to the farm to restore order and ensure the safety of the veterinarians who were testing cattle.

The National Guard treated the Lenker farm as a war zone. At 5:00 a.m., squads of soldiers set up machine guns and blocked the roads on three sides of the farm. At 6:00 a.m., an infantry unit arrived in eight trucks at the front of the farm. The troops were accompanied by the state veterinarian and his staff of veterinarians. Mr. Lenker represented that he had sold the cattle. However, when he could not produce a bill of sale, Mr. Lenker was placed under arrest. His cattle were eventually tested with no reactors. The veterinarians subsequently tested the herds of the other objectors under the protection of the National Guard. Because of the involvement of the National Guard and the manner in which they operated, this episode has been called the "Cow War."

During the second area test in Meeker County, 141 cattle owners refused to allow their

[12] A factor that made dairy farmers sign the petition to area test for tuberculosis was an ultimatum from eastern butter markets. The farmers were told that after a certain date, they would buy butter only from tuberculosis-free cattle.

animals to be tested on the advice of an attorney. These farmers sought and obtained an injunction. The matter was eventually appealed to the Minnesota Supreme Court, where the injunction was dissolved and the cattle owners were told that they had to submit to the testing. Notwithstanding the Court's decision, some farmers still refused to allow their cattle to be tested. Evidence of the noncompliance was obtained and four of these farmers were arrested. All four pled guilty and were fined. Two of them decided to be martyrs and went to jail. However, after eight to ten days in jail, they changed their mind and paid the fine. One of the four also pled guilty to importing a bull into the county without a tuberculin test. After the four leaders had been arrested, resistance to the test faded and all 141 herds in Meeker County were tested.

In 1931, the legislature repealed the authority of the county commissioners to vote 25 cents per head for a tuberculin test when presented with the proper petition to the county commissioners. This amendment removed one of the means used to prevent or delay the test.

PROBLEMS IN IDENTIFYING REACTORS AND TESTED CATTLE

When the tuberculin test came into use on cattle, a significant problem involved the identification of reactors. Originally, veterinarians used ear tags. The 1895-1898 Report of the State Board of Health prepared by Dr. C. E. Cotton indicated that a cattle owner had removed the ear tags from animals that had reacted to the tuberculin test. Apparently, there was no regulation explicitly prohibiting the removal of ear tags. Some cattle dealers took advantage of this omission in the law by removing the official ear tag that indicated the animal had been tested for tuberculosis. In 1934, the Board issued a regulation prohibiting the practice without written approval of the Board.

The 1899-1900 report noted that, in cooperation with the health departments of Minneapolis and St. Paul, the Board had decided that reactors would be branded on the left hip with the capitol letter "T." Dr. Reynolds, head of the veterinary section, had six such branding irons made and distributed. However, he later reported that he did not believe that any of the branding irons had been used. There were extensive objections from the owners of dairy cattle to branding because of the bawling, odor of burning hair and skin, and the general commotion that it produced in the herd.

Area Test Act Sustained by Supreme Court

OBJECTORS HAVE LOST ON EVERY POINT

The appeal taken by certain Meeker county objectors to the area test law, and which litigation has hampered the testing campaign here and prevented this county being put in the accredited list of tuberculosis free areas, was decided by the Minnesota supreme court in a decision handed down last Friday.

The area test law was attacked by the attorneys hired by the Meeker county objectors on the ground that it was unconstitutional. The court rules squarely against this contention, and upholds the area test law and the earlier enactment providing that the state live stock sanitary board was empowered to institute criminal proceedings if necessary to enforce the regulations.

At the last complete test, taken last fall, there were 141 cattle owners who refused to have their herds tested, and the first step will be to complete the test as to these herds and release them from quarantine. We do not see what further legs the opposition has to stand on in the campaign of objection. We hope the decision will end the opposition and that they will decide to obey the law now that it has been declared valid by the highest court in the state.

From Litchfield Independant, March 4, 1925.

Big Crowd at T. B. Area Test Meeting Monday

OBJECTORS GETTING READY FOR TESTING

A meeting of those who refused to test their cattle under the area plan was held at the court house Monday afternoon. Sheriff Anderson made a trip to St. Paul to see Dr. Cotton of the Sanitary Live Stock Board and got a promise from him to come and attend the meeting, which was set by Mr. Anderson for Monday afternoon. There were fifty or sixty farmers present, mostly those who had refused to test. William Schulte of Cedar Mills was named as chairman, and Dr. Cotton explained the situation. He said the objectors would be obliged to make the test at their own expense, and that the state indemnity would be paid, but that the objectors had forfeited their chance to get the federal portion of the indemnity. A general discussion followed, which was somewhat acrimonious at times.

The question of the legal action that had been taken and the restraining order that was issued, and the quarantine that had been put on the herds of the objectors, was discussed.

The meeting was an afterclap of arrests that had been made of certain objectors who had broken the quarantine. Complaints had been made last August or September against certain of the objectors who had ignored the quarantine, but they were held up pending the appeal to the state supreme court as to the constitutionality of the area test law. This was decided a couple of weeks ago upholding the act, whereupon warrants were issued for Gunder Draxten, L. M. Jensen, Peter Pehle, Ole Nordgard and Alfred Schultz. On coming before Justice Hanson all plead guilty and were given the minimum fine, which is $25 or 30 days in jail. Schultz and Pehle paid their fines, or arranged to do so, the others deciding to serve time instead of paying the fine and costs. They seemed a little bit peeved because they were made the goats, while others of the objectors, who had probably broken the quarantine also, would get off by subjecting their herds to the test.

Mr. Pehle, for instance, had been in hard luck for some time. Abortion got in his herd some time ago, and he was obliged to get rid of the cows and under the area test he had lost most of the cows in the herd that he had built up. Then on top of that to be subjected to a fine was piling it on pretty thick he thought. Those who had elected to serve time instead of paying their fines have not been subjected to rigid cell life in our bastile. They were at the meeting in company with the sheriff. No one wants to see these men in jail, and many offered to contribute to pay their fines, though they are not in such circumstances that they are unable to raise the sum needed to release themselves. A neighbor offered to pay the fine of one of them who was before the court Saturday, but he declined. He was then told to go home and think it over and come back Monday. All the men are substantial farmers, but were given bad advice in the matter and acted on it.

There were in all 143 who refused to submit to the last test that was made, Cedar Mills town holding the largest number of any of the three or four towns that contained objectors. Most of the towns cleaned up without a single objector.

The arrests made were for breaking the quarantine, and not for refusing to test. There is no penalty for refusing to test, but such herds are put under quarantine.

The sentiment of the meeting was apparently for submission to the test, and many have already made arrangements for testing their cattle. They will be obliged to have the testing done at their own expense and will lose the government portion of the indemnity paid for any cattle that are condemned, but will be paid the state portion.

From Litchfield Independant, March 11, 1925.

Ear tags continued to be removed and exchanged, and reactors were removed from the herd and reported slaughtered when, in fact, they may have been sold to an unsuspecting buyer. In 1919, the Board made another attempt to correct the problem of identifying reactors. The Board decided that the letter "T" would be branded in the cow's right ear to denote that the animal had been tested, and the letter "C" would be branded in the cow's left ear if it reacted. However, this method was not used to any significant extent. During the same year, Dr. C. E. Cotton was instructed to purchase 100 neck chains to mark reacting cattle that would be shipped into the stockyards.

On June 16, 1920, the Board promulgated regulations for marking reactors to the tuberculin test that have remained in effect ever since. Reactors were branded on the left jaw with the letter "T" three inches high, and a metal tag bearing a serial number with the inscription Minnesota Live Stock Sanitary Board would be either attached to the cow's left ear or placed on a chain around the cow's neck. The advent of modified

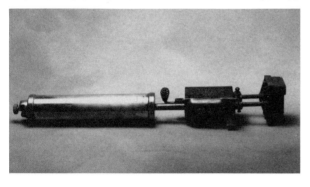

Early self heating branding iron for T.B.

blow torches as a means of heating branding irons made branding easier. Subsequently, caustic paste was used in place of branding irons to mark the reactors.

SWINE A SOURCE OF INFECTION IN CATTLE

The presence of tuberculosis in swine was another factor that made it difficult to control and eliminate the disease in cattle. Pigs could be infected with the bovine, avian, or human strain of the tuberculosis organism. In 1904, according to Dr. J. Arthur Myers, 78 hogs were shipped to South St. Paul stockyards for slaughter. Fifty-two of the carcasses were condemned as unfit for food

because of tuberculosis. Over half of the cattle on the farm of origin reacted to the tuberculin test.

When cattle were confined to a lot and fed corn, it was common to place hogs in the same lot to feed on the undigested corn that has passed through the digestive tract of the cattle. This is how the hogs were exposed to tuberculosis.

Cream separators were not common on dairy farms. Thus, the whole milk was taken to the creamery where the cream was removed and skim milk was a by-product. About this time, the Board recognized that the skim milk returned from creameries to the farm to feed hogs constituted another source of infection. The Board issued an order that skim milk had to be pasteurized before it was returned to the farm. The enforcement of the order came under the jurisdiction of the State Dairy and Food Department, which did not have sufficient personnel to give the order very high priority. In 1909, the order was revised to make it more effective.

In 1920, the Board noted that most dairy farms now had cream separators, and that cream was being shipped to the creameries while the skim milk remained on the farm. The by-product of manufacturing dairy products from cream, which was buttermilk, was not expressly covered by the previous orders, which were limited to skim milk and cheese by-products. The Board therefore amended the order to include buttermilk.

In the early 1920s, chickens were recognized as another significant source of tuberculosis. Many hogs were found to be infected with the avian type of the disease. While authorities had known for several years that tuberculosis existed in poultry, this fact was not considered to be of any great economic importance because of the small size of the numerous farm flocks at the time. In 1925, the Board of Animal Health unsuccessfully attempted to persuade the legislature to appropriate funds to test poultry for certain diseases, including tuberculosis. The Board also assigned a field veterinarian, Dr. L. E. Jenkins, to work full time on the elimination of avian tuberculosis. Dr. Jenkins was instructed to test poultry in counties that had been officially designated as modified tuberculosis-free areas. After a period of training, Dr. Jenkins began testing poultry flocks in Meeker, Traverse, and Red Lake Counties in July of 1926. He later performed tests in Murray County.

By the end of 1927, Dr. Cotton reported that, while the disease had "been practically eliminated" in four townships in Murray County, he doubted the cost-effectiveness of the program. The average cost of testing a flock was $14.36, and the average cost of testing each bird was eight cents. Additionally, Dr. Jenkins was having trouble getting flock owners to cooperate in cleaning and disinfecting their property after disposal of the diseased birds so that new flocks could be placed on clean ground.

In early 1928, the Board decided that the results of tuberculin testing of poultry did not justify the expense. The Board directed the secretary to develop a plan whereby Dr. Jenkins would visit each accredited county and promote cleanliness, sanitation, and flocks made up of only young poultry. Tuberculosis in poultry under a year of age was rare except in heavily infected flocks. The limitation of flocks to poultry that had only been through the first laying period was promoted as the most economical way to eliminate tuberculosis in poultry. Testing was limited to where it was necessary to determine whether a flock was infected or to test valuable breeding birds. In the later part of 1929, Dr. Jenkins was reassigned and the program was dropped altogether.

In 1928, the Bureau of Animal Industry began a national study to determine if there was a correlation between tuberculosis in hogs and poultry. As a cooperative project, the BAI offered to detail two veterinarians if the Board would also furnish two veterinarians to conduct the study. The offer was accepted and Freeborn and Mower Counties were selected for the study. The Wilson Packing Plant in Albert Lea and the Hormel Packing Plant in Austin agreed to mark hogs that were slaughtered so that animals with lesions of tuberculosis could be traced back to the farm of origin. The poultry owners signed an agreement whereby their birds would be slaughtered for a postmortem inspection.

The plan was not enthusiastically received by the owners of the poultry flocks. Only twenty percent of the birds in all of the poultry flocks in the two counties were tested. When the birds were marketed in this manner, the farmers received little or nothing for the birds and received no indemnity. In 1938, the BAI withdrew their last veterinarian and the project ceased. From this testing, approximately half of the poultry flocks in the two counties were determined to have tuberculosis.

In 1929, the Board began writing letters to notify owners of hogs with lesions that tuberculosis had been discovered at South St. Paul's stockyards. If the hogs had generalized lesions, the infection was of bovine origin. If the lesions were confined to the lymph nodes of the neck, the infection was considered to be of avian origin. When the infection was considered to be of avian origin, the Board sent directions to owners for ridding their herd of the disease. The Board reported that it received good cooperation from the owners who received these letters.

In the meantime, word spread that the best way to rid poultry of tuberculosis was to keep birds only for the first laying season and to raise them on clean ground. This information was disseminated by extension people, county agents, veterinarians, and the Board of Animal Health. Due to changes in the poultry industry that occurred later when large laying houses were built and large broiler establishments came into use, the farm flock largely disappeared as eggs and broilers could be produced more cheaply in large flocks. With the small farm poultry flock passing out of existence, chickens were no longer a source of infection of tuberculosis for swine.

MINNESOTA BECOMES A MODIFIED ACCREDITED TUBERCULOSIS-FREE AREA AND ERADICATES THE DISEASE

The program to control and eradicate tuberculosis in cattle moved forward on all fronts, including swine and poultry, until all 87 counties signed the agreement to test. In 1934, all 87 of these counties were approved as modified accredited tuberculosis free counties.

The declaration that Minnesota was a modified accredited tuberculosis free area was celebrated in November of 1934 with a banquet at the West Hotel in Minneapolis. Dr. C. P. Fitch was the toastmaster. The banquet was a spirited occasion of historical significance. Governor Floyd B. Olson saluted the vision that reached back a quarter of a century. Dr. C. E. Cotton toasted the many veterinarians who had spent time away from their homes and businesses for weeks at a time in order to test the animals. He also praised the county agents for their part in "lining up" the herds and recruiting men to help with the menial duties involved in completing this project. Dr. W. J. Fretz toasted the legislators for funding the program. Finally, Dr. A. J. Chesley spoke on behalf of the medical profession and Mr. W. S.

Moscrip paid tribute on the part of the dairy and livestock associations.

After Minnesota became a modified accredited tuberculosis-free state, continued surveillance of the disease was essential in order to maintain this status. There were still some farms with tuberculosis in cattle. The source of the reinfection of these herds was particularly difficult to identify. Sometimes the disease was contracted from humans with tuberculosis who were caring for the cattle. On other farms, there were aged chickens in the barn such as bantams, roosters, or laying hens that infected the cattle with tuberculosis. Surveillance of the situation was performed by area testing each county every six years. In 1967, area testing was replaced by the so-called slaughter detection plan. This is a "trace-back" arrangement whereby cattle that move into the public market for slaughter are "back tagged" with a number through which they can be traced to the herd of origin. Should tuberculous lesions be found at slaughter, the herd of origin is tested and re-tested until the herd is free of tuberculosis.

In 1976, another milestone in the fight against tuberculosis was reached when tuberculosis was declared eradicated from cattle in Minnesota. To make certain that tuberculosis does not again become a problem, the Veterinary Services of the Department of Agriculture continues to "back tag" cattle. The Food Safety and Inspection Service of the Department of Agriculture inspects the carcasses for signs of tuberculosis.

ERADICATION OF BRUCELLOSIS

Over the years, the name used to refer to brucellosis has undergone several changes. In the late 1800s and the early 1900s, it was called "contagious abortion," "infectious abortion," and "abortion disease." When Dr. Bang of Denmark appeared to have discovered the etiological agent, it was called "Bang's disease." When Dr. Bruce actually discovered the etiological agent, the disease was finally referred to as brucellosis.

In 1907, the Board became concerned enough about brucellosis that it disseminated suggestions for the control of brucellosis in herds. In 1913, the Board reported on a treatment that had been used successfully in Montana. The treatment consisted of large doses, given either hypodermically or orally, of a 4 percent solution of carbolic acid. The Board stated that as much as 750 c.c. could be administered on a daily basis.

The Board also advised that this level of dosage could cause dilation of the pupils and staggering. In 1916, the Board issued directions for treating bulls to prevent the spread of brucellosis in herds. The treatment consisted of infusing 4 to 8 ounces of a 1.5 percent creolin or lysol solution or a 2 percent solution of carbolic acid solution into the sheath.

Brucellosis nonetheless spread rapidly. The 1917 annual report stated: "This disease is probably the most dreaded by stockman because he sees and experiences actual financial loss." However, the Board of Animal Health decided not to issue any regulations to control infectious abortion disease because there was "no absolute way to determine if an animal has aborted or is likely to in the near future."

In 1922, the Board reported that losses from the disease had been increasing during the previous ten years. The Board decided to prohibit the movement of recently aborted cattle. This directive relied on the owner of these animals to voluntarily abide by the regulation because detection by an officer of the Board was difficult.

AGGLUTINATION TEST AND BRUCELLOSIS CONTROL PROGRAM

In the early 1920s, the agglutination test for brucellosis also came into use. Blood samples from cattle that were tested were sent to the laboratory at the University of Minnesota. The 1922-1924 report of the Board called attention to the increasing number of blood samples received by the laboratory. At the end of 1926, the Board issued regulations for certification of an "abortion-free accredited herd." To obtain this status, the herd must have had three negative tests of all cattle over six months of age over a 180-day period. By 1928, there were only seven herds in the accreditation program, and only one herd — the herd owned by St. Mary's College in Winona — had actually been accredited. The other six herds in the program were the herds at the Minnesota State Prison and the University of Minnesota.

Late in 1928, with the assistance of cattle associations, the Board revised the regulations to make the regulations more attractive to farmers. By 1930, 18 herds were in the program. The Board transferred Dr. L. S. Englerth to brucellosis control duties. Reactors were marked with a special reactor tag in the left ear. The regulations were issued in 1941 that called for the branding of reactors with the letter "B" on the left jaw. The signing of

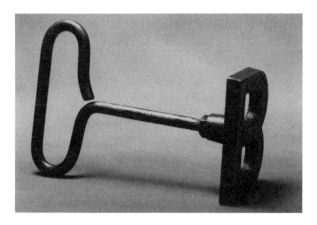

Brucellosis branding iron.

the revised agreement proceeded at a rapid pace. By 1931, 1,234 herds were in the program, and 125 herds were officially approved as free of brucellosis.

RAPID PLATE TEST AREA CONTROL PROGRAM

The diagnosis of brucellosis was made easier with development of the rapid plate test that could be conducted by veterinarians in the field. By using this test, the number of persons running the test increased, and it was no longer necessary to send the samples to the laboratory at the University of Minnesota. During the 1934-1935 fiscal year, 140 veterinarians received laboratory instruction on how to conduct the rapid plate test.

In 1939, the legislature enacted a law that provided a plan for area control of brucellosis. The plan was patterned after the tuberculosis program that used the test and slaughter method. The testing took place on a countywide basis and began in the northern counties where the cattle population was low and the rate of infection was believed to be minimal. The Board of Animal Health and the BAI furnished veterinarians to test all of the cattle over six months of age in Pennington, Red Lake, and Hubbard Counties. The rate of infection in Pennington and Red Lake Counties was low enough that these counties could have been declared modified brucellosis accredited areas. However, the Board had not adopted the rules and regulations necessary for such a declaration.

Early in 1940, the Board adopted the proper rules and regulations for a county to be declared a modified brucellosis free area. The regulations were later changed to require testing of

Bangs Disease Area Test To Be Given Here

Last Monday, August 30, Dr. Ralph West, Executive secretary of the State Live Stock Sanitary Board, was here and held a public hearing in the courthouse in Glenwood on the Bangs disease area test petition, which had been signed by over 1000 cattle owners in the county.

The petition was not challenged and Dr. West stated that the county test would be initiated as soon as funds and personnel to carry on the work becomes available and proper notices have been published as prescribed by law.

The state law requires that in any county a petition requesting the county to area test for bangs disease in cattle must be signed by 67 per cent of the cattle owners before the state Live Stock Sanitary Board can start an area test in the county.

The Pope County Farm Bureau started circulating a petition this spring and now have more than the 67 per cent of the cattle owners signatures required by law.

Through an area test of all cattle in the county and the elimination of infected animals this disease can be reduced to a minimum as well as the public health and economic losses associated with the disease.

From Pope County Tribune, September 2, 1948.

all cattle regardless of age. This amendment of the regulations lowered the infection rate as calves usually tested negative.

USE OF BRUCELLOSIS VACCINES

The Board proceeded cautiously with the use of vaccines to produce resistance against brucellosis. During the 1934-1935 fiscal year, the Board authorized the administration of the brucellosis vaccine to 13 herds on a trial basis. This trial occurred before Strain 19 of the organism was available and, apparently, the trial was not satisfactory.

In 1938, the Board reported on the experimental use of Strain 19. The new strain of the organism showed great promise as a vaccine. The Board began to relax its control slightly on the use of Strain 19 and allowed the strain to be administered on written permission. To obtain a permit, applicants had to supply evidence that there was a high rate of infection in their herds. All vaccinated animals were to be quarantined until they had passed a negative test for brucellosis.

In 1941, a calfhood vaccination agreement was prepared for owners to sign before any vaccination for brucellosis could be performed. The agreement only allowed vaccination of calves between the ages of 4 and 8 months.

OBJECTIONS TO AREA TEST

In the early spring of 1941, Clarence Converse, William Van Sant, Clyde Stowell, and August Kuschel of Crow Wing County obtained a temporary injunction to prevent the testing of their cattle for brucellosis. They contended that names on the test petition, which had been submitted to the Board by Crow Wing County on December 11, 1940, had been forged. They also contended that several of the signers were not cattle owners. At the subsequent hearing, the presiding judge ordered plaintiffs' attorney, M. Eleanor Nolan, to obtain affidavits to support her clients' contentions. She later had to admit to the court that she was unable to obtain the affidavits and consented to the voluntary dismissal of the action.

Soon after the case was dismissed, State Representative Halstad and County Commissioner Schwanke traveled to St. Paul with a number of cattle owners to meet with Dr. Cotton. They told Dr. Cotton that the Board had failed to consider the objections that had been raised concerning the petition that had been the subject of the lawsuit. The Board subsequently met with attorney Nolan and her clients. Nolan argued that many of the signers of the petition had changed their mind. However, she apparently could offer little evidence to support these allegations. After the meeting, the Board decided to proceed with the test in Crow Wing County.

Problems continued to arise in Crow Wing County. In early 1942, Theodore Nesser of Fort Ripley refused to allow his cattle to be tested. He was arrested and taken before a local court where he pled guilty and was fined $100. The fine was suspended providing that he submitted his cattle for testing within ten days. Nesser appealed the sentence. As there would be considerable delay before the next term of court could hear his appeal, the court ordered officials to go forward with the testing of Nesser's cattle. The court determined that to delay testing Mr. Nessor's cattle would endanger his neighbor's animals in ordering the test.

The court order was obtained on May 11, 1942, and two days later Dr. L. E. Clausen of the Bureau took blood samples from Nessor's herd. Mr. Nessor insisted that the blood samples be sent to the laboratory at the university farm for diagnosis. However, when the test results showed five reactors, Mr. Nessor refused to allow the cattle to be tagged and branded as reactors. He was again taken to court where his attorney attempted a novel argument to prevent the test results from being entered as evidence. Counsel argued that there were no witnesses who could establish the test was made on blood samples from his client's cattle. The court rejected the argument and ordered Mr. Nessor to allow his cattle to be branded. A number of other cattle owners with reactors in Crow Wing County had refused to allow their cattle to be branded pending disposition of Mr. Nessor's case. When he was ordered to allow his cattle to be branded, these farmers also decided to submit their cattle to branding.

In 1947, the opposition to the test in Aitkin County was led by Mr. Robert Boyer and his two brothers, who refused to allow their cattle to be tested. Rather than relying on local officials to handle the prosecution, the attorney general appointed a special prosecutor, Mr. Harrison B. Sherwood of St. Cloud, to represent the state. Sherwood instructed Dr. H. G. McGinn, the Board's field veterinarian; Mr. Lester Tate, the Board's law enforcement officer; and Dr. L. E. Clausen, the B.A.I. veterinarian, to call on the farm owned by Robert Boyer on November 20, 1947, to test his cattle. Mr. Boyer ordered them all off the premises, and forcibly ejected Dr. Clausen from the farm.

A complaint was issued against Boyer for interfering with a federal officer. The state also sought to obtain a court order to prohibit Boyer from any further interference with agents of the Board who were conducting the tests. Joseph J. Ryan, Boyer's attorney, conferred with Sherwood and agreed that Boyer would submit his cattle to a test after the first of the year. This delay only encouraged other cattle owners who were inclined to object to the test in Aitkin, Crow Wing, and Cass Counties.

In another instance, an editorial by Mr. C. E. Muns of Chaska appeared in the *Minnesota Guernsey News* that was very critical of the brucellosis program. The editorial greatly disturbed the members of the Board and they invited Mr. Muns to a meeting. In their subsequent discussion, Mr. Muns admitted that the editorial only represented his opinion and did not necessarily reflect the opinions of the Guernsey breeders. However, the Board was not able to convince Mr. Muns that his views were wrong.

Early in 1942, J. Russell Gute and Cletus Murphy, the county agents in Steele and Waseca Counties, respectively, appeared to register complaints about the lack of cooperation of veterinarians and their assistants in the testing. The agents reported they were receiving the complaints from the farmers. For example, veterinarians did not provide the farmers with enough advance notification to allow them to confine their cattle. Some veterinarians did not disinfect their needles. Other veterinarians mixed up blood samples. The agents were told to report all such complaints immediately to the veterinarians in charge of the test in their respective counties.

The brucellosis eradication program was completed in 1954. Since then, prevention activities have been limited to surveillance. During this period of time, only one cattle owner successfully avoided compliance with the state brucellosis eradication regulation. This particular farmer was much ahead of his time. In the early 1950s, he grew a beard, had a live-in girl friend, and was a serious dissenter. Although he was very intelligent, he was also unstable and did not believe in the program. At times, one could have a rational conversation with him. However, he could become violent when pressured to comply with

the regulations concerning brucellosis. He said that he kept a loaded shotgun behind the barn door and would not hesitate to use it if an agent of the Board of Animal Health tried to carry out a rule that was not to his liking.

This farmer moved his home frequently. He first lived in Cass County, later in Carver County, still later in McLeod County, and, finally, he returned to Cass County. He usually rented farms with rundown buildings. The stalls in his dairy barn were often tied up with twine string. However, the farmer had good cows and took good care of his animals, and his cattle produced well.

The farmer was prosecuted on several occasions for violating the regulations. While he sometimes was represented by an attorney, in most cases the farmer served as his own lawyer. Some of the cases were dismissed; others were won by the state; and a few were won by the farmer. Even when the state won, it did no good because the sentence was too light to deter the farmer from further violations.

At times, it seemed as though the local law enforcement officers and the courts sympathized with the farmer's cause. Several of the judges complimented him on his ability to represent himself in court. These compliments caused him to continue to violate the regulations so that he could continue to represent himself in court.

The last time the state sought to obtain compliance from the farmer in court occurred in McLeod County. A municipal judge found the farmer not guilty and warned the state never to bring this man back to his court again. The farmer's herd eventually became brucellosis-free through his own culling of the diseased animals. In this case, time healed the problem without help from the court. The farmer will be remembered as the only person in Minnesota who consistently got away with violating the rules.

Another difficult situation arose in Watonwan County when it became the first county in that part of Minnesota to sign the agreement to area test for brucellosis. When the first test was undertaken, the infection rate in the county was 4.7 percent of the cattle and 28 percent of the cattle herds. Opposition to the program grew and the county commissioners asked to be released from the brucellosis testing agreement. The commissioners feared violence would occur if the second test was undertaken. The attorney general determined that the county could not back out of the agreement to test. The second test results demonstrated that only 1.19 percent of the cattle and 7.8 percent of the herds were infected.

Watonwan County had difficulty lowering the rate of infection to qualify as a modified brucellosis-accredited county, which requires nor more than one percent of the cattle and no more than five percent of the herds be infected. As opposition to the test continued, officials found it difficult to prevent the importation of untested cattle into Watonwan County from the adjacent counties that were not being area tested. Officials admitted privately that it had been a mistake to try to accredit an isolated area like Watonwan County.

The Board was also concerned by the promotion of brucellosis vaccination by certain biologic houses. These companies advertised their vaccination as a more effective and less costly method to control brucellosis. These biologic houses caused many cattle owners to believe the Board of Animal Health should abandon the area test plan and adopt vaccination to control brucellosis.

In an effort to combat the efforts by the biologic houses, the Board strengthened the regulations regarding the sale of *Brucella abortus* vaccine and other biologics containing active infectious agents. However, the Board had trouble monitoring the sales of the biologic houses who shipped *Brucella abortus* vaccine directly to farmers and druggists from out of state. In addition, farmers would cross the border into the next state to purchase the vaccine. Along the borders, druggists would advertise in local newspapers that they carried *Brucella abortus* vaccine. If they were located in a Minnesota town and were taken to task about the advertisement, the druggist would argue that the advertisement was aimed at the subscribers who lived across the border in the adjacent state.

The Board eventually concluded that a national law was necessary to control the sale of *Brucella abortus* vaccine. The secretary of agriculture signed an amendment effective January 1, 1942, requiring all licensed biologic houses and distributors to keep detailed records of shipments and sales of viruses, serums, or analogous products including *Brucella abortus* vaccine, and anthrax, from one state to another. The sales of such products had to be reported to the proper livestock sanitary officials in the state or territory to which it was being consigned, as well as the

BAI. Unfortunately, the regulation was not vigorously enforced in Minnesota due to the shortage of personnel.

"CURES" FOR BRUCELLOSIS

At this time, the promotion of cures and preventatives for Bang's disease was at its height. The most aggressive promoters in Minnesota were Bowman's Abortion Remedy, 3-V Tonic, and Dr. David Robert's Abortion Medicine. Other cures or preventatives that were promoted involved feeding minerals and iodine preparations. In addition, some farmers continued to use the carbolic acid treatment publicized earlier by the Board. The promoters of the remedies for brucellosis were aided by the nature of the disease. Approximately 75 percent of the animals that aborted from brucellosis would not abort again during the next pregnancy. Of those that did abort again, approximately 75 percent would not abort a third time. Although some animals were left sterile by the disease, the averages greatly favored the animals regardless of the treatment that was given.

Those persons and companies that guaranteed their product to work would usually replace the product if it failed to work rather than refunding the purchase price. Some of the promoters of these products made flamboyant claims. They also threatened any official who disputed their claims. As proof, they often used testimonials that were fabricated.

Mr. Eric Bowman owned Bowman Laboratory in Owatonna. He became displeased when the Board of Animal Health and the Bureau of Animal Industry refused to approve his product. On August 3, 1935, Mr. Bowman organized a campaign of letters to United States Senator Schall condemning the Board of Animal Health and the Bureau of Animal Industry. Senator Schall promptly introduced Mr. Bowman's letter, as well as other letters he had received on the subject, into the *Congressional Record*.

The Board and the Bureau were greatly disturbed by this action. Dr. Cotton wrote a letter replying to the charges published in the *Congressional Record*, and sent the letter to Senator Schall and U S Representative Elmer J. Ryan. He asked that the letter also be placed in the *Congressional Record*. Although Congressman Ryan promptly placed the letter in the *Record*, Senator Schall ignored the request. After several additional letters, Senator Schall referred the letter to a committee and had them place it in the *Record*.

Through articles that appeared in the veterinary literature and in farm magazines, the Bureau of Animal Industry and state animal disease control agencies all pointed out the ineffectiveness of these "cures" and "preventatives" for the control of brucellosis. However, farmers continued to spend large sums of money for these products due in large part to the effective sales methods of their promoters. The claims of these promoters, which were supported by testimonials, generated political pressure on Congress.

Because of the large sums of money farmers spent on "cures" and preventatives of brucellosis, Congress passed an amendment to the Agricultural Administration Act authorizing funds to test various proprietary products alleged to be "preventatives" or "cures" for brucellosis. The available funding that was made available was enough to test two products. The tests were carried out as a cooperative project between the University of Wisconsin and the Bureau of Animal Industry. Bowman's Abortion Remedy and 3-V Tonic were selected as these products were believed to be the most widely advertised and used products of this type.

The 3-V Tonic that was tested in 1936-1937 was obtained from Mr. T. E. Crawford of the Crawford Company, in Winona. Analysis of 3-V Tonic by the U.S. Food and Drug Administration showed that it was primarily composed of lime, magnesium carbonate, charcoal, a soluble compound of sulfur and calcium, and smaller proportions of ferrous sulfate, sulfur, powdered linseed, and ginger. The tests used 60 heifers and showed that 3-V Tonic was ineffective in preventing pregnant heifers from becoming infected with brucellosis or from aborting after having acquired the disease.

Bowman's Abortion Remedy was tested in 1937 using 40 heifers. Analysis of the product showed that it was composed of over 90 percent sugar, a trace of creosote and ash, with water making up the remainder of the compound. The test demonstrated that the product was ineffective in either preventing or curing brucellosis.

The results of the tests of 3-V Tonic and Bowman's Abortion Remedy were published in 1940. These tests offered proof that the products were worthless in the control of brucellosis. The tests also provided evidence that enabled the Federal Trade Commission to prosecute for false advertising those who marketed the "cures" and remedies.

While sales of these products did decline after the tests, the use of the "cures" and remedies did not disappear altogether. Some of the promoters changed the wording of their advertisements and word of mouth was still used for promotion of the products. Some farmers remained convinced that the products were effective. For example, as noted above, Bowman's Abortion Remedy was composed mainly of sugar that was brown in color. In fact, some farmers assumed the product was brown sugar. For several years thereafter, there were farmers in the Owatonna area who on occasion would feed their cows brown sugar as protection against brucellosis. As area testing progressed, the demand for the "cures" and remedies lessened, and these products gradually disappeared.

CONTROL OF BRUCELLOSIS GIVEN IMPETUS

Public support for the control of brucellosis was mobilized by a 1945 report that indicated 78-80 percent of undulant fever (brucellosis) cases in humans were caused by the etiological agent of brucellosis in cattle, *Brucella abortus*. Undulant fever was a relatively new disease to physicians in Minnesota. When they learned to diagnose it, the disease was found to be quite common. When it was learned that one of the main sources of human infection was brucellosis in cattle, support for programs to eliminate the disease in cattle grew substantially.

The control of brucellosis was further aided by the passage of a law in 1945 requiring all cattle to be tested for brucellosis before they could be offered for sale. This law closed a loophole in the regulations through which infected cattle had been dispersed and the disease had been spread.

SHORTAGE OF VETERINARIANS FOR CONTROL PROGRAMS

During World War II, most veterinary students were deferred from the military draft to get their degree. Veterinary positions in the military services were soon filled. Meanwhile, newly graduated veterinarians, most of whom were unmarried, were coerced to join state disease control agencies. Their work consisted mostly of making countywide tests for tuberculosis and brucellosis. One county was tested at a time. Fifteen or twenty young veterinarians would be assigned to each county. When a county test was completed, the group would proceed to the another county.

Government-owned cars were assigned to these veterinarians. These vehicles were to be used for business only. However, the veterinarians were permitted to tow their private cars when they moved into a new county. It was quite a spectacle to see nearly twenty government cars driven by young men move into these small towns towing private cars.

The local people were not sure they wanted their cattle tested during this war period when agriculture products were in great demand. They did not realize that in the long run, disease control would increase productivity. Moreover, they were concerned their daughters and young women would be threatened by the influx of so many young, unmarried veterinarians. Marriages did take place, and some of these couples have celebrated their fiftieth anniversary.

In 1945, the Board encountered difficulties in hiring staff veterinarians and veterinarians for per diem testing. In addition, the Bureau reduced its staff from 45 to 9 veterinarians in Minnesota, and placed these remaining veterinarians on a 40-hour workweek. In tuberculosis testing, this lowered by one-third the number of animals that they could test in a week. By 1947, the Board was a year behind schedule in testing for brucellosis and tuberculosis. Because of this delay, some counties were in danger of losing their accreditation.

The Board of Animal Health appealed to Dr. Sims, chief of the Bureau of Animal Industry, to assign more veterinarians to Minnesota. Dr. Sims instead suggested that laymen be hired to do the bleeding. The Board objected to this solution and called an emergency meeting of veterinarians on July 25, 1947. Dr. E. H. Gloss, a member of the Board, presented the problem to the veterinarians in a very lucid manner and asked for their help. After some discussion, the 133 veterinarians present pledged 520 weeks of assistance. This pledge eased the situation considerably.

In 1950, a renewed inability to hire veterinarians caused Dr. Fred Driver, Inspector in Charge of the Bureau of Animal Industry in Minnesota, to request approval to hire veterinary students to draw blood for brucellosis tests. The Board approved the request as did the Veterinary Examining Board, and students were hired to work that summer.

The students were paid $252.00 per month plus $5.00 per day for room and board, plus 6 cents per mile. They were to test a minimum of 100 head per day, or at least seven herds of cattle. They were assigned to an area where the cattle population on the farms was small. Some had only four or five animals. Groups of four or five students would work under the supervision of a veterinarian. Some of the students involved were John Eckstein, Larry Algiers, Eiler Fredericksen, Verdie Gysland, Ray Hanson, Elmer Hokkanen, Lyle Klein, Harvard Larson, Maurice Palmer, Glen Schubert, and Edward Usenik.

In the early 1950s, the cattle owners in many counties had signed petitions requesting the countywide or area test for brucellosis. The shortage of veterinarians to do this testing was partially solved after the state started paying veterinarians and their assistants on a per head basis. At the start, veterinarians were paid 40 cents per head and assistants were paid 10 cents per head. The Board of Animal Health soon found that the per head incentive caused many veterinarians to test four times as many cattle in a day as one would expect a salaried veterinarian to test. Some of them tested around 3,000 head per week to gross $1,200 for the week. To earn this amount, they worked six or seven days a week from early morning to late evening.

About 20 veterinarians followed the per head testing on a full-time basis. They called themselves "per headers." The Board called them "contract veterinarians." Those people who did not like them referred to these veterinarians as "itinerant cow testers." These contract veterinarians served a very valuable purpose. Their excellent public relations skills made it possible for them to line up large numbers of heads to test. Without their help, the Board would not have been able to keep up with the demand for tests.

One contract veterinarian had the habit of skipping the small scattered herds in a county and then starting a new assignment in another county. There was little profit in testing small herds so he skipped them. The Board, however, required testing of all herds. At the organizational meeting, the veterinarian in charge of the test, George C. Keller, refused to give the uncooperative veterinarian his assignment until he had completed the tests on all herds in the previous county. This veterinarian took the assignment anyway without permission. When this was discovered by Dr. Keller, he and the veterinarian got into an unintended wrestling match. Although he recovered

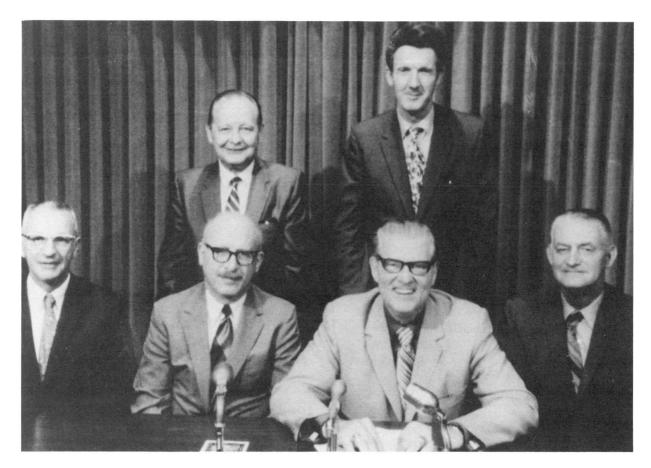

Minnesota Brucellosis Free declaration in Governor LeVander's office, 1970. Seated, left to right, Dr. John P. Arnold, pres. M.V.M.A., Dr. Jack G. Flint, exec. sec'y Board of Animal Health, Gov. LeVander, Mr. Paul Pierson, pres. Board of Animal Health, standing, Dr. Daniel Werring, veterinarian in charge, U.S.D.A., Minnesota, Dr. George Keller, Board of Animal Health, incharge of Brucellosis Division

the test assignment, Dr. Keller was very embarrassed by the episode. When he was teased about this incident in future years, Dr. Keller always said, "This was a demonstration of how not to do things."

RING TEST

A test developed in Germany that used the milk instead of blood serum and was called the "ring test" became a great aid in the surveillance of brucellosis. The test was improved by Dr. Martin Roepke of the University of Minnesota. After a few field trials, a program was established to use the ring test on a county-wide basis. By June of 1949, the ring test was used in a systematic manner in all of the counties in the area testing program. In conducting the ring test, herd samples of milk were taken at milk-collecting stations. The test determined whether there was infection in the herd. If the sample indicated infection, the animals in the herd were tested for brucellosis by drawing blood samples and performing the plate test. The ring test enabled the Board to keep more current on the status of dairy herds, was less

expensive than testing by drawing blood samples, and was more convenient for the dairy herd owners.

CHANGE IN VACCINATION PROGRAM: PROBLEMS WITH OVERAGE VACCINATION

Use of the *Brucella abortus* vaccine was limited to calves that were between three and seven months of age as of July 1, 1969. Further, dairy cattle under 20 months of age and beef cattle under 24 months of age that had been officially vaccinated by July 1, 1969, were exempt from the brucellosis test.

There were problems in reducing the rate of infection due to the persistence of the vaccination titer. The vaccination titer normally disappears in a few months in calves vaccinated at the proper age. However, it occasionally persists for years in calves vaccinated after they were over the age limit.

Brucella abortus vaccine could be obtained from one of the biologic houses or druggists referred to above that sold pharmaceuticals directly to laymen. These untrained professionals often would vaccinate animals well over the age limit. As these animals were not officially vaccinated, the Board had no record of their vaccination and they were given no grace period to lose their vaccination titer. These animals were tested along with the other members of the herd. If they reacted to the test, the cattle were branded as reactors. In that situation, they may not actually have been infected with brucellosis. Consequently, the rate of infection was artificially raised and this caused consternation on the part of both the owners and the Board of Animal Health.

MINNESOTA "BRUCELLOSIS FREE" IN CATTLE AND SWINE

Regardless of the problems and setbacks, the testing proceeded and, in July 1970, Minnesota was declared brucellosis free. This meant that the herd infection rate was one percent or less, and individual cattle infection rate was 0.2 percent or less over an 18-month testing period.

On July 27, 1973, the Board provided for a swine brucellosis program to enable Minnesota to obtain a validated status. On May 1, 1975, Minnesota was validated as swine brucellosis free.

On October 1, 1984, Minnesota had gone one full year without a single brucellosis reactor diagnosis. Therefore, on November 29, 1984, the state was declared an area in which brucellosis had been eradicated.

The eradication of brucellosis does not mean that there is no need for surveillance to prevent the return of the disease. All cattle sold in Minnesota either at auction or private sale must be tested. Dairy cattle are ring tested quarterly, and all breeding cattle two years of age and older are blood tested when they are sent to slaughter. Testing at slaughter is to monitor beef herds. They would not be monitored in the ring test on milk.

AVIAN DISEASE CONTROL

The first reference to the control of poultry diseases by the Live Stock Sanitary Board occurred in 1925 when a request was made to the legislature for appropriations to test poultry for certain diseases, including tuberculosis. In the control of tuberculosis, authorities had realized that chickens were a source of infection, especially in swine. However, the legislature declined to appropriate the funds.

Although it had failed to convince the legislature of the serious problem of tuberculosis in

chickens, the Board assigned Dr. L. E. Jenkins to full time duty on the elimination of avian tuberculosis. He began by attacking the problem with flock testing. However, in 1928, the Board decided that flock testing was not an economical way to eliminate tuberculosis in poultry. Although some sampling continued, the program was changed to emphasize education.

CONTROL OF POULTRY DISEASES IN CHICKENS

PULLORUM DISEASE

Pullorum disease, or bacillary white diarrhea, became a state-wide problem in the raising of chicks. In 1929, the Board voted to assign two veterinarians to control the disease. One of these veterinarians was to be a specialist in poultry diseases. The work was delayed due to difficulty in filling the low paying position of the poultry disease expert. Finally, Dr. H. D. Osborn of LeRoy, Minnesota, was hired. Dr. Osborn began work on October 1, 1929, only to resign on May 17, 1930. Dr. L. E. Jenkins, who had been assigned to assist Dr. Osborn, filled the gap created by Dr. Osborn's departure.

A program was developed to accredit flocks for pullorum disease. Five hatcheries signed the initial agreement for the program. Testing began in the fall of 1929 with 112 flocks consisting of 39,000 chickens. The rate of infection in these tests was 10 percent of the birds.[13]

As the testing continued, the incidence of the disease dropped dramatically in those flocks in which use of sanitary measures such as the immediate disposal of deceased birds was followed by cleaning and disinfection.

In 1930, a committee of the Minnesota Cooperative Baby Chick Association met with the Board of Animal Health to discuss when and how poultry flocks should be deemed "accredited." A committee was composed of President E. B. Anderson, Secretary Gregorson, Messrs. Ernest, Dyer, Baumgartner, and Tullock, and others whose names were not recorded.

Mr. W. T. Foley of the Farmer made the presentation to the Committee. He stated that the hatcheries in the state of Minnesota were using the term "accredited" to denote culling from the standpoint of type, breed and, to some extent, performance. The hatcheries in the East and

[13] For more on testing for pullorum and other *Salmonella*, see Table III-5.

Southeast were using the term "accredited" only to indicate control. The states in the central part of the United States were using accreditation much as it was used in Minnesota. Meanwhile, the members of the Board of Animal Health objected to accreditation except as it would relate to disease control.

Dr. John R. Mohler, chief of the Bureau of Animal Industry, proposed that "accredited" status be used to denote both culling and disease control. Dr. Mohler further stated that, if 15 states accepted the definition that he proposed, the federal government would cooperate and supply funds to assist in disease control. The Board eventually adopted the "Mohler Plan" in early 1934, and the cooperative agreement was signed sometime thereafter.

In 1931, the legislature became more concerned by the problems with poultry disease and created the Poultry Improvement Board. The board was composed of the "Commissioner of Agriculture, Executive Officer of the Board of Animal Health, Chief of the Poultry Division of the College of Agriculture, University of Minnesota and two experienced poultrymen who were owners and operators of commercial hatcheries." The legislature authorized the board to adopt and enforce rules and regulations for the control and elimination of certain communicable diseases in poultry.

In July of 1931, the Board of Animal Health adopted the rapid whole blood plate test for pullorum. This test could be conducted in the field and only required one-time testing of the birds. However, the test did not come into widespread use until later. In the meantime, veterinarians continued to send blood samples to the laboratory for the pullorum test.

The Board of Animal Health arranged for veterinarians to receive instructions on how to conduct the rapid whole blood plate test for pullorum at the laboratory at the University of Minnesota. During the 1931-1932 fiscal year, 91 veterinarians took the course. Twenty-five of those who took the course also received additional instruction in the field from the Board's veterinarians and were approved to conduct the test.

A plan was prepared whereby the Board of Animal Health would supervise the flock owners and hatcheries in their effort to obtain accreditation for pullorum disease. Under the agreement, the flock owners and hatcheries employed veterinarians to draw the blood and submit the samples to the laboratory. In addition, all reactors were removed from the premises. During the 1932-1933 fiscal year, 28 hatcheries with 401 flocks consisting of 107,000 chickens were tested. The rate of infection from these tests was 8 percent.[14] The agreement was changed the following year to require removal of all reacting birds from the premises as soon as the report of the test was received and the cleaning and disinfecting of the premises within 20 days of the date of the test.

Minnesota regulations provided that custom hatching could be carried out in the same room in a separate incubator. In December 1934, Mr. W. K. Dyer, secretary and executive officer of the Minnesota Poultry Improvement Board, informed the Board of Animal Health that the National Baby Chick Association Code prohibited the performance of custom hatching unless maintained in separate and distinct rooms. Mr. Dyer further stated that, if Minnesota adopted the national code, it would be financially impossible for hatchery owners in Minnesota to comply with the law, and they would be forced to drop out of the testing program administered by the Board. The Board waited until October of 1935 before amending the regulation to conform with the national code so as to require that eggs from flocks not tested for pullorum be hatched in separate and distinct rooms.

In January 1937, the Board of Animal Health and the Minnesota Poultry Improvement Board entered into a cooperative agreement with the Bureau of Animal Industry for the control of pullorum disease. Under the agreement, the Bureau provided coordinators who would supervise and administer the National Poultry Improvement Plan in Minnesota. The Bureau paid the salary and expenses for these personnel.

There were three classifications under the National Poultry Improvement Plan:

U.S. Pullorum Tested;

U.S. Pullorum Passed; and

U.S. Pullorum Clean.[15]

The regulations were amended in October 1938 to allow trained laymen to conduct the rapid whole blood plate test on flocks with the U.S.

---

[14] For more on testing see Table III-5.
[15] No reactors in two consecutive tests not less than six months apart.

Pullorum Tested classification. Thirty-nine laymen received training and were approved to conduct the test during the 1938-1939 fiscal year. Forty-eight more were approved to conduct the test the following year. During this time, there still were 67 veterinarians conducting pullorum tests.

During the 1939-1940 fiscal year, the Board of Animal Health reached an agreement with the Minnesota Poultry Improvement Board wherein testing services would not be furnished to new hatcheries unless they signed up with both of the boards under the national plan. The following year, the regulations were changed so that hatcheries registered under the national plan also came under the supervision of both the Board of Animal Health and the Minnesota Poultry Improvement Board. Additionally, the regulations allowed the establishment of the U.S. Controlled Pullorum classification for flocks with less than 2 percent infection.

In 1948, the Snow Hatcheries in Sleepy Eye, which also had branch hatcheries in Albert Lea, St. Cloud, and Worthington, was charged with irregularities in the pullorum testing of flocks that supplied eggs for their hatcheries. According to the allegations, some of the flocks were tested by persons not approved by the Board to conduct the test while the results were signed by other persons who had been approved to conduct the test. At the hearing, the hatchery was unable to absolve itself of the charges and was dropped from the program.

In 1949, the Beaudry Hatchery in Albertville was dropped from the program for hatching eggs from an unapproved source. The Battle Lake Hatchery was also dropped from the program for hatching eggs supplied by the Loose Hatchery at Boyd, a source that was not in the pullorum program.

In April 1957, testing for pullorum-typhoid became compulsory for all hatcheries and breeding flocks selling chicks and hatching eggs. Chicken flocks had to meet U.S. Pullorum-Typhoid Passed or Clean classification, or its equivalent. Rules were established requiring all hatching eggs and day old chicks imported into Minnesota to meet U.S. Pullorum-Typhoic Clean status or its equivalent.

Pullorum disease and fowl typhoid were made reportable diseases during the 1957-1958 fiscal year. Infected flocks were quarantined and marketed under supervision of the Board. Although exempted during the 1959-1960 fiscal

year, waterfowl were later required to be tested. In 1963, poultry for exhibition were required to be tested for pullorum-typhoid.

The rate of infection with pullorum-typhoid continued to drop until no reactors were found during the 1965-1966 fiscal year. See Table III-5. No reactors have been found in chickens since that time. In August 1975, Minnesota received the U.S. Pullorum-Typhoid Clean State classification from the U.S. Department of Agriculture for all poultry, including turkeys.

TABLE III-5

DATA ON PULLORUM-TYPHOID TESTING OF CHICKENS AT FIVE YEAR INTERVALS

Fiscal Year	No. of Hatcheries	No. of Flocks	No. of Birds	Percent Infected
1930-1931	—	256	81,000	12.0
1935-1936	42	840	194,275	3.9[a]
1940-1941	91	2,071	568,731	5.7
1945-1946	173	5,497	1,918,371	2.0
1950-1955	249	5,271	2,044,351	0.8
1055-1956	208	3,302	1,639,107	0.2
1960-1961	215	1,746	1,503,142	0.007
1965-1966	138	597	745,685	No reactors
1970-1971	85	185	494,474	No reactors
1975-1976	42	98	371,483	No reactors
1980-1981	24	54	353,512	No reactors
1985-1986	13	30	635,703	No Test[b]
1989-1990	9	36	498,180	No Test[c]

[a]   Testing for S. pullorum started under Board of Animal Health official program in 1931-1932.

[b]   Partial testing for birds listed.

[c]   Because Minnesota has a U.S. Pullorum-Typhoid Clean State Classification, hatcheries can participate in the program without testing. In 1989-90, 3,300 birds were tested as part of the S. enteritidis program. All were negative.

Source: Data courtesy of Dr. Harry R. Olson, Board of Animal Health

NEWCASTLE DISEASE

Newcastle disease, or avian pneumoencephalitis, made its appearance in the eastern states while the Board of Animal Health and the Minnesota Poultry Improvement Board were trying to eliminate pullorum-typhoid disease. Newcastle disease spread rapidly, and in June 1946, Dr. Ruel Fenstermacher of the University of Minnesota Diagnosis Laboratory reported that he had diagnosed Newcastle disease. The diagnosis was confirmed by serum neutralization test at the Pathology Division of the Bureau of Animal Industry.

Drs. L. E. Jenkins and O. B. Gochnauer were assigned to visit the farms and quarantine those flocks from which the birds with Newcastle disease had originated. They were also instructed to check other flocks in the neighborhood to learn the source of the infection. As a further measure to prevent the spread of the disease, all poultry exhibits were banned from county and state fairs. From January 1, 1947, to May 28, 1947, 33 positive cases of the disease were found in 21 Minnesota counties. By July 11, 1947, 98 flocks in 50 counties had been infected.

While a vaccine was available for Newcastle, the Board was not sure of the vaccine's effectiveness. The poultry industry pressured the Board to allow the use of these vaccines. The Board voted to issue permits for the purchase of specified amounts of vaccine by veterinarians, hatchery owners, and poultry growers. Fifteen permits were issued in 1948. The permits were issued on the condition that users would report the results of the vaccination to the Board on special forms. In this way, the poultry industry was testing the effectiveness of the vaccine for the Board.

While the vaccine generally proved effective in controlling the disease, the vaccines that did not contain a killed virus failed to eliminate the disease. The disease continued to spread. As a result, the restriction on the use of vaccines was lifted and Newcastle now is controlled by vaccination.

INFECTIOUS BRONCHITIS

In the late summer and fall of 1952, there was a severe outbreak of infectious bronchitis in chickens in southern Minnesota. The special committee that had been appointed to study means of controlling diseases of poultry recommended limited use of a virulent vaccine for preventing bronchitis.

At this time, an attenuated vaccine for infectious bronchitis was developed by Salsbury Laboratories, in Charles City, Iowa. Salsbury was granted a special license by the Bureau of Animal Industry to manufacture and distribute the vaccine. The Board of Animal Health approved the use of the vaccine on an experimental basis under the direction of Dr. B. S. Pomeroy of the University of Minnesota's Division of Veterinary Medicine. Although the vaccine was only to be used on young chicks, the Board received complaints from the industry and others that some hatchery operators were using the vaccine on adult birds. The Board had not received a copy of the provisions that had accompanied the special license granted to the Salsbury Laboratories by the Bureau, and apparently assumed that the Bureau was controlling the sale of the product. Following the use of the vaccine in the spring, the Board received a notice from the Bureau in mid-summer stating that, pursuant to the special license issued to the laboratory, the vaccine could be shipped interstate under restrictions that may be imposed by the state. The Board closed this loophole by requiring distribution of the vaccine in Minnesota only under special permit for each shipment and mandating that it had to be administered by a veterinarian to young birds on the farm.

On February 10, 1954, the Board voted to allow wider use of the vaccine in hatcheries. All vaccinated birds had to be kept in special chick battery hatcheries for at least four weeks following vaccination, the birds had to be inspected by a qualified veterinarian, and purchasers had to be given a statement pointing out that the birds' immunity was only temporary and they had to be revaccinated with a modified live virus or a virulent virus to obtain permanent immunity.

In 1955, restrictions on the sales of modified live virus vaccines for infectious bronchitis were lifted when the manufacturer was licensed by the Agricultural Research Service of the Department of Agriculture. The following year, the Board approved the sale of a combination vaccine composed of live viruses of infectious bronchitis and Newcastle disease. Both diseases are now controlled by the use of vaccines and are no longer considered reportable diseases.

MYCOPLASMA INFECTIONS

Mycoplasma infections in chickens, or chronic respiratory disease ("CRD"), were recognized in the 1950s. Chronic respiratory disease is caused by *Mycoplasma gallisepticum* and affects feed conversion, growth of chicks, egg production, and egg hatchability. This disease was shown to be egg-transmitted. The mortality rate is low unless the disease is complicated by another disease.

The National Poultry Improvement Plan (NPIP) developed a program for the control of *Mycoplasma gallisepticum* in meat-type and egg-type primary and parent chicken breeding flocks. In 1977, the Board amended the mycoplasma rule for turkeys so as to cover all poultry effective June of that year. The program provided for voluntary participation in *Mycoplasma gallisepticum* (MG) and *Mycoplasma synovia* (MS) programs. However, no chicken hatcheries elected to take part in the MS program.

Generally, there has been little enthusiasm for the mycoplasma control program among Minnesota chicken hatcheries. The first chicken hatchery took part in the MG program in fiscal year 1979. Four more hatcheries took part in the program the following year. Seventeen chicken hatcheries were operating in the state in fiscal year 1984, and only three of these hatcheries actually participated in the MG program. In the 1990s all three chick hatcheries are under the MG program.

CONTROL OF POULTRY DISEASES IN TURKEYS

PULLORUM DISEASE

The testing of turkeys for pullorum disease started during the 1933-1934 fiscal year when nine flocks consisting of 2,600 birds were tested. The infection rate in this group was 2.35 percent. Because the rapid whole blood test used in chickens proved unreliable, the tube agglutination test for pullorum was recommended for use with turkeys. These tests were conducted at the University of Minnesota's Diagnostic Laboratory. The laboratory also conducted a bacteriological examination of the reactors. The number of turkey flock owners and turkey hatcheries requesting tests has gradually increased over the years. See Table III-6.

TABLE III-6

DATA ON TESTING TURKEYS FOR PULLORUM-TYPHOID AND S. TYPHIMURIUM

Fiscal Year	No. of Hatcheries	No. of Flocks	No. of Birds	% Infected Pullorum-Typhoid	% Infected S. typhimurium
1935-1936	—	32	3,948	0.46	—
1940-1941	—	93	21,896	0.9	—
1945-1946[a]	77[b]	380	167,496	3.7	—
1950-1951	63[b]	485	247,629	0.43	—
1955-1956	49[b]	539	432,199	0.09	—
1960-1961	56[b]	798	948,142	0.009	0.04
1965-1966	42[b]	631	700,353	0.021	0.56
1970-1971	26[b]	256	527,572	0.02	0.02
1975-1976[c]	14	147	596,319	[d]	1 flock
1985-1986	9	112	635,703	[d]	None
1989-1990	9	100	923,175	[d]	None

[a] Official Minnesota pullorum program started in 1943-1944.
[b] Some official hatcheries combined chicken and turkey testing.
[c] Official *S. typhimurium* control program began in 1971-1972.
[d] Minnesota recognized U.S. pullorum-typhoid free in 1973.

Note: 1985-1986 and 1989-1990 data from commercial flocks. Exhibition flocks are required to have part of the flock tested.

Source: Data courtesy of Dr. Harry R. Olson and Keith Friendshuh, Board of Animal Health.

Diagnostic Laboratory reports indicated that pullorum disease in turkeys was on the increase and had become established in Minnesota turkey breeding flocks. The infection in other states was also high, and Minnesota imported a high percentage of its hatching eggs from West Coast states. In 1943, the Minnesota Turkey Growers Association, in cooperation with the Board of Animal Health and the University of Minnesota, requested $10,000 from the legislature for laboratory testing and supplies. The legislature eventually appropriated $6,000 for the Diagnostic Laboratory and $4,000 for the Board to support this program.

Mobile Testing Units. A mobile unit was equipped and used on a trial basis to facilitate the tube agglutination test for pullorum in turkeys. The unit proved successful, so it was no longer necessary to transport blood samples to the university for testing. The Department of Diagnostic Investigation furnished the technicians and laboratory supplies while the Board furnished supervising veterinarians and paid travel expenses for the mobile unit. Miss Florence Jones was the first technician involved in the program. She continued in that capacity until her retirement. Dr. L. E. Jenkins supervised the first mobile unit and the poultry programs for the Board. When he retired, Dr. Harry Olson became supervisor of the programs.

The original mobile unit proved practical and, during the 1947-1948 fiscal year, a second unit was added to handle the increased number of turkeys that could be tested. The state was divided into a northern and southern area with Highway 12 serving as the dividing line. Each year, the mobile unit in the north set up in Detroit Lakes twice and once each in Little Falls and Thief River Falls. The unit in the south was stationed as a semipermanent laboratory in a building rented in Mankato.

During the 1950-51 fiscal year, Swift & Company began to furnish permanent space for the north mobile laboratory at Detroit Lakes free of charge. This arrangement continued until the 1961-62 fiscal year when the laboratory moved into the Korinta Building in Detroit Lakes and the Minnesota Turkey Growers Association assumed the cost. During the 1954-55 year, the laboratory at Mankato was closed. A laboratory was subsequently created in Rochester during the 1961-62 fiscal year when the Minnesota Turkey Growers Association rented space in the Bathke Animal Hospital. This laboratory was later moved to the Olmsted County Fairgrounds. Meanwhile, the laboratory at Willmar was moved to the Pfizer Diagnostic Laboratory Building, which had been purchased by the University of Minnesota in 1968. During the 1977-1978 fiscal year, the laboratories at Detroit Lakes and Rochester were closed and all of the testing was done at the Willmar Laboratory under the direction of Dr. L. T. Ausherman.

PULLORUM CONTROL PROGRAM ADOPTED.

In October 1943, the Board adopted rules and regulations to control pullorum in turkeys. Under the plan, there were four classifications of flocks:

1. Minnesota Pullorum Tested;

2. Minnesota Pullorum Controlled;

3. Minnesota Pullorum Passed; and

4. Minnesota Pullorum Free.

In 1945, these rules and regulations were amended so as to qualify Minnesota for a cooperative agreement with the Bureau of Animal Industry under the National Turkey Improvement Plan.

Considerable progress was made in reducing pullorum disease in turkeys, and during the 1948-1949 fiscal year the industry requested an amendment to the regulations to remove the "tested" classification and the requirement that no flocks could have over 2 percent infection and still be under supervision.

The Board subsequently amended the rules during the 1953-1954 fiscal year so as to delete the "tested" and "controlled" classifications. In April 1957, poultry testing for pullorum-typhoid became compulsory. The hatcheries and breeding flocks selling poults and hatching eggs were required to meet the same U.S. Pullorum-Typhoid Clean classification as day-old poults and hatching eggs imported from other states.

During the 1957-1958 fiscal year, pullorum disease and fowl typhoid were made reportable diseases. Infected flocks were quarantined and marketed under supervision of the Board. In August 1965, the Board received a request from the Minnesota Turkey Growers Association to develop a Pullorum-Typhoid Eradication Program. The Department of Agriculture began to develop criteria for states to qualify for U.S. Pullorum-Typhoid Clean state classification. In June 1966, the National Poultry Improvement Plan proposed a program for turkeys. The Board was notified in February 1968 that Minnesota met all of the requirements for a U.S. Pullorum-Typhoid Clean State for turkeys. Minnesota was the first state to receive this classification.

MINNESOTA A PULLORUM-TYPHOID FREE STATE.

There was no isolation of *S. pullorum* or *S. gallinarium* (causative organisms of pullorum disease and fowl typhoid) from turkeys in Minnesota from 1956 to 1975. Consequently, Minnesota received from the U.S. Department of Agriculture the U.S. Pullorum-Typhoid Clean State classification, which covered commercial flocks.

The turkey industry as a whole cooperated in the programs to control diseases. However, there were exceptions to this cooperation. One example involved the Mixa Turkey Hatchery at Redwood Falls. During a routine inspection, turkey eggs from an infected flock were found in the hatchery. Mr. Mixa, the owner, was directed to immediately retest the flock from which the eggs had originated or remove the eggs from the hatchery. Mr. Mixa refused to do either of these options on the grounds that he could not afford the expense of compliance. Mr. Mixa's hatchery was subsequently dropped from supervision.

SALMONELLA TYPHIMURIUM

In 1950, an unofficial typhimurium program was initiated. Earlier that year, the Minnesota Turkey Growers Association established the Breeder Hen Committee, which was primarily concerned with supporting turkey disease control programs and establishing an unofficial *Salmonella typhimurium* or paratyphoid control program. The Breeder Hen Committee collected fees from the cooperating hatcheries and flock owners to finance the increased cost of the testing program at the mobile laboratories. The flocks were tested using pullorum and typhimurium as separate test tube antigens. The laboratory prepared the antigens. During the 1950-1951 fiscal year, 63 hatcheries involving 485 flocks and 247,629 birds cooperated in the pullorum and typhimurium programs. As soon as they were diagnosed, the reactors were removed from the flock. Breeding flocks that had the reactors were retested until no reactors to the serological test were found or the serological reactors were negative to bacteriological examination.

Official S. Typhimurium Control Program. In 1970, the Minnesota Turkey Growers Association requested the development of an official *S. typhimurium* control program. The association also requested amendment of the rules on importation of day old poults and hatching eggs from other states to require that these poults and eggs originate from *S. typhimurium* negative or "clean" flocks.

The official Minnesota Typhimurium Control Program for turkeys began in the 1971-1972 fiscal year. The program modified the testing procedure so that, instead of testing the entire flock, 500 blood samples and 500 cloacal swabs were taken from each flock. The blood samples were tested using a combination antigen containing *S. pullorum* and *S. typhimurium* (P10) killed organisms. The cloacal swabs were cultured in enriched media and plated to identify the presence of any *Salmonella*. If *S. typhimurium* was recovered, the flock was considered infected. If other serotypes of *Salmonella* were recovered, no

official action was taken. During the 1971-1972 fiscal year, nine out of 201 flocks were infected. The hatcheries with the infection elected to drop the typhimurium program. During the 1972-1973 fiscal year, three typhimurium infected flocks were identified. The hatcheries with those flocks were eliminated from the program. Since 1980, the average number of infected flocks identified each year has been one.

Salmonella Program Enlarged. In 1981, turkey industries in California and Minnesota initiated a cooperative *Salmonella* program. Under the program, the *Salmonella* profile of the turkey flocks owned by cooperating California primary breeders was relayed to cooperating Minnesota hatcheries.

In addition, the Minnesota turkey industry began a program with animal protein providers to reduce *Salmonella* contamination of animal by-products used in turkey breeder feeds.

The Minnesota Breeder Hen Committee recommended to the turkey industry use of one of the following feeding programs for breeder candidates:

1. No animal by-products may be used and feed must be pelletized;

2. No animal by-products may be used and mash feed must be used;

3. Animal by-products may be used and feed must be pelletized; or

4. Animal by-products from Salmonella-clean source may be used and mash feed must be used.

One hundred percent of the industry complied to the recommendations when feeding breeders in lay. However, 15 percent of the industry used animal by-products in mash feed to young breeder replacements. An intensified environmental monitoring system has been added to the program. In 1981, 35 percent of the breeder flocks aged 16-20 weeks were found to be *Salmonella* clean at the time of the official test. By 1984, this figure had climbed to 72 percent.

Mycoplasma Control Programs / Mycoplasma gallisepticum. Infectious sinusitis in turkeys became a serious problem in the 1950s. *Mycoplasma gallisepticum* ("MG") was determined to be egg transmitted. A pilot testing program that started in the fall of 1956 was later enlarged to test 10 percent of the serum samples from all turkey flocks. This was modified to limit the test to 100 samples taken at the time of the official pullorum-typhoid test. During the 1960-1961 fiscal year, because there were outbreaks of the disease following the partial flock tests, the Board started an unofficial *Mycoplasma gallisepticum* program to test all of the birds in the flock. In an effort to fine tune the test, selected reactors were sent to the University of Minnesota's laboratory for retesting and bacteriological examination to recover the organism. At the request of the turkey industry, the Board adopted the examination as an official program in July of 1963. Any flock found to be infected with the disease was eliminated from the program.

During the 1966-1967 fiscal year, the National Poultry Improvement Plan added an official *Mycoplasma gallisepticum* testing program, and the test was reduced to 500 samples per flock. All flocks that were tested that year were negative for the disease. That number has been maintained through the present time. In 1980, Minnesota was one of the first states to obtain the U.S. Department of Agriculture requirements for *Mycoplasma gallisepticum* Clean State for turkeys.

Mycoplasma meleagridis. In the 1960s, Dr. Pomeroy and his co-workers began research on *M. meleagridis* ("MM") which involved a lesion known as air sacculitis. This research had great economic importance because this disease was one of the major causes of condemnations of fryer-roaster turkeys in Minnesota. For several years, turkey flocks were monitored for *M. meleagridis* and *M. synoviae*. However, it was not until the 1979-1980 fiscal year that negative flocks for *M. meleagridis* were identified. In July 1980, the National Plans Conference adopted a U.S. *Mycoplasma meleagridis* Clean Flock Program that became effective January 1, 1983. The testing for *M. meleagridis* was intensified during the 1980-1981 fiscal year when 60 percent of the flocks were negative on the initial test. During the 1983-1984 fiscal year, all hatcheries participated in the official *M. meleagridis* program. Of these, five hatcheries qualified all breeding flocks, and three hatcheries had at least some positive flocks.

Mycoplasma Synoviae. Mycoplasma synoviae produces soft enlargements of joints and tendon sheaths, interferes with growth, and causes lameness. Flocks were tested for both *M. synoviae* and *M. meleagridis* on a monitoring basis. During the 1979-1980 fiscal year, the Board started an unofficial *M. synoviae* program for turkeys. During the 1983-1984 fiscal year, the flocks under the official *M. meleagridis* program were also tested for *M. synoviae*, and no infected flocks were identified. In 1984, the National Plans Conference approved the *M. synoviae* program.

DR. FLINT RETIRES; DR. HAGERTY NEW EXECUTIVE SECRETARY

Dr. Jack G. Flint retired as the Board's executive secretary[16] on January 1, 1985. Dr. Flint will be remembered as a very able administrator who used common sense and persuasion to bring about the accomplishments of his term of office. He was a modest, unassuming person who had a good sense of humor. Much was accomplished in Minnesota disease control during Dr. Flint's 24-year tour of duty. The following are some of the disease control efforts that came to completion in Minnesota during this period:

- 1963 Sheep scabies was declared eradicated.
- 1972 Minnesota became hog cholera free.

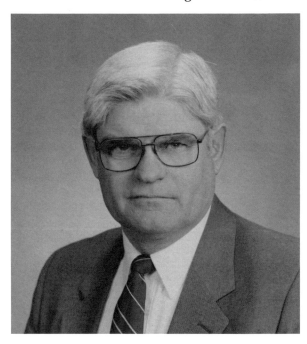

Dr. Thomas J, Hagerty, executive secretary, Jan. 1, 1985-present

16/ The title, secretary and executive officer, did not fit into the Board's computer and was changed on July 6, 1984, to executive secretary.

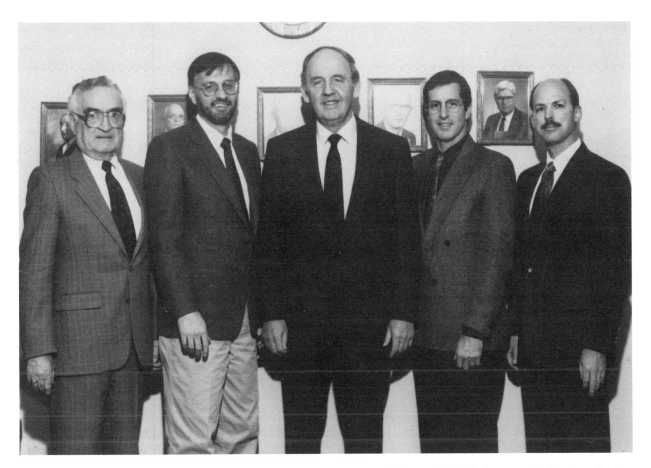

Professional staff, Board of Animal Health, 1992; left to right, Drs. Walter J. Mackey, William L. Hartman, John Landman, Keith Friendshuh, Paul Anderson.

- 1975 Minnesota was declared swine tuberculosis free.
- 1975 Minnesota was declared pullorum-typhoid clean.
- 1976 Minnesota was declared bovine tuberculosis free.
- 1980 Minnesota was recognized as Mycoplasma galisepticum clean in turkeys.
- 1984 Brucellosis was eradicated in Minnesota.

The period from 1960 through 1984 was a very productive period of disease control thanks to the leadership of Dr. Flint, as well as the efforts of his predecessors and colleagues.

Dr. Thomas Hagerty of St. Michael was selected by the Board of Animal Health to succeed Dr. Flint. Dr. Hagerty had practiced in St. Michael for 26 years, was a past president of the Minnesota Veterinary Medical Association, and had been chairman of the St. Michael Albertville school board. He joined the staff on October 1, 1984, and had the opportunity to work with Dr. Flint before his retirement. He is only the sixth secretary and executive office of the Board since its beginning in 1903.

MEMBERS OF THE BOARD OF ANIMAL HEALTH

Many distinguished citizens of the state have served on the Board of Animal Health. They have given freely of their time in the interest of the livestock and poultry industries. In the control of diseases, they have been obliged to occasionally make unpopular decisions that have subjected them to severe criticism by the public. The names of those dedicated individuals with their years of service are recorded below in Exhibit III-2.

EXHIBIT III-2

MEMBERS OF THE BOARD OF ANIMAL HEALTH

Name	Address	Years of Service
W. W. P. McConnell	Mankato	1904-1909
Forest Henry	Dover	1903-1905
Dr. Charles E. Cotton	Minneapolis	1903-1905
Dr. M. H. Reynolds	St. Paul	1903-1922
J. J. Furlong	Austin	1903-1908
Wm. Timpane	Waterville	1905-1910
C. A. Nelson	Fridley	1908-1923
P. H. Grogan	St. James	1909-1914

(Exhibit III-2 continued on next page)

(Exhibit III-2 continued)

Name	Address	Years of Service
Carl Sholin	Milaca	1910-1915
H. R. Smith	St. Paul	1904-1917
W. S. Moscrip	Lake Elmo	1917-1949
T. C. Hovde	Hanska	1915-1920
Dr. J. N. Gould	Worthington	1918-1926
Col. C. H. Marsh	Litchfield	1920-1930
Dr. C. P. Fitch	St. Paul	1922-1940
O. W. Healy	Mapleton	1923-1938
Dr. H. A. Greaves	Glenwood	1926-1931
P. O. Holland	Northfield	1930-1940
Dr. W. A. Anderson	Sleepy Eye	1931-1941
Charles Ewald	Waldorf	1939-1958
A. L. Sayers	Hastings	1940-1948
Dr. W. L. Boyd	St. Paul	1940-1956
Dr. E. H. Gloss	Gaylord	1946-1956
Dr. G. F. Ghostley	Anoka	1948-1955
E. H. Knodt	Rosemount	1949-1964
Dr. E. J. Kerr	Minnesota	1956-1961
Dr. J. B. Flanary	St. Charles	1957-1961
C. C. Chase	Pipestone	1958-1961
Dr. H. J. Ruebke	Ada	1955-1961
Dr. R. S. Kufrin	Benson	1961-1964
Dr. Glen H. Nelson	New Richland	1961-1961
Graydon McCulley	Maple Plain	1961-1972
Dr. L. H. Pint	Austin	1961-1965
Charles Hartung	Bertha	1964-1969
Dr. J. J. Kelley	Marshall	1964-1967
Dr. John Fogarty	Belle Plaine	1965-1967
Dr. R. J. Tabola	Jackson	1967-1978
Dr. A. B. Magnusson	Blooming Prairie	1967-1978
Paul Pierson	Lake Elmo	1969-1979
Dr. A. O. Setzepfandt	Bird Island	1972-1975
Alvin Offerman	Montevideo	1972-1981
Dr. Robert Mersch	Fairfax	1975-1984
Odell Christianson	Wendell	1976-1978
Dr. E. K. Karnis	Alexandria	1978-1981
Lois Elaine Lindberg	Miltona	1978-1981
Jerry Rypka	Owatonna	1979-1983
Dr. C. H. Contag	New Ulm	1981-1985
Robert J. Barton	Silver Lake	1981-1983
Kenneth E. Neeser	St. Cloud	1981-1985
Jack Delaney	Lake Benton	1983-1991
Herbert Halverson	Hanska	1983-1988
Dr. Sharon Hurley	New Ulm	1984-1992
Dr. Henry Banal	Sauk Centre	1985-1992
Theodore Huisinga	Wilmar	1986-
Allan Routh	Owatonna	1988-2-3 mos.
Patricia Christensen	Milroy	1991-
Russell J. Wirt	Lewiston	1991-
Dr. John Howe, Jr.	Grand Rapids	1992-
Dr. Joni Scheftel	Watertown	1993-

FEDERAL VETERINARIANS IN CHARGE FOR MINNESOTA

The valuable assistance of the U.S. Department of Agriculture, Bureau of Animal Industry, and Animal and Plant Health Inspection Service has been referred to above. However, the authors would be remiss if they did not name the federal veterinarians in Minnesota who super-

vised the important role the U.S. Department of Agriculture played in the control of animal and poultry diseases in Minnesota. See Exhibit III-30. These men gave unselfishly of their time and effort, cooperated with the Board of Animal Health, and used sound judgment and leadership in administering the programs.

EXHIBIT III-3

FEDERAL VETERINARIANS

Name	Title	Date of Service
Dr. M. O. Anderson	Chief Inspector	1918
Dr. W. J. Fretz	Chief Inspector	1919-1945
Dr. Fred C. Driver	Chief Inspector	1946-1959
Dr. Daniel Werring	Veterinarian in Charge	1960-1971
Dr. Robert Morgan	Veterinarian in Charge	1971-1973
Dr. E. M. Joneschild	Veterinarian in Charge	1974
Dr. Basil Ward	Veterinarian in Charge	1975-1980
Dr. Donald Luchsinger	Veterinarian in Charge	1980-1985
Dr. Page E. Eppele	Veterinarian in Charge	1985-1988
Dr. Donald H. Person	Veterinarian in Charge	1988

Minnesota over the years has developed the enviable record of having very progressive disease control programs. This success is no doubt due to the splendid spirit of cooperation that has existed between the disease control officials, the practicing veterinarians, the veterinary college staff, and the livestock owners. The spirit of cooperation continues to exist to this day.

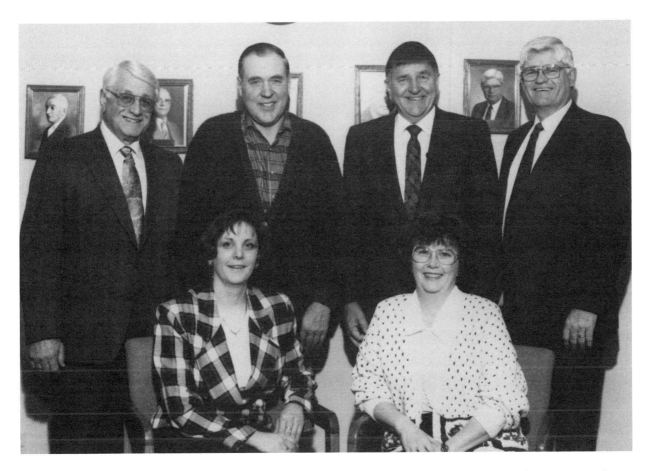

Members of the Board of Animal Health, 1992; left to right. seated, Dr. Sharon Hurly, chm., Mrs. Patricia Christenson, standing, Dr. Henry Banal, Mr. Russell Wirt, Mr. Ted Huisinga, Dr. Thomas J. Hagarty, exec. sec'y.

CHAPTER IV

State and Regional Associations

It is important in any profession for members to meet, exchange ideas, discuss problems and learn of new developments. These activities usually begin with a group of a few members of the profession who are particularly interested in these issues. This group eventually grows larger until a formal organization is formed.

MINNESOTA VETERINARY MEDICAL ASSOCIATION

In the late 1880s, some of Minnesota's more progressive graduate veterinarians saw the need for a state-wide forum to exchange information and to promote the veterinary profession. Two veterinary organizations had been formed previously but neither covered the entire state. One of these organizations was the short-lived Northwestern Veterinary Medical Association formed in 1888, and the other was the Southern Minnesota Veterinary Medical and Dental Association.[1]

A small group of veterinarians headed by Drs. C. C. Lyford, Richard Price, and M. H. Reynolds called a meeting for January 28, 1897, at the Merchant's Hotel in St. Paul to start a state-wide veterinary organization. Dr. Reynolds, who was the only veterinarian employed at the time by the University of Minnesota, sent the notice of the meeting to the graduate veterinarians in Minnesota. Because he had lectured at short courses throughout the state, Dr. Reynolds was well-known and well-liked among Minnesota's veterinarians.

Thirteen of the 87 graduate veterinarians then practicing in Minnesota attended the meeting, and a new veterinary association was formed.[2] In the January 29, 1897, issue of the St. Paul Pioneer Press, the initial meeting was described as follows:

The Minnesota State Veterinary Medical Association is one day old. It was born yes-

terday afternoon at the Merchant's Hotel while a dozen veterinary surgeons gathered in answer to a call for the organization of a veterinary society . . . for the diffusion of knowledge; the extension of professional acquaintances; for pleasant reunions; for the stimulation of professional study and investigation, and especially at this time, of considering the advisability of trying to improve the condition of our state veterinary legislation . . . .

After Dr. N. S. Erb of Faribault had been made temporary chairman and Dr. Richard Price of this city, temporary secretary, the surgeons speedily resolved to organize under a permanent charter. Dr. Price was made a committee of one to secure an appropriate charter, while the following officers were named: Dr. S. D. Brimhall of Minneapolis, president; Dr. J. P. Anderson of Rochester, first vice-president; Dr. A. Youngberg of Lake Park, second vice-president; Dr. L. Hay of Faribault, secretary and Dr. K. J. McKenzie of Northfield, treasurer.

Committees appointed yesterday were: on infectious diseases, Doctors Reynolds, Gould, Sr., and Youngberg; on finances, Doctors Anderson, Eddy and Dallimore; on education, Doctors Ward, Gould and Anderson; and on legislation, Doctors Lyford, Price and Erb.

The surgeons present at yesterday's meeting were Doctors N. S. Erb of Faribault; H. L. Eddy, C. C. Lyford, S. D. Brimhall of Minneapolis; Richard Price, G. A. Dallimore, L. Adamson of St. Paul; J. P. Anderson of Rochester; M. H. Reynolds of the state agricultural experiment station at St. Anthony Park; L. Hay of Faribault; A. Youngberg of Lake Park; K. J. McKenzie of Northfield; J. N. Gould of Worthington and S. Ward of St. Cloud.

The Articles of Incorporation for the new association were drawn, signed, and filed with the secretary of state on February 23, 1897. The Articles of Incorporation stated:

---

[1]. The only reference found on the Southern Minnesota Veterinary Medical and Dental Association stated that group was to meet in Owatonna, Minnesota, on July 12, 1897, and that it had been in existence for several years. The proceedings were not mentioned in the Owatonna newspaper of that date.

[2] Because all of the older records of the association were destroyed in the 1943 fire at the University of Minnesota's Veterinary Building, much of the information about the early history of the association must be taken from newspapers.

The purpose and objective of this association shall be the cultivation of the science and art of comparative medicine; the promotion of animal industry as a branch of agriculture; the interchanging of professional experiences and encouragement of professional zeal; the promotion of friendly feeling and cooperation in the entire medical profession, and the maintenance and care of such apartments as are provided for the society; the preservation of all specimens, books and other articles which may come into its possession; and obtaining necessary and proper legislation, and to this end and purpose may acquire, buy, sell, hold, lease and mortgage all sorts of property, real, personal or mixed, and may do such other things as shall be necessary and convenient for the promotion of said purpose and objectives.

In addition to the persons named above, Drs. J. G. Annand of Lake City, E. N. Chute of Fairmont, J. A. Hanish of Zumbrota, B. Lambrechts of Montevideo, and H. Langevin of Crookston also signed the articles. The membership fee was originally set at $2.00 and the annual dues were set at $1.00.

On September 1, 1927, the Minnesota State Veterinary Medical Association reincorporated as the Minnesota Veterinary Medical Society. The reincorporation documents were signed by Drs. C. E. Cotton of Minneapolis, Harry Evenson of Sacred Heart, C. P. Fitch of St. Paul, H. A. Greaves of Glenwood, William McLaughlin of Rush City, C. A. Nelson of Brainerd, B. A. Pomeroy of St. Paul, A. C. Spannaus of Waconis and A. J. Thompson of Hutchinson. The constitution was amended on January 10, 1930, and filed with the attorney general on January 29, 1938. In 1957, the Minnesota Veterinary Medical Society again changed its constitution and renamed itself the Minnesota Veterinary Medical Association.

ANNUAL MEETINGS OF THE MVMA.

The MVMA's annual meetings were held in St. Paul until 1911 when they began to alternate the location between St. Paul and Minneapolis. In 1973, Radisson South Hotel in Bloomington entered the rotation. Over the years, the attendance and exhibits have increased to the point where it is difficult to find a hotel with facilities large enough to house the annual meeting. For that reason, no meetings have been held in St. Paul since 1979. Most of the recent meetings have been held at the Radisson South Hotel because it has the requisite physical space and parking and it is more convenient for most Minnesota veterinarians.

The scientific program at the early meetings consisted of papers and demonstrations, known as "wet clinics," presented by members of the association. The demonstrations would take place at the Agricultural Experiment Station at the University Farm, located on the University of Minnesota's St. Paul Campus. Dr. Reynolds and his staff would act as hosts for these demonstrations. Wet clinics were also held at the infirmaries of Twin Cities practitioners. The presenters for the next program were chosen before adjournment of each annual meeting.

More of the papers presented at the early MVMA meetings were subsequently published in the *American Veterinary Review* (later the *Journal of the American Veterinary Medical Association*) than from any other veterinary association in the country.

As the association grew in size, speakers from outside the MVMA were invited to appear on the annual programs. It was considered an honor to be invited from out of state to present a paper before the association. These presentations brought more recognition to the individuals and their practice or institution.

Until the 1940s, topics at the early meetings centered on horses, cattle, swine, and, to a lesser extent, sheep. Small animals only held a small part of the program. However, the small animal part of the program steadily increased and in 1943, the annual meeting was extended from two to three days to accommodate the additional papers and demonstrations on small animals. In 1962, programs on large and small animals were held simultaneously. Public health and regulatory medicine programs were subsequently added and the length of the meeting extended to four days. The meeting also expanded to include programs oriented to species such as equine, bovine, porcine, canine, and feline.

Initially, the business portion of the annual meeting was incidental to the regular meeting and was fit into the program where possible. Business was later conducted during the first morning of the meeting when the committee reports were given and the other business of the association was presented. The procedure was

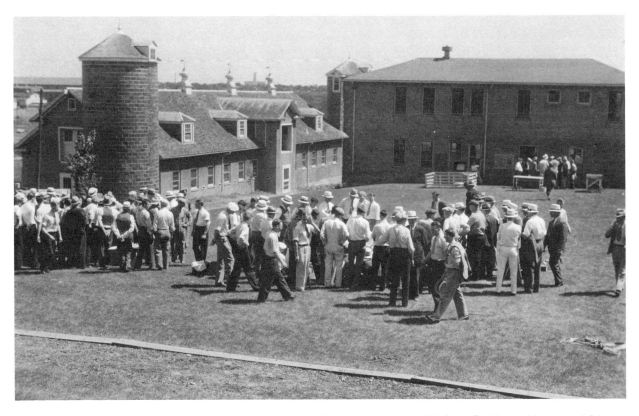

Veterinary Short Course, 1932, on the St. Paul Campus; building on the right is the Old Serum Building building on the left is Unit III.

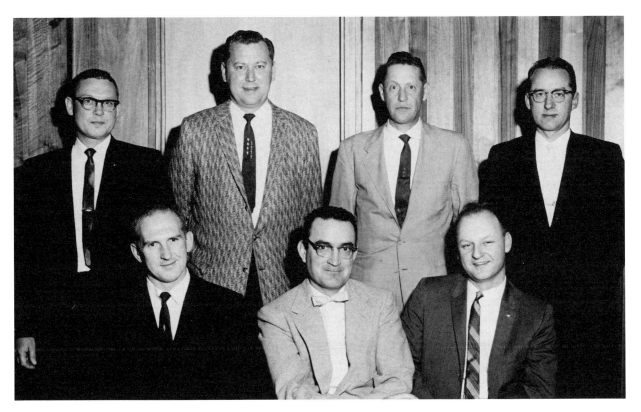

Summer clinic Committee, Owatona, 1961, left to right, seated, Drs. Dean Kingrey, Walter J. Mackey, Bruce Hohn, standing, Drs. Paul Cox, Glen Nelson, A.B. Magnusson, C.H. Schlauderaff.

once again changed so that committee reports were given in the morning with some of the business of the association, and then a final business meeting was held on the afternoon of the last day of the meeting. This procedure proved unsatisfactory as many practitioners timed their arrival for after the business session on the first morning. In 1961, in an effort to educate members on the contents of the various committee reports, the association began to publish these reports and handed them out during registration. Practitioners nonetheless left the meeting early to go home rather than staying for the final business session on the last afternoon. Consequently, only a handful of members—often as few as five or six—would make the business decisions affecting the entire membership. In 1970, the time of the business meeting was changed to a noon luncheon and the luncheon ticket was included in the registration fee. Since then, the business meeting has been very well attended.

SEMIANNUAL MEETINGS OF THE MVMA

The first Semiannual meeting of the MVMA was held only a few months following its date of organization. On the evening of July 13, 1897, members met at the Steele County Court House in Owatonna. The following day, the members attended demonstrations at Dr. W. Amos' infirmary. The Semiannual meetings were held in different cities around the state with the local practitioner or practitioners serving as hosts. In addition to Owatonna, these meetings took place in such locations as Austin, Brainerd, Duluth, Faribault, Hutchinson, Litchfield, Mankato, Minneapolis, Northfield, Stillwater, St. Cloud, and St. Paul.

Over time, it became increasingly more difficult to find a practitioner who was willing to host the Semiannual meeting. The last such meeting was held at Hutchinson in 1921. Beginning in 1922, the semiannual meeting was held jointly with the Agricultural Extension Division of the University of Minnesota as a two day short course. It was held at the Division of Veterinary Medicine Building on the St. Paul Campus of the University of Minnesota. This arrangement continued until 1942 when the course was terminated because of World War II.

After a lapse of 19 years, the semiannual meeting was revived in 1961 as the Practitioners Clinic in Owatonna where the original semiannual meeting had been held in 1897. The

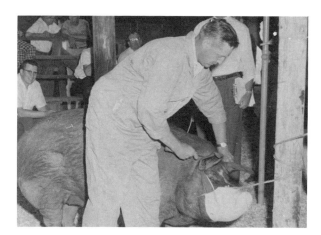

Dr. A.B. Magnusson anesthetizing a boar at the summer clinic in Owatonna, 1961.

Practitioners Clinic was sponsored jointly by the South Central Minnesota Veterinary Medical Association and the MVMA. Dr. Paul Cox was chairman of the local committee. The success of this meeting has resulted in several subsequent clinics (see Exhibit IV-1).

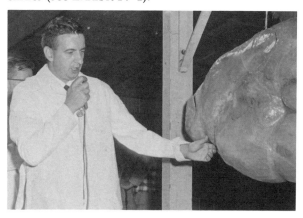

Dr. E.A. Usenik discussing four divisions of the stomach of the bovine at the summer clinic in Owatonna, 1961.

EXHIBIT IV-1

MEETING PLACES OF THE PRACTITIONERS CLINIC

Year	City	Local Host
1961	Owatonna	South CentraAssociation
1962	New Ulm	Minnesota ValleeMedical Association
1963	Willmar	Central Minneseteedical Association
1964	Wayzata	Suburban VeterinaryMedical Association
1965	Rochester	S. E. Minnesota Veterinary Medical Association
1966	College of Veterinary Medicine, St. Paul	Twin City Veterinary Medical Association

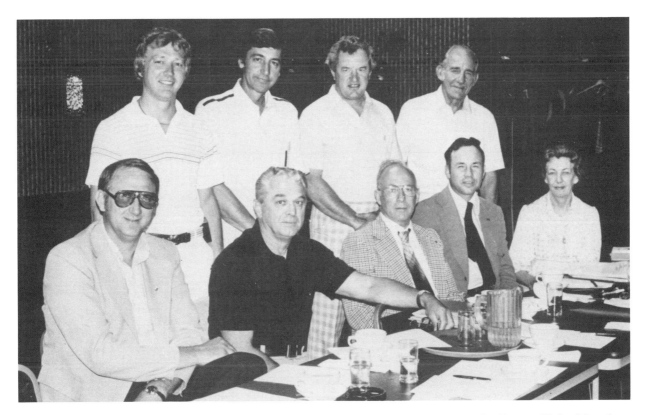

Summer clinic at a northern resort, left to right, seated, Drs. Ron Kuecker, Tony Zehrer, Walter Bonnett, Wesley Schroeder, Ms. Dorothy Gustafson, standing, Drs. Jerry Sprau, Leslie Butman, Robert Martens, James Karcher.

By 1967, no local associations volunteered to host the clinic. The name of the program was changed to Summer Clinic and the meetings were moved to resorts in Northern Minnesota where veterinarians could enjoy an outing with their entire family while attending the meetings.

CODE OF ETHICS

The MVMA originally issued a Code of Ethics in 1911, and subsequently published revised Codes in 1920, 1927, and 1942. The Code of Ethics established rules for the proper conduct of a veterinary practice in regard to the public and fellow practitioners. Professionalism is stressed throughout the Code.

OFFICERS OF THE MVMA

PRESIDENT

The MVMA has been graced by the service of many of Minnesota's most prominent and well respected veterinarians as its president. These men have been instrumental in providing the enthusiasm, vision, and dedication that have helped make the MVMA one of the most accomplished state veterinary medicine associations in the nation. See Exhibit IV-2.

EXHIBIT IV-2

PRESIDENTS OF THE MVMA

1897-98	S. D. Brimhall	1898-99	N. S. Erb
1899-00	M. H. Reynolds	1900-01	S. H. Ward
1901-02	J. N. Gould	1902-03	C. C. Lyford
1903-04	K. J. McKenzie	1904-05	Leopold Hay
1905-06	A. F. Lees	1906-07	Richard Price
1907-08	George McGillivary	1908-09	Walter Amos
1909-10	Charles E. Cotton	1910-11	J. P. Anderson
1911-12	C. A. Mack	1912-13	C. J. Sigmond
1913-14	M. R. Higbee	1914-15	M. R. Higbee
1915-16	C. S. Shore	1916-17	W. C. Bromaghin
1917-18	E. T. Frank	1918-19	R. R. Donaldson
1919-20	C. A. Nelson	1920-21	H. A. Greaves
1921-22	H. C. Lyon	1922-23	W. L. Boyd
1923-24	R. J. Coffeen	1924-25	Ralph L. West
1925-26	B. L. Cook	1926-27	W. C. Prouse
1927-28	Wm. McLaughlin	1928-29	A. J. Thompson
1929-30	Harry Evenson	1930-31	J. X. Parent
1931-32	John N. Campbell	1932-33	D. B. Palmer
1933-34	A. C. Spannaus	1934-35	P. H. Radford
1935-36	P. H. Riede	1936-37	R. A. Merrill
1937-38	A. H. Schmidt	1938-39	B. A. Pomeroy
1939-40	Guy Van Duzee	1940-41	G. S. Failing
1941-42	H. G. McGinn	1942-43	F. W. Hansen

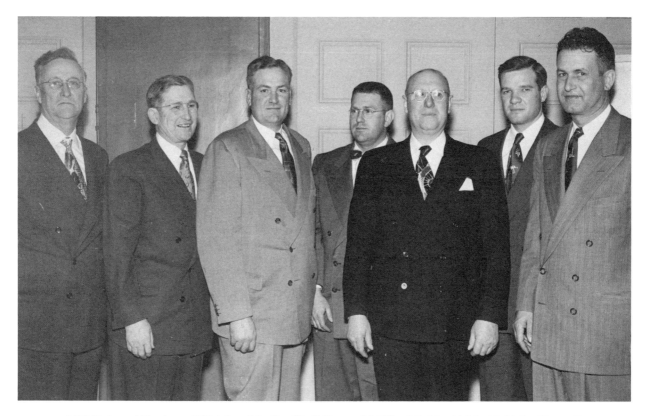

MVMA Annual Meeting, c. 1950, left to right, Drs. Wm.F. Flanary, J.J. Kelly, C.E. Schrafel, John M. Higbee, Henery E. Schwermann, W.M. Lawson, L.H. Pint.

(Presidents of the MVMA continued)

1943-44	D. L. Halver	1944-45	J. S. Dick, Jr.
1945-46	C. F. Schlotthauer	1946-47	Carl H. Hansen
1947-48	E. H. Gloss	1948-49	R. Fenstermacher
1949-50	C. H. Haggard	1950-51	J. J. Kelly
1951-52	W. F. Flanary	1952-53	George A. Larson
1953-54	E. G. Hughes	1954-55	Don Spangler
1955-56	H. C. H. Kernkamp	1956-57	L. H. Pint
1957-58	H. E. Schwermann	1958-59	George Hartle
1959-60	Glen Nelson	1960-61	R. S. Kufrin
1961-62	Fred Gehrman	1962-63	V. L. Dahl
1963-64	James Karcher	1964-65	L. T. Christensen
1965-66	T. P. Nankervis	1966-67	A. B. Magnusson
1967-68	V. K. Jensen	1968-69	James O. Hanson
1969-70	W. Clough Cullen	1970-71	John P. Arnold
1971-72	Elmer Hokkanen	1972-73	Stanley Held
1973-74	Milton Stensland	1974-75	Thayer E. Porter
1975-76	Al J. Kunkel	1976-77	Paul J. Cox
1977-78	Sanford B. Wilson	1978-79	Benjamin S. Pomeroy
1979-80	Wesley G. Schroeder	1980-81	Walter A. Bonnett
1981-82	Robert Wescott	1982-83	Ronald D. Kuecker
1983-84	Thomas Hagerty	1984-85	James A. Libby
1985-86	Walter J. Mackey	1986-87	Gene R. Kind
1987-88	Kenneth Greiner	1988-89	Jerry Sprau
1989-90	Ralph Molnau	1990-91	Peter Poss
1991-92	Richard Olson	1992-93	Gary D. Neubauer

1993-94 Keith Friendshuh

1994-present Dr. Barbara O'Leary

SECRETARY-TREASURER

The office of secretary-treasurer may be the most important position in the operation of the MVMA. When the MVMA was formed, the positions of secretary and treasurer were separate offices. Dr. K. J. McKenzie served as the first treasurer from 1897 to 1900. When Dr. McKenzie was elected secretary in 1900, the offices of secretary and treasurer were combined.

The MVMA has been fortunate to have competent, dedicated, and loyal persons as secretary-treasurers. These individuals deserve much credit and recognition for their great contributions. Their names and dates of office are given in Exhibit IV-3.

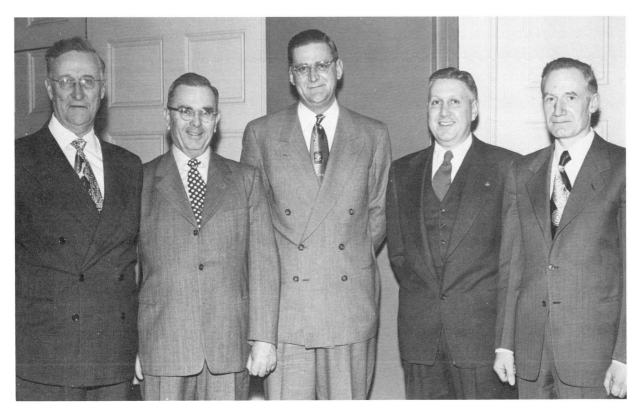

MVMA officials c. 1953, left to right, Drs. Wm. F. Flanary, George Larson, E.G. Hughes, Don Spangler, B.S. Pomeroy.

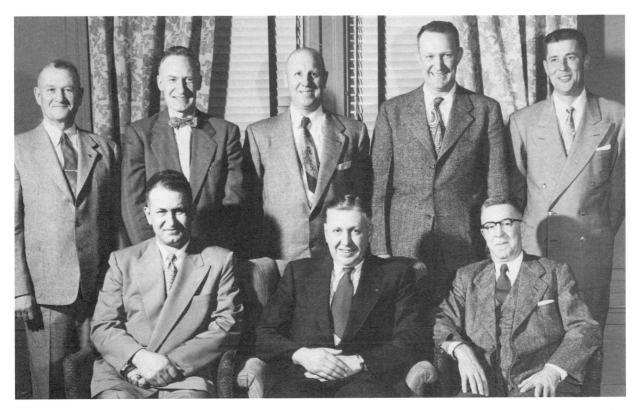

MVMA Board of Directors and officers, 1954, left to right, seated, Drs. L.H. Pint, Don Spangler, H.C.H. Kernkamp, standing, D.E. Trump, B.S. Pomeroy, Henery E. Schwermann, Raymond Tobola, R.S. Kufrin.

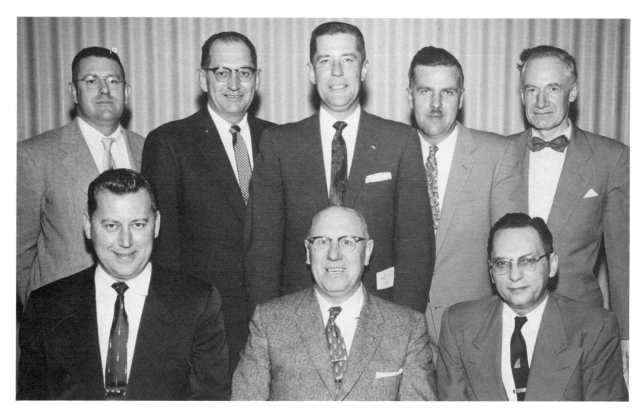

MVMA Board of Directors and officers, 1958, left to right, seated, Drs. Glen Nelson, Henry E. Schwermann, George Hartle, standing, Drs. John M. Higbee, V.K. Jensen, R.S. Kufrin, Vern L. Dahl, B.S. Pomeroy.

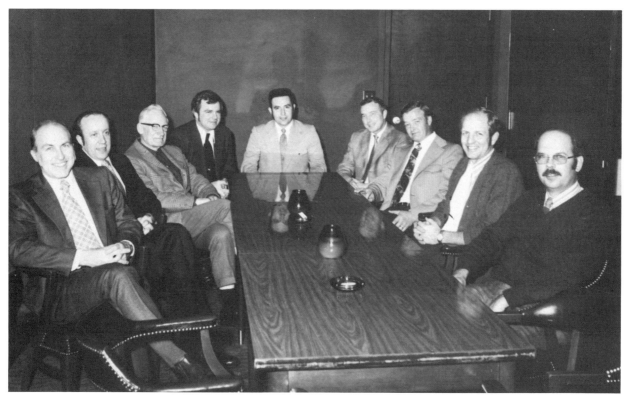

MVMA Board of Directors and officers, 1972, left to right, Drs. Conway Rosell, Elmer Hokkanen, B.S. Pomeroy, Thayer Porter, Stanley E. Held, Miltkon Stenland, Al Kunkel, Kenneth Magnuson, Charles Schlotthauer.

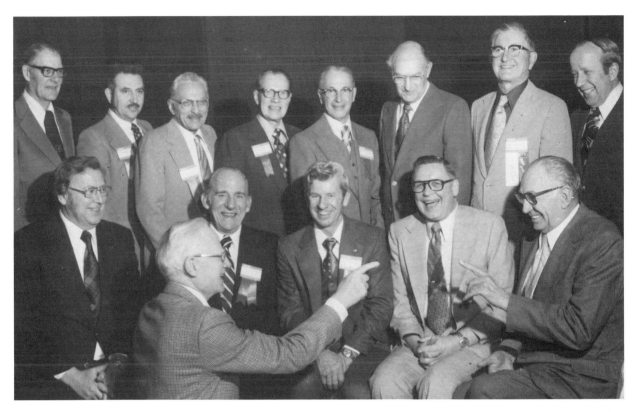

MVMA past president's breakfast, 1977, kneeling, Dr. B.S. Pomeroy, left to right, seated, Drs. Glen Nelson, James Karcher, Sanford Wilson, Paul Cox, V.K. Jensen, standing, Drs. L.T. Christensen, Stanley E. Held, George G. Hartle, James O. Hanson, John P. Arnold, W. Clough Cullen, Fred Gehrman, Elmer Hokkanen.

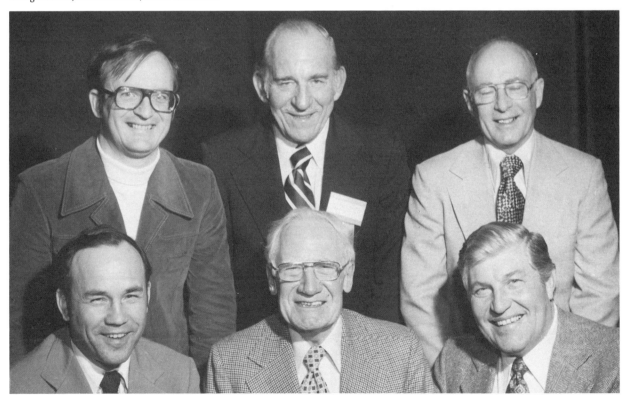

MVMA officials, 1978, left to right, seated, Drs. Wesley Schroeder, B.S. Pomeroy, Robert Wescott, standing, Drs. Robert Dietl, James Karcher, Walter Bonnett.

Presidents of the MVMA

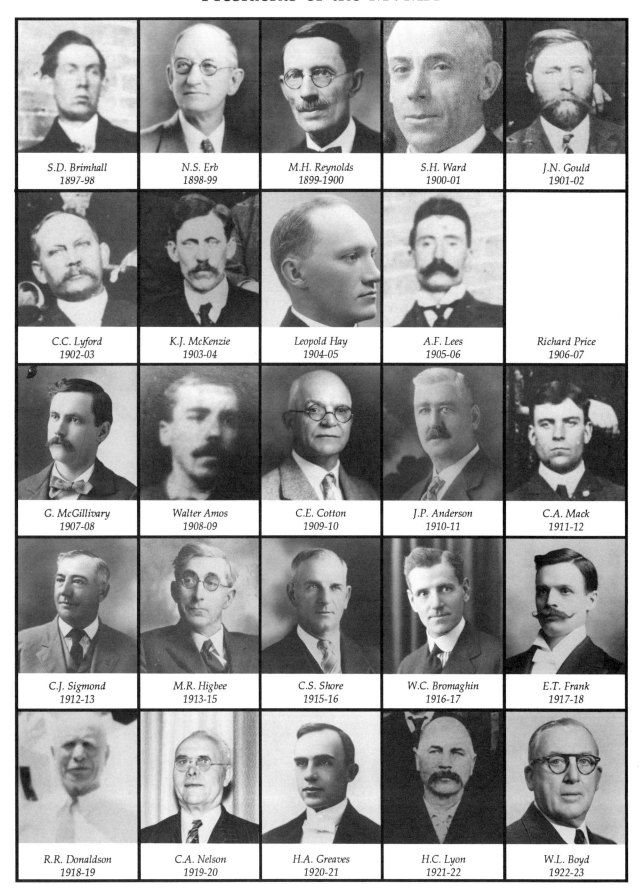

S.D. Brimhall *1897-98*	*N.S. Erb* *1898-99*	*M.H. Reynolds* *1899-1900*	*S.H. Ward* *1900-01*	*J.N. Gould* *1901-02*
C.C. Lyford *1902-03*	*K.J. McKenzie* *1903-04*	*Leopold Hay* *1904-05*	*A.F. Lees* *1905-06*	*Richard Price* *1906-07*
G. McGillivary *1907-08*	*Walter Amos* *1908-09*	*C.E. Cotton* *1909-10*	*J.P. Anderson* *1910-11*	*C.A. Mack* *1911-12*
C.J. Sigmond *1912-13*	*M.R. Higbee* *1913-15*	*C.S. Shore* *1915-16*	*W.C. Bromaghin* *1916-17*	*E.T. Frank* *1917-18*
R.R. Donaldson *1918-19*	*C.A. Nelson* *1919-20*	*H.A. Greaves* *1920-21*	*H.C. Lyon* *1921-22*	*W.L. Boyd* *1922-23*

Photos courtesy of the MVMA.

Presidents of the MVMA

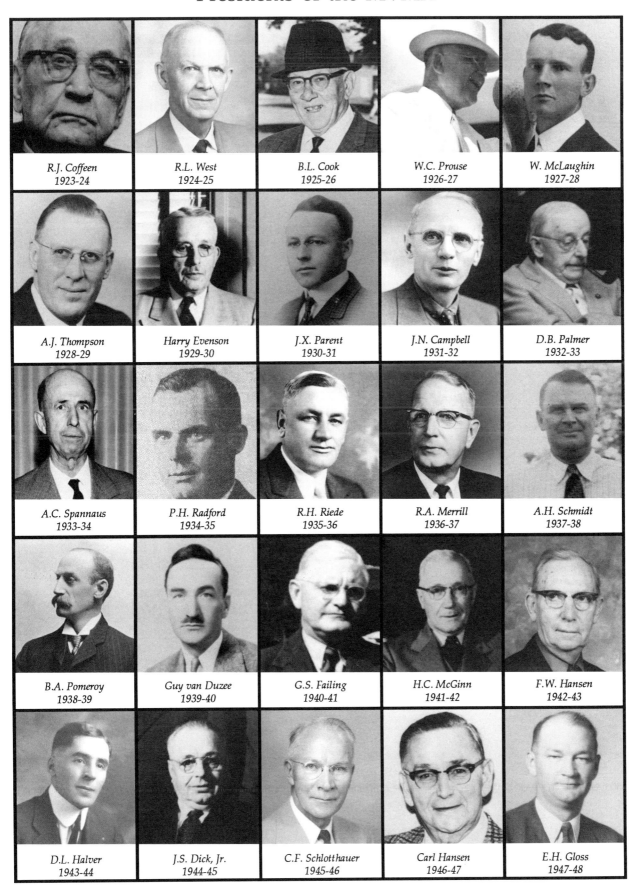

R.J. Coffeen 1923-24	R.L. West 1924-25	B.L. Cook 1925-26	W.C. Prouse 1926-27	W. McLaughin 1927-28
A.J. Thompson 1928-29	Harry Evenson 1929-30	J.X. Parent 1930-31	J.N. Campbell 1931-32	D.B. Palmer 1932-33
A.C. Spannaus 1933-34	P.H. Radford 1934-35	R.H. Riede 1935-36	R.A. Merrill 1936-37	A.H. Schmidt 1937-38
B.A. Pomeroy 1938-39	Guy van Duzee 1939-40	G.S. Failing 1940-41	H.C. McGinn 1941-42	F.W. Hansen 1942-43
D.L. Halver 1943-44	J.S. Dick, Jr. 1944-45	C.F. Schlotthauer 1945-46	Carl Hansen 1946-47	E.H. Gloss 1947-48

Photos courtesy of the MVMA.

Presidents of the MVMA

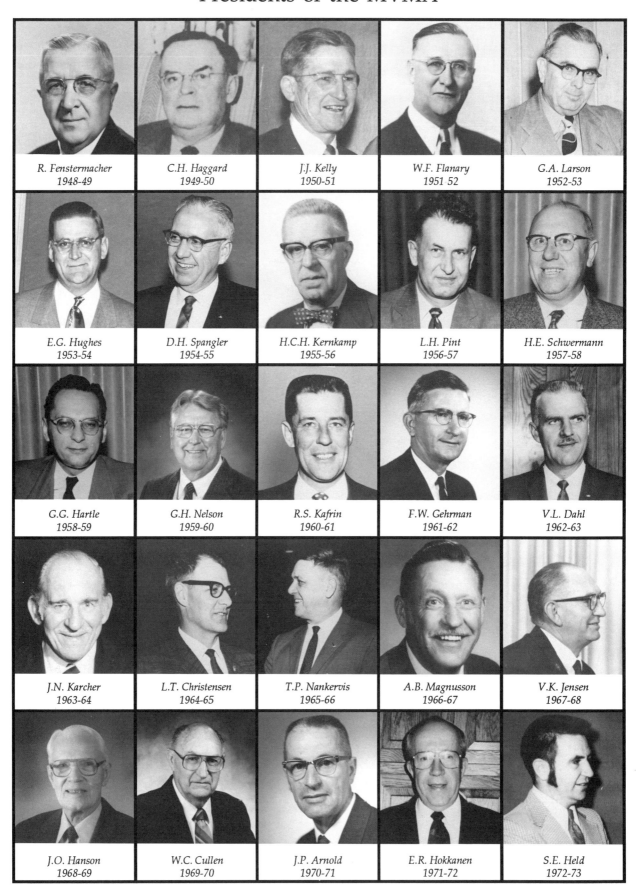

R. Fenstermacher
1948-49

C.H. Haggard
1949-50

J.J. Kelly
1950-51

W.F. Flanary
1951 52

G.A. Larson
1952-53

E.G. Hughes
1953-54

D.H. Spangler
1954-55

H.C.H. Kernkamp
1955-56

L.H. Pint
1956-57

H.E. Schwermann
1957-58

G.G. Hartle
1958-59

G.H. Nelson
1959-60

R.S. Kafrin
1960-61

F.W. Gehrman
1961-62

V.L. Dahl
1962-63

J.N. Karcher
1963-64

L.T. Christensen
1964-65

T.P. Nankervis
1965-66

A.B. Magnusson
1966-67

V.K. Jensen
1967-68

J.O. Hanson
1968-69

W.C. Cullen
1969-70

J.P. Arnold
1970-71

E.R. Hokkanen
1971-72

S.E. Held
1972-73

Photos courtesy of the MVMA.

Presidents of the MVMA

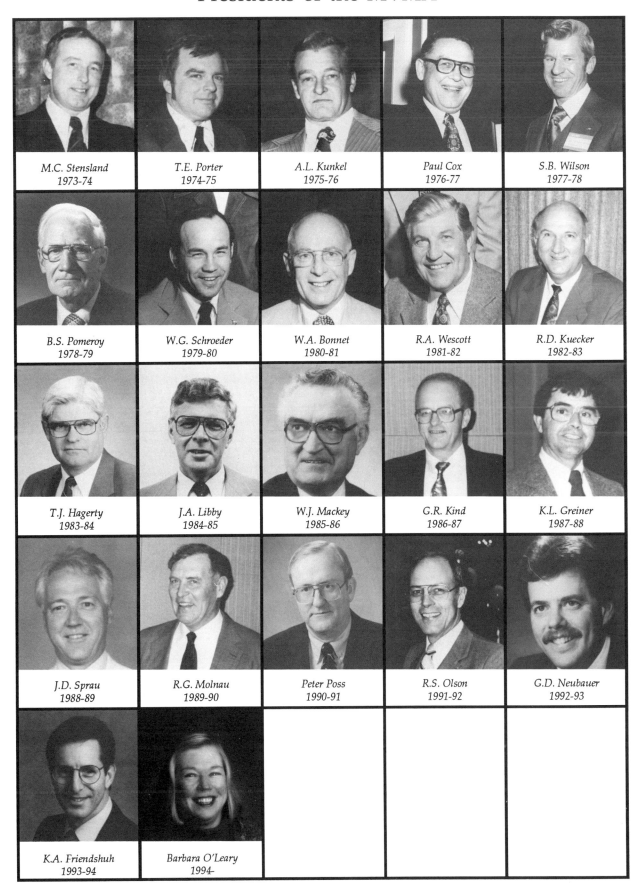

M.C. Stensland
1973-74

T.E. Porter
1974-75

A.L. Kunkel
1975-76

Paul Cox
1976-77

S.B. Wilson
1977-78

B.S. Pomeroy
1978-79

W.G. Schroeder
1979-80

W.A. Bonnet
1980-81

R.A. Wescott
1981-82

R.D. Kuecker
1982-83

T.J. Hagerty
1983-84

J.A. Libby
1984-85

W.J. Mackey
1985-86

G.R. Kind
1986-87

K.L. Greiner
1987-88

J.D. Sprau
1988-89

R.G. Molnau
1989-90

Peter Poss
1990-91

R.S. Olson
1991-92

G.D. Neubauer
1992-93

K.A. Friendshuh
1993-94

Barbara O'Leary
1994

Photos courtesy of the MVMA.

EXHIBIT IV-3

SECRETARY-TREASURERS OF THE MVMA

Date	Name	City
1897-1900	Leopold Hay	Faribault
1900-1903	K. J. McKenzie	Northfield
1903-1904	J. S. Butler	Minneapolis
1904-1906	J. G. Annand	Wabasha
1906-1909	C. A. Mack	Stillwater
1909-1917 or 1918	G. Ed Leech	Winona
1918-1935	C. P. Fitch	St. Paul
1935-1950	H. C. H. Kernkamp	St. Paul
1950-1975	B. S. Pomeroy	St. Paul
1975-1987	James Karcher	Burnsville
1987-	Mary Olson	Mora

EXECUTIVE SECRETARY-EXECUTIVE DIRECTOR

The membership and activities of the MVMA grew as the number of veterinarians in Minnesota increased. This increase in membership added to the work and responsibilities of the secretary-treasurer until it was difficult for the person holding that position to perform the other necessary duties of that office. At the MVMA's annual meeting in 1930, discussion focused on the importance of having a full-time person to carry out these duties. A special committee was appointed to survey the problem and report at the next annual meeting. At the 1931 meeting, the committee recommended hiring a full-time secretary who would take on the additional duties of "representing the veterinary profession at other professional, commercial and livestock meetings, keep close contact with legislation derogatory to the veterinary profession and take an active part in the prosecution of illegal veterinary practitioners." The committee pointed out that, in order to hire a full-time secretary, it would be necessary to increase the annual dues to $25.00. The committee proposed to submit that question to the members by a mail vote. The proposal was accepted and the mail vote yielded a resounding defeat of the proposal to hire a full-time secretary.

In the succeeding years, the question of employing a full-time secretary was raised at various meetings. However, the MVMA took no action until 1968 when Dr. B. S. Pomeroy, the MVMA's secretary-treasurer, brought the matter to a head by informing the Board of Trustees that the office had become so extensive that he could no longer perform all of his appointed duties. Dr. James O. Hanson, president of the MVMA, promptly appointed a committee to study the situation.

The committee eventually recommended that the Board of Trustees hire a full-time executive secretary to take over many of the responsibilities of the office. The report was accepted, and Drs. Stanley Held, Elmer Hokkanen, and John P. Arnold were appointed to a committee to select an executive secretary.

Dorothy Gustafson of the Gramont Corporation in Minneapolis was selected as the MVMA's first full-time executive secretary. Ms. Gustafson assumed the office on January 1, 1970, and served until ill health forced her retirement early in 1982. With the hiring of Ms. Gustafson, the MVMA had an office that members could contact on a daily basis. Ms. Gustafson brought to bear her experience in other organizations and with the press, and she updated the association's business procedures. She will be remembered as a hard working, dedicated, and competent officer who worked with loyalty and pride beyond the limits of her health.

Following the resignation of Dorothy Gustafson, the MVMA contracted with Office Enterprises, Inc., in Roseville for secretarial services. Under the contract, Office Enterprises made an executive secretary and additional secretarial services available as needed. The MVMA paid the executive secretary and the assistant executive secretary for the use of business and office machines other than typewriters and telephones owned by the association. The MVMA also rented the office space.

Deborah Melton was selected by the Board of Trustees to succeed Dorothy Gustafson. The title of the office was changed after her selection to executive director. Deborah Melton served a few months, only to resign effective September 30, 1982.

Carol Sutton replaced Deborah Melton as executive director and served until mid-1986 before she resigned. Ms. Sutton was a conscientious, competent, and caring person who was sensitive to the needs and wishes of the members. Through her untiring efforts, the number of exhibitors and the attendees greatly increased at the annual meeting.

Linda Lacher succeeded Carol Sutton in July 1986 as executive director. She had previous-

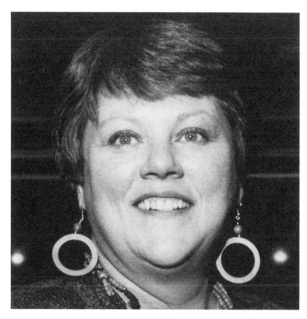

Linda Lacher, Executive Director.

ly served as Director of Specialty Services of the Minnesota Medical Association, and had spent six years on the staff of the Minnesota Senate. Ms. Lacher has very ably served this organization and has greatly expanded its activities.

MVMA AND GROUP INSURANCE

Prior to 1949, the MVMA had endorsed a group health and accident program that was underwritten by a casualty insurance company. Complaints were lodged by members who were disappointed with the way their claims were settled.

The MVMA's Insurance Committee investigated the matter and decided that the complaints had merit. The committee proposed to study the possibility of developing the MVMA's own group health and accident program. The MVMA engaged John Zimdars, an insurance broker in Milwaukee, to assist the committee in the study. The committee eventually recommended a Group Disability Income and Family Health policy underwritten by the Time Insurance Company of Milwaukee, a company that Zimdars happened to represent. The MVMA adopted the recommendation and member enrollment began in 1950.

The Insurance Committee revised and expanded the insurance program in 1968. Even with these improvements, some members of the MVMA preferred the policy developed by the

American Veterinary Medical Association (AVMA). With the assistance of John Zimdars, the Insurance Committee made several studies of the two programs. Each time, Zimdars convinced the committee with a masterful presentation that the Time Insurance Company policy was superior. In 1970, the AVMA hired an independent insurance consultant, Robert Provost, to evaluate the two programs. After Zimdars again gave a masterful presentation to demonstrate the Time Insurance Company policy best met the needs of the membership, he was excused and Provost began unraveling the insurance terms and fine print in the programs and put them in common English. When the two programs were compared in this way, it was apparent that the AVMA program was much better than the policy underwritten by the Time Insurance Company. The Insurance Committee, chaired by Dr. W. F. Schwartze of Lester Prairie, subsequently recommended to the Board of Trustees "that the present plan be discontinued and the MVMA switch to the National Insurance Trust with the AVMA." The Board of Trustees accepted the committee's recommendation.

The MVMA entered into negotiations with the AVMA to effect the change-over of the policies. The parties agreed to an open enrollment period. During this period, all veterinarians who were members of both the MVMA and the AVMA would, upon application, be accepted without requiring evidence of insurability. Payments would continue as before for members who were collecting disability payments at the time of the change-over. The parties set February 1, 1971, as the target date for the change-over of insurance programs.

President Elect Dr. Elmer Hokkanen of Minneapolis served as chairman of a special committee to oversee the transition. The committee started an extensive effort to educate members as to the terms of the program and the details for enrollment to the MVMA's members. A series of constituent groups and regional meetings were held. Printed materials explaining the change were sent to all members. The transition was very smooth due to the fine efforts of the special committee.

In 1953, the MVMA officially endorsed a group life insurance policy for its members under 60 years of age. Several hundred members took advantage of this program. The policy is underwritten   by the Union Central Life Insurance

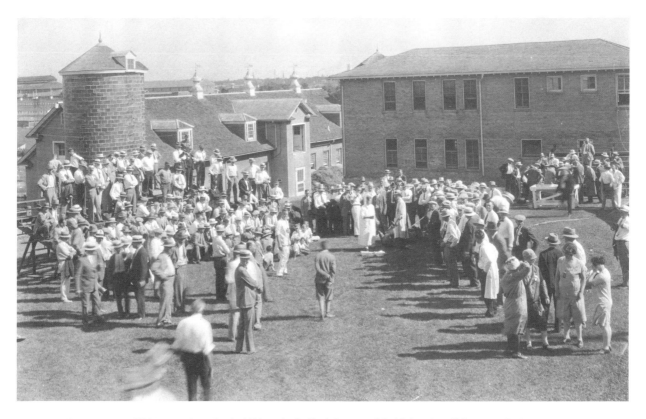

Clinic during AVMA annual meeting in 1928 on the St. Paul Campus of the University of Minnesota. Building on the right is the Old serum Building used to produce hog cholera anti-serum.

Company of Cincinnati, Ohio. Robert D. Davis, an insurance counselor, administered this life insurance program.

MVMA HOSTS AVMA

ANNUAL CONVENTION

The MVMA has hosted the annual convention of the American Veterinary Medical Association in 1902, 1928, 1955, 1969, and 1993. The conventions have all been held in Minneapolis with the exception of the first one.

In 1902, the scientific and business sessions of the convention were held in the West Hotel, and the clinic session took place in the Veterinary Division Buildings on the St. Paul Campus of the University of Minnesota. Nearly 200 veterinarians registered for these meetings. Entertainment included an afternoon at the State Fairgrounds watching horse racing and a trip by rail to Spring Lake where the conventioneers boarded a paddle-wheel steamer, the Puritan, for a boat ride on Lake Minnetonka. The cruise was followed by a banquet at Hotel De Lotero and a ride back to Minneapolis by rail.

Dr. M. H. Reynolds was chairman of the committee in charge of local arrangements. The efforts of the committee were greatly appreciated,

as reflected in an editorial in the American Veterinary Review that read: "The Association contains upon its rolls no more able, enthusiastic and energetic members than hail from the State of Minnesota. From a glance at the pictures (veterinary building and clinic amphitheater) it will at once be seen that the A.V.M.A. has never enjoyed such privileges."

In 1928, the Nicollet Hotel served as convention headquarters. Dr. C. E. Cotton chaired the committee on local arrangements for veterinarians and Mrs. Willard L. Boyd took charge of arrangements for the women's activities. A record number of 1,500 persons attended the meetings. The scientific program was divided up among general practice, small animal medicine and surgery, education and research, and sanitary science and public health. A comprehensive and interesting clinic session was held in the Division of Veterinary Medicine of the university under the direction of Dr. Willard L. Boyd.

In 1955, Hotel Radisson was the official headquarters for the convention, but the business and section meetings were held in the Minneapolis Auditorium. Dr. Fred Gehrman was chairman of the local arrangements and Mrs. Robert Merrill chaired the arrangements by the Women's Auxiliary. Closed circuit television was used to enable more persons to clearly view medical and surgical demonstrations. The small animal procedures were performed in the Small Animal Clinic at the College of Veterinary Medicine, and the large animal demonstrations were carried out at the Minneapolis Auditorium. The large animals were transported from the College of Veterinary Medicine to the auditorium using a shuttle system. Dr. Harvey Hoyt was in charge of transporting the animals, and veterinarians attending the convention were obliged to be present at 4:00 a.m. to help in the transportation.

The closed circuit television worked very satisfactorily and received compliments for its excellence. The family night program included a Civic Opera and Ice Show in the St. Paul Auditorium. Approximately 1,700 of the 2,715 registrants were transported by buses to the St. Paul Auditorium and back to their hotel in Minneapolis. Many had never seen figure skating before and were greatly impressed by the skill of the youngsters who performed in the show. The local arrangements were so well organized and executed that the AVMA headquarters requested a copy of the plans for use in future conventions.

In 1969, the official headquarters for the convention was the Lemington Hotel. The meetings were held at the Minneapolis Auditorium, which had been rebuilt and refurbished to accommodate large and small conventions. Dr. B. S. Pomeroy was chairman of the local committee and Mrs. B. S. Pomeroy chaired the program prepared by the Women's Auxiliary. The family night activities greatly resembled the program that had received so much praise in 1955. Approximately 2,200 conventioneers were transported by buses to the St. Paul Auditorium for the evening shows. Closed circuit television was again used successfully for demonstrations.

The 1928 and 1969 conventions set records for attendance, thus evidencing the popularity of Minnesota and the recognition that the Minnesota veterinarians are gracious hosts.

LIGHTNING STRIKE

In 1966 the MVMA was asked by the Associated Insurance Companies of Minnesota, 241 strong, to set up a program called "Lightning Strike in Livestock." The Insurance Companies claimed they were tired of paying false claims to livestock owners, hence the request. By various schemes it was rather easy for unscrupulous animal owners to claim lightning strike as the cause

of death and collect from the Insurance Companies. At this time, there was no standard program in Minnesota for determining cause of death.

Dr. Ray Solac, Dr. B. S. Pomeroy, and Dr. Jay H. Sautter paid a visit to the Veterinary School in Ames, Iowa, where a similar program had been established.

In 1967, Dr. Jay H. Sautter together with Dr. Ray Solac, a representative of the Insurance Companies, and a representative of the local insurance agency set up a series of meetings in the state, especially where the livestock population was the most dense. At the meetings the program was explained. These programs were well attended, attracting up to 200 people at a single meeting.

The plan was simple. If a farmer submitted a claim, a veterinarian was called to conduct a necropsy to establish the cause of death. The veterinarian was paid for his services and sent a report of his findings, and the farmer was paid according to the results.

Copies of the findings were submitted to the Diagnostic Laboratory where they were tabulated and reported to the Insurance Companies at their annual spring meeting. They were delighted with the results and presented a plaque to Dr. Sautter for his efforts in the program.

AWARDS

Each year the MVMA gives special recognition to persons who have made outstanding contributions to veterinary medicine or to their community in a way that reflects favorably upon veterinary medicine.

The award of Veterinarian of the Year is the highest honor that the MVMA can bestow upon any of its members. This honor is awarded in recognition of acts and deeds above and beyond the call of their vocation of veterinary medicine. The recipients of this award (see Exhibit IV-4) have made significant contributions to the betterment of their community and, in some cases, the advancement of state and national affairs. These persons have given of themselves unselfishly to help others. The award was given for the first time in 1965.

EXHIBIT IV-4

VETERINARIANS OF THE YEAR

1965	Arnold J. Thompson
1977	Robert K. Anderson
1966	Don Spangler
	James V. Bundy
	R. S. Kufrin
1978	Sanford B. Wilson
1967	Thomas J. Nankervis
1979	A. O. Setzepfandt
1968	LeRoy T. Christensen
1980	Milton Stensland
1969	Vernon K. Jensen
1981	Robert Martens
1970	Benjamin S. Pomeroy
1982	James A. Libby
1971	Herbert H. Kanning
1983	Stanley E. Held
1972	Fred W. Gehrman
1984	Charles Casey
1973	George G. Hartle
1985	Thomas Hagerty
1974	George W. Mather
1986	William Funk
1975	Clarence H. Schlauderaff
1987	Thomas Wetzel, Sr.
1976	B. Robert Lewis
1988	Ronald D. Kuecher
1989	Gene R. Kind
1990	Michael F. McMemony
1991	Paul E. Zollman
1992	Martin Bergeland
1993	Ralph Molnau
1994	Richard Olson

The Distinguished Service Award is made in the form of a citation for outstanding contributions, life-time service, and dedication to the welfare of the animal and poultry industries and veterinary medical science. (See Exhibit IV-5.)

EXHIBIT IV-5

DISTINGUISHED SERVICE AWARD

John P. Arnold	H. C. H. Kernkamp
Donald Barnes	Walter J. Mackey
Willard L. Boyd	Michael F. McMemony
John Campbell	Arthur Magnusson
Robert Dunlop	Glen Nelson
Jack G. Flint	T. P. O'Leary
Harold Fuglsang	Carl A. Osborne
Fred Gehrman	D. B. Palmer
Henry J. Griffiths	L. H. Pint
Griselda (Bee) Hanlon	Benjamin S. Pomeroy
James O. Hanson	Henry Schwermann
Stanley L. Hendricks	Donald L. Sime
Robert M. Hardy	Dale K. Sorensen
Vernon K. Jensen	W. T. S. Thorp
James Karcher	Darrell E. Trump
George E. Keller	Ralph L. West
J. J. Kelly	Charles W. Wetter

The MVMA has awarded honorary memberships to persons who have made outstanding contributions to veterinary medicine. (See Exhibit IV-6.) Some honorary members have worked in allied fields such as human medicine, livestock and poultry industries, pet animals, humane societies, and zoos. Members of the press and legislative bodies have also received honorary memberships.

EXHIBIT IV-6

HONORARY MEMBERS

Gaylord Anderson	Frank Martin
Martin Annexstad, Jr.	August Mueller
Henry Bauer	Roy C. Munson
Neal K. Black	J. Arthur Myers
Harold Brunn	Ancher Nelson
Norris K. Carnes	James Olson
Clyde Christensen	John L. Olson
Wendell DeBoer	Lloyd Peterson
Rollin Donnistown	Carol Plager
Ruth Duschene	William Rempel
Sidney Ewing	Robert Rupp
Rosemary Finnegan	Max Schultze
John Fletcher	Maynard Speece
Richard Goodrich	Wesley Spink
Hubert Humphrey	Alfred Stedman
Sally E. Jorgensen	Allan Stensrud

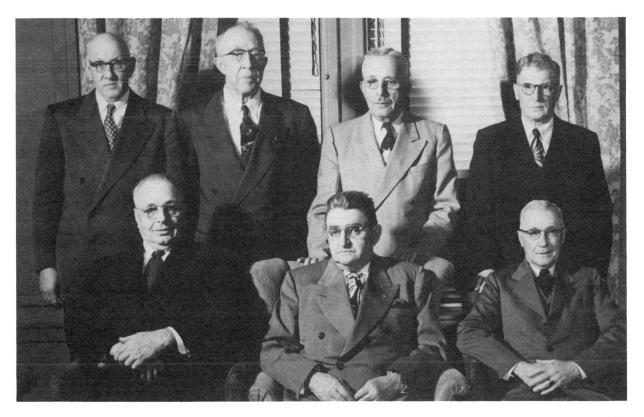

Members of the "40 Year Club", left to right, seated Drs. John S. Dick, R.W. Kiebel, H.G. McGinn, standing, Drs. B.L. Cook, W.M. Bolstad, Harry Evanson, J.W. Kummer.

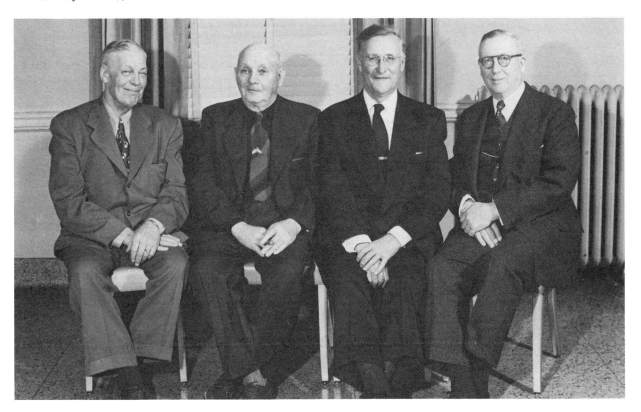

Members of the "40 Year Club", left to right, Drs. Elmer W. Berg, E.T. Phelps, Wm. F. Flanary, Willard L. Boyd.

(Continuation of Honorary Members)

Rose Kenaley   David Stone
William Kircher   Raymond Wolf
Lyle Lamphere   Dave Locey
Harold Macy

Beginning in 1946, all active members who had graduated from a veterinary college at least 50 years previously were made life members. Life membership was later expanded to include retiring veterinarians who are at least 65 years of age and have been a member for 25 years, or persons who have been a member for at least 40 years. Life members enjoy all of the privileges of active membership without the obligation of paying dues and assessments.

Since the early 1950s, the MVMA has made a cash award to the outstanding senior student in clinical veterinary medicine. In 1986, the terms of the award were changed to a cash gift based on need to a second- or third-year student.

MINNESOTA ACADEMY OF VETERINARY MEDICAL PRACTICE

In the late 1960s, consumer groups began to question the competency of professionals in the veterinary field. They believed that some unqualified professionals had received a license to practice and that many of the older practitioners had not kept up with advances in their field. They felt that, as a result, many professionals were rendering substandard service to their clients.

The consumer groups pressed for public representation on licensing boards and demanded continuing education courses as a prerequisite for license renewal. Consequently, laypersons were appointed to the Board of Veterinary Examiners in Minnesota and some states adopted the requirement of continuing education or "C.E." credits for license renewal.

Many veterinarians feared that laypersons would administer the C.E. credit requirements. The concern over the possibility of mandatory C.E. courses and credits for license renewal in Minnesota caused the Committee on Education to take action in 1971. The committee proposed that the MVMA's bylaws be amended to provide for the establishment of an Academy of Veterinary Medical Practice. The proposal was adopted and the committee was authorized to proceed with the arrangements.

The committee began obtaining copies of the constitutions and bylaws of veterinary medical practice academies in other states to use as guides. The materials from Iowa proved to be the most useful. In 1974, the Minnesota Academy of Veterinary Medical Practice was formally organized with 102 charter members. The first officers of the academy are given in Exhibit IV-7 and the presidents in Exhibit IV-8.

EXHIBIT IV-7

FIRST OFFICERS OF THE MINNESOTA ACADEMY OF VETERINARY MEDICAL PRACTICE

President	Dr. James O. Hanson	St. Peter
President Elect	Dr. Ronald F. Dubbe	Waconia
Secretary	Dr. Wesley Schroeder	Maple Plain
Board of Directors		
	Dr. John F. Anderson	Cannon Falls
	Dr. Robert A. Dietl	Bloomington
	Dr. Walter A. Bonnett	Edina
	Dr. Charles A. Pieper	Clarissa

The academy developed guidelines for assigning C.E. credits to courses, meetings, self study, seminars, and conferences, and established the requirements to become a full member and to maintain that membership. To record credits, the academy prepares a form each year on which each member is to list the veterinary courses, conferences, seminars, and meetings that he or she has attended over the year.

The formation of the Academy of Veterinary Medical Practice defused the movement to require accumulation of continuing education credits as a prerequisite for license renewal. The advocates of such a requirement decided that the veterinary medicine profession was making responsible efforts to keep their members abreast of recent developments in their field.

Each year, as a service to its members, the academy sponsors a conference or seminar related to practice management. Those members who have maintained the required credits are provided with a plaque suitable for framing to hang on the wall of their clinic or office as evidence to their clients that they have kept abreast of recent developments in veterinary medicine.

EXHIBIT IV-8

PRESIDENTS OF THE ACADEMY

Dr. James O. Hanson	St. Peter	1974-76
Dr. Ronald F. Dubbe	Waconia	1976-77
Dr. Wesley Schroeder	Maple Plain	1977-78
Dr. John P. Arnold	White Bear Lake	1978-79
Dr. Glen Zebarth	Buffalo	1979-80
Dr. Keith Friendshuh	Annandale	1980-81
Dr. William Funk	Brooklyn Park	1981-83
Dr. Kenneth Detlefsen	Red Wing	1983-84
Dr. Milton Stensland	Austin	1984-85
Dr. Charles Gehrman	Minnetonka	1985-86
Dr. Richard Olson	Arden Hills	1986-88
Dr. Robert Lorenz	Alexandria	1988-89
Dr. Holly Neaton	Waterson	1989-90
Dr. John F. Anderson	Cannon Falls	1990-91
Dr. Larry Anderson	Duluth	1991-93
Dr. Wade Himes	International Falls	1993-

WOMEN'S AUXILIARY TO THE MINNESOTA VETERINARY MEDICAL ASSOCIATION

For several years, veterinarians and their wives discussed the need of an auxiliary of the Minnesota Veterinary Medical Association. In 1934, Mrs. P. H. Radford of Slayton attended a meeting of the Women's Auxiliary of the American Veterinary Medical Association in New York City where the president, Mrs. T. H. Ferguson from Lake Geneva, Wisconsin, encouraged Mrs. Radford to start an auxiliary in Minnesota. With the help of her husband, who was then president of the MVMA, and Dr. C. P. Fitch, the MVMA's secretary, the women who attended the banquet at the MVMA's 1935 annual meeting were asked to discuss whether the MVMA should form an auxiliary. Approximately 25 women attended the meeting. Mrs. C. P. Fitch of St. Paul was chosen to serve as chairman pro tem and Mrs. J. S. Dick of Minneapolis was selected secretary pro tem. The group voted to form an auxiliary. Mrs. Fitch appointed a membership committee headed by Mrs. L. E. Jenkins, a constitution committee headed by Mrs. P. H. Radford, and a nominating committee.

The organizational meeting was held that summer during the July 11-12, 1935, Veterinary Short Course on the St. Paul Campus of the University of Minnesota. Because neither Mrs. Fitch nor Mrs. Dick was present, Mrs. H. C. Butler of Madelia was chosen temporary chairman, and Mrs. H. C. H. Kernkamp of St. Paul acted as secretary pro tem. The officers elected during the organizational meeting are shown in Exhibit IV-9 and the presidents in Exhibit IV-10.

EXHIBIT IV-9

FIRST OFFICERS OF THE WOMEN'S AUXILIARY

President	Mrs. C. E. Cotton, Minneapolis
1st Vice President	Mrs. C. P. Fitch, St. Paul
2nd Vice President	Mrs. J. X. Parent, Foley
Corresponding Secretary	Mrs. G. S. Failing, Winona
Secretary-Treasurer	Mrs. P. H. Riede, Mabel

The auxiliary had 58 charter members and the dues were set at 50 cents. The auxiliary decided that the wife of the incoming president of the MVMA would be responsible for hospitality at the annual meetings.

In January of 1936, the auxiliary adopted the following objectives:

1. To help the schooling of boys studying veterinary medicine, worthy boys who are high in scholastic standing and also are in need of financial aid to further this study.

2. To interest the wives of veterinarians in furthering publicity through this auxiliary.

3. That each member should try to help raise funds for the Auxiliary in any way she might favor.

Membership in the auxiliary was open to all wives, daughters, mothers, and sisters of members of the Minnesota Veterinary Medical Association.

Social and educational programs have always been an important part of the annual meetings of the auxiliary. These programs have taken the form of luncheons, lectures, style shows, demonstrations, and trips or excursions.

In 1945, the time of the annual meeting was changed from the summer during the Veterinary Short Course to the winter during the annual meeting of the MVMA. No meeting was held in 1944 because of World War II.

Since 1949, the auxiliary has supported the College of Veterinary Medicine at the university by donating funds to its library or to scholarships.

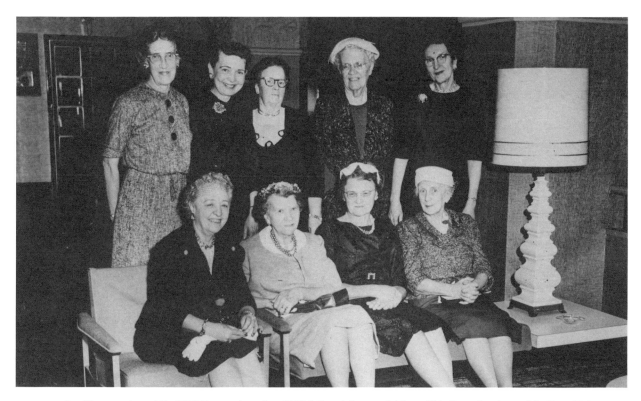

Auxiliary members at the MVMA annual meeting, 1960, left to right, seated, Mmes. Nels Runquist, Annandale, Peter H. Riede, Mabel, Albert C. Spannaus, Waconia, Bessie Brown, Atwater, standing, Mmes. H.C.H. Kernkamp, St. Paul, Ellis Gloss, Gaylord, Willard L. Boyd, St. Paul, Charles N. Carl, Clinton, Oscar Gochnauer, Minneapolis.

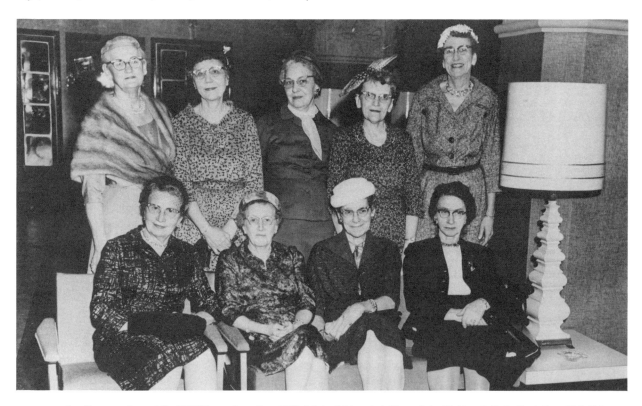

Auxiliary members at the MVMA anual meeting, 1960, left to right, seated, Mmes. John N. Campbell, St. Paul, Donald B. Palmer, Wayzata, John S. Dick, Anoka, Vincent J. Robinson, Minneapolis, standing, Mmes. Fred Driver, Mendota Heights, Leo S. Englerth, St. Cloud, Georgte A. Larson, Breckenridge, Ralph L. West, St. Paul, Robert A. Merrill, St. Paul.

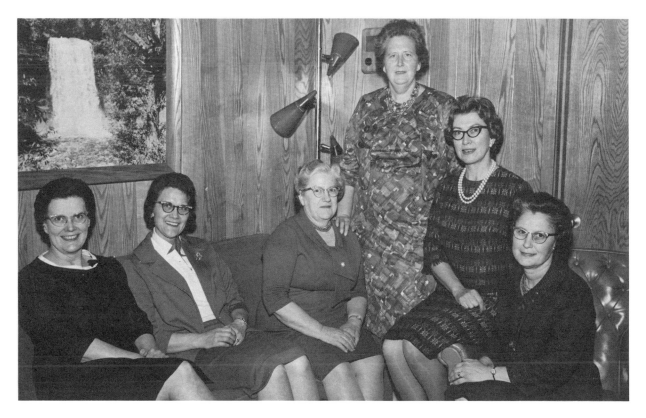

Past presidents of the MVMA Auxiliary, left to right, Margaret Arnold, Isabelle French, Mildred Chapin, Mary Magnusson, Dorothy Christensen, Peg (Margaret) Sautter.

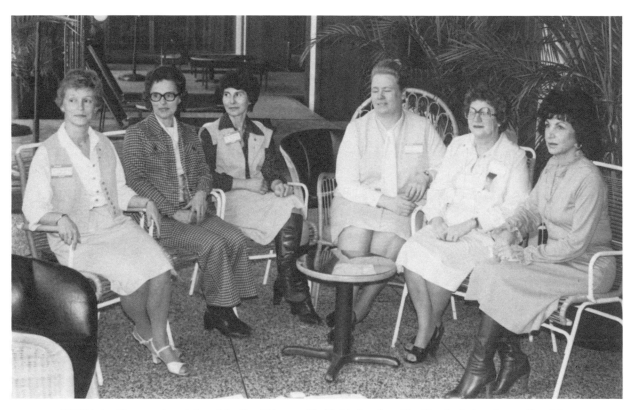

MVMA Auxiliary members, left to right, Carol Martens, Phyllis Mackey, Jacquiline Stensland, Ann Contag, Rose Johnson, Rosemary Butman.

Presidents of the MVMA Auxiliary

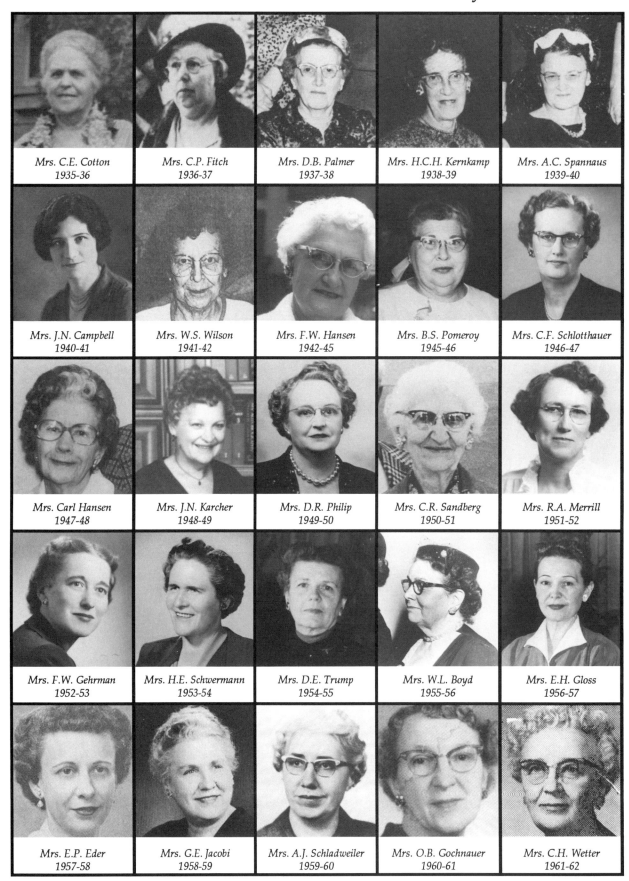

Mrs. C.E. Cotton 1935-36	Mrs. C.P. Fitch 1936-37	Mrs. D.B. Palmer 1937-38	Mrs. H.C.H. Kernkamp 1938-39	Mrs. A.C. Spannaus 1939-40
Mrs. J.N. Campbell 1940-41	Mrs. W.S. Wilson 1941-42	Mrs. F.W. Hansen 1942-45	Mrs. B.S. Pomeroy 1945-46	Mrs. C.F. Schlotthauer 1946-47
Mrs. Carl Hansen 1947-48	Mrs. J.N. Karcher 1948-49	Mrs. D.R. Philip 1949-50	Mrs. C.R. Sandberg 1950-51	Mrs. R.A. Merrill 1951-52
Mrs. F.W. Gehrman 1952-53	Mrs. H.E. Schwermann 1953-54	Mrs. D.E. Trump 1954-55	Mrs. W.L. Boyd 1955-56	Mrs. E.H. Gloss 1956-57
Mrs. E.P. Eder 1957-58	Mrs. G.E. Jacobi 1958-59	Mrs. A.J. Schladweiler 1959-60	Mrs. O.B. Gochnauer 1960-61	Mrs. C.H. Wetter 1961-62

Photos courtesy of the MVMA Auxiliary.

Presidents of the MVMA Auxiliary

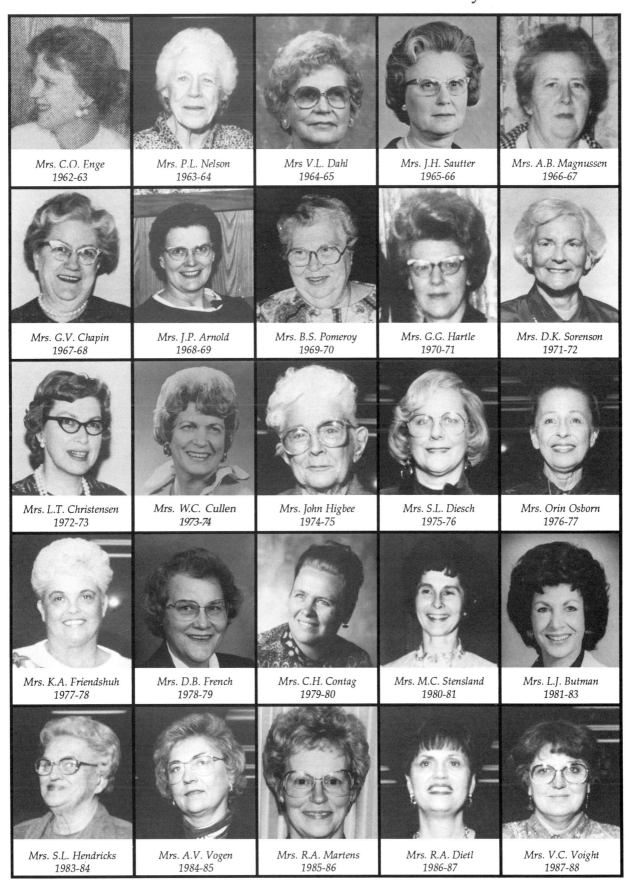

Mrs. C.O. Enge
1962-63

Mrs. P.L. Nelson
1963-64

Mrs V.L. Dahl
1964-65

Mrs. J.H. Sautter
1965-66

Mrs. A.B. Magnussen
1966-67

Mrs. G.V. Chapin
1967-68

Mrs. J.P. Arnold
1968-69

Mrs. B.S. Pomeroy
1969-70

Mrs. G.G. Hartle
1970-71

Mrs. D.K. Sorenson
1971-72

Mrs. L.T. Christensen
1972-73

Mrs. W.C. Cullen
1973-74

Mrs. John Higbee
1974-75

Mrs. S.L. Diesch
1975-76

Mrs. Orin Osborn
1976-77

Mrs. K.A. Friendshuh
1977-78

Mrs. D.B. French
1978-79

Mrs. C.H. Contag
1979-80

Mrs. M.C. Stensland
1980-81

Mrs. L.J. Butman
1981-83

Mrs. S.L. Hendricks
1983-84

Mrs. A.V. Vogen
1984-85

Mrs. R.A. Martens
1985-86

Mrs. R.A. Dietl
1986-87

Mrs. V.C. Voight
1987-88

Photos courtesy of the MVMA Auxiliary.

Presidents of the MVMA Auxiliary

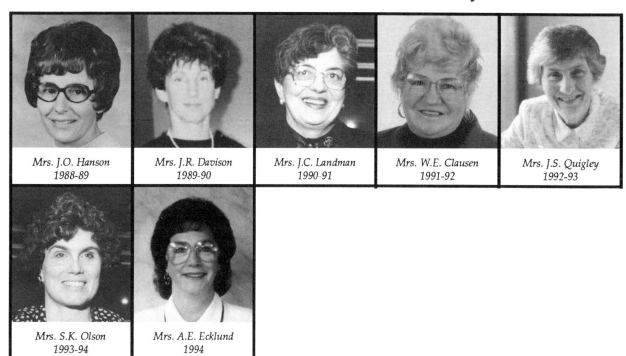

Mrs. J.O. Hanson
1988-89

Mrs. J.R. Davison
1989-90

Mrs. J.C. Landman
1990-91

Mrs. W.E. Clausen
1991-92

Mrs. J.S. Quigley
1992-93

Mrs. S.K. Olson
1993-94

Mrs. A.E. Ecklund
1994

Photos courtesy of the MVMA Auxiliary.

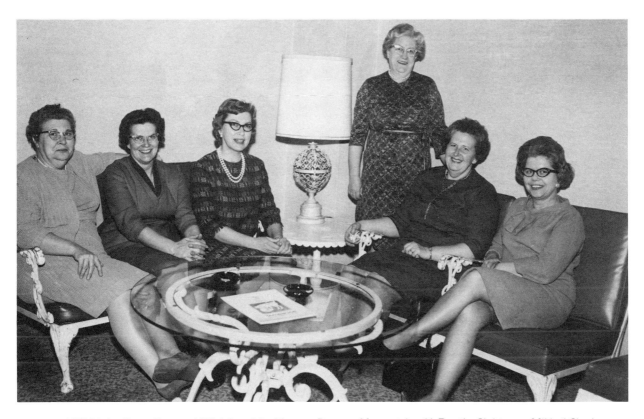

MVMA Auxiliary officers, c. 1968, left to right, Margaret Pomeroy, Margaret Arnold, Dorothy Christensen, Mildred Chapin, Mary Magnusson, LaVerne Schaefer.

In 1976 the Student Loan Fund was established. This was designed to be an emergency loan in time of desperate need. The auxiliary uses fund raising projects to obtain money for the loans and averages about 15 loans per year.

Loans are made for up to $500 at 3 percent interest. If the student is unable to repay the loan before graduation, the rate of interest becomes 8 percent and it is due one year after graduation.

EXHIBIT IV-10

AUXILIARY PRESIDENTS

1935-36	Mrs. C. E. Cotton	Minneapolis
1936-37	Mrs. C. P. Fitch	St. Paul
1937-38	Mrs. D. B. Palmer	Wayzata
1938-39	Mrs. H. C. H. Kernkamp	St. Paul
1939-40	Mrs. A. C. Spannaus	Waconia
1940-41	Mrs. John N. Campbell	Truman
1941-42	Mrs. W. S. Wilson	Buffalo
1942-45	Mrs. F. W. Hansen	South St. Paul
1945-46	Mrs. B. S. Pomeroy	St. Paul
1946-47	Mrs. Carl Schlotthauer	Rochester
1947-48	Mrs. Carl Hansen	Faribault
1948-49	Mrs. J. N. Karcher	Minneapolis
1949-50	Mrs. D. R. Philip	Mankato
1950-51	Mrs. C. R. Sandberg	Zumbrota
1951-52	Mrs. R. A. Merrill	St. Paul
1952-53	Mrs. F. W. Gehrman	Minneapolis
1953-54	Mrs. H. E. Schwermann	New Ulm
1954-55	Mrs. Darrell E. Trump	Owatonna
1955-56	Mrs. W. L. Boyd	St. Paul
1956-57	Mrs. E. H. Gloss	Gaylord
1957-58	Mrs. E. Paul Eder	Blue Earth
1958-59	Mrs. G. E. Jacobi	Minneapolis
1959-60	Mrs. A. J. Schladweiler	Madison
1960-61	Mrs. O. B. Gochnauer	Minneapolis
1961-62	Mrs. C. H. Wetter	Princeton
1962-63	Mrs. C. O. Enge	St. James
1963-64	Mrs. Paul L. Nelson	Minneapolis
1964-65	Mrs. V. L. Dahl	Arlington
1965-66	Mrs. Jay H. Sauter	St. Paul
1966-67	Mrs. A. B. Magnusson	Blooming Prairie
1967-68	Mrs. G. V. Chapin	Kasson
1968-69	Mrs. John P. Arnold	White Bear Lake
1969-70	Mrs. B. S. Pomeroy	St. Paul
1970-71	Mrs. George G. Hartle	Minneapolis
1971-72	Mrs. Dale K. Sorensen	St. Paul
1972-73	Mrs. L. T. Christensen	Hancock

(Exhibit IV-10 Continued)

1973-74	Mrs. W. Clough Cullen	Mankato
1974-75	Mrs. John Higbee	Marine on the St. Croix
1975-76	Mrs. Stanley L. Diesch	Roseville
1976-77	Mrs. Orin Osborn	Le Sueur
1977-78	Mrs. Keith Friendshuh	Annandale
1978-79	Mrs. Donald French	Chatfield
1979-80	Mrs. Carlos H. Contag	New Ulm
1980-81	Mrs. Milton Stensland	Austin
1981-83	Mrs. Leslie Butman	Minnetonka
1983-84	Mrs. Stan Hendricks	Watertown
1984-85	Mrs. Alan Vogen	Apple Valley
1985-86	Mrs. Robert Martens	Nicollet
1986-87	Mrs. Robert Dietl	Richfield
1987-88	Mrs. Virgil Voigt	Hutchinson
1988-89	Mrs. James O. Hanson	St. Peter
1989-90	Mrs. J. Robert Davison	Farmington
1990-91	Mrs. John Landman	Arden Hills
1991-92	Mrs. William Clauson	Perham
1992-93	Mrs. Joseph Quigley	Fridley
1993-94	Mrs. Steven Olson	Austin
1994-present	Mrs. Allen Eklund	Askov

MINNESOTA ASSOCIATION OF VETERINARY TECHNICIANS

Practitioners have used assistants since the early days of the veterinary profession in Minnesota. The early assistants were hired on a part-time basis and helped during a certain season of the year or on specific cases. For example, horses are customarily castrated in the springtime. Practitioners would schedule to perform castrations over a period of two weeks. During this period, the practitioner would hire a person who was good at handling horses and "dependable with the twitch" to assist him to perform the castrations. Many of the colts that were castrated were not accustomed to being restrained and the owner was either not able or not inclined to restrain the animal, thus necessitating the help of an assistant.

Some assistants were hired on a full-time basis to operate the office while the veterinarian was away, clean equipment, and replenish drugs used by the veterinarian on calls. In small animal practices, assistants would often be trained to perform tasks during surgery, including the application of ether or chloroform for anesthesia. These persons had no special training in veterinary medicine or laboratory techniques other than that given by the veterinarian.

As the practice of veterinary medicine advanced and became more scientific in techniques and laboratory tests, the persons assisting veterinarians received better training and became known as "technicians." Nonetheless, these assistants were not regulated, and some veterinarians had their assistants perform duties in violation of the Practice Act.

The increase in the number of veterinary technicians, establishment of training programs and institutions, and concern over regulation led to the creation of the MVMA's Animal Technicians Committee. The members of the committee were appointed in 1969 with Dr. Robert Wescott of Elgin designated as chairman.

In its first report, the committee noted the veterinary technician training schools then in the planning stages in Minnesota. The committee recommended that the administration of the training programs include doctors of veterinary medicine, and that programs be developed with the assistance of the Animal Technicians Committee.

In 1973, the Animal Technicians Committee implemented a procedure for registering veterinary technicians. By the end of that year, 78 veterinary technicians had been registered. In the same year, guidelines were developed listing the duties that could be performed by veterinary technicians.

The Animal Technicians Committee presented programs for the veterinary technicians at the 1974 and 1975 annual meetings of the MVMA. In 1974, 130 veterinary technicians attended the annual meeting.

At the 1975 annual meeting, the veterinary technicians formed the Minnesota Association of Veterinary Technicians, or MAVT. (See Exhibit IV-11 for the presidents and secretaries of MAVT.) Since then, MAVT has organized annual programs and held their annual meeting in conjunction with the annual meeting of the MVMA.

A credential committee was established in 1983 to develop a certification program for veterinary technicians. The original members of the committee included Ms. Nanette Malcomson, Ms. Nancy Henne, Dr. Vic Perman, Dr. W. Clough Cullen, Dr. Janet Donlin, and Dr. David Fell. The first Annual Certification Examination was given to 167 veterinary technicians on June 23, 1984.

EXHIBIT IV-11

PRESIDENTS AND SECRETARIES OF MAVT

Year	President	Secretary
1975	Anthony Crimi	—
1976	Greg Huffman	—
1977	Rebecca Schultz	Jane Rathje
1978	Betty Covinton	Deb Zwart
1979	Vicki Wilcox-Waltz	Colleen Sauber
1980	Claudia Durand	Deb Young
1981	Nancy Hennen	Adel Boeschler
1983	Nanette Malcomson	Deb Bemder
1984	Nanette Malcomson	Katie Decosse
1985	Ann Zimmerman-Hohn, CVT*/	Chris Drum, CVT
1986	Katie Decosse, CVT	Sandy Schweich, CVT
1987	Katie Decosse, CVT	Sandy Schweich, CVT
1988	Sandy Schweich, CVT	Marlys Korn, CVT
1989	Mary Lund, CVT	Laurie Fleming, CVT
1990	Andrea Johnson, CVT	Patti Christie, CVT
1991	Andrea Johnson, CVT	Bernetta Siewert, CVT
1992	Bernette Siewert, CVT	Kay Penning-Pehrson, CVT
1993	Bernette Siewert, CVT	Kay Penning-Pehrson, CVT

*/ The CVT title does not appear with the names of the officers elected before 1985. The first certification examination for the CVT title was given in mid-1984. Those officers did take the examination when given and received the CVT designation.

REGIONAL ASSOCIATIONS

In the early newspapers, there is a brief reference to two regional veterinary associations. The first was the Northwestern Veterinary Association, which originated from a banquet and smoker held in conjunction with the 1885 commencement exercises for the first graduating class from the Northwestern Veterinary College. Veterinarians from the Twin Cities and the surrounding area were invited to this event. During the evening of good fellowship, the group decided to form a veterinary association. They proceeded to elect a slate of officers and the Northwestern Veterinary Medical Association was formed. Unfortunately, there are no records of any subsequent meetings of this organization.

The other early veterinary association was the Southern Minnesota Veterinary and Dental Association. The term "Dental" referred to equine dentistry which was an important part of veterinary practice during that era. This association was referred to in a newspaper article on the formation of the Minnesota Veterinary Medical Association. No further evidence of its existence has been found.

ARROWHEAD VETERINARY MEDICAL ASSOCIATION

The Arrowhead Veterinary Medical Association was formed during the spring of 1964 in Duluth, Minnesota. Arrowhead's original officers were Dr. M. D. Fetters, Barnum, president; and Dr. Mark Field, Duluth, secretary. Arrowhead's membership is composed of veterinarians from Northeastern Minnesota extending south and west of Duluth to include the Iron Range and the Canadian border, as well as Northwestern Wisconsin.

CENTRAL VETERINARY MEDICAL ASSOCIATION

The Central Veterinary Medical Association was organized in 1982 and covers an area in Central Minnesota that includes the cities of St. Cloud, Alexandria, Brainerd, Milaca, and Elk River. Dinner meetings are held on a quarterly basis with a scientific presentation as the centerpiece of three of the four programs. One meeting a year is a social event to which the members' spouses are invited.

An unusual event led to the formation of this group. The St. Cloud Chamber of Commerce issued a directory that listed veterinarians with tradesmen rather than with professional people. This disturbed Dr. Kallestad who, along with other St. Cloud veterinarians, questioned the persons responsible for the listings. It soon became evident that the Chamber had little knowledge of the veterinary profession or the education required to become a veterinarian. Consequently, the veterinarians made a presentation to the Chamber about the veterinary profession. The chamber members were impressed by the presentation and asked if there was a society or association of veterinarians in St. Cloud that could represent the profession. This was an embarrassing question as there was no such association. To fill this void the Central Veterinary Medical Association was formed and it has proved to be a very successful association.

CHAIN OF LAKES VETERINARY ASSOCIATION

The Chain of Lakes Veterinary Association was formed at Fairmont, Minnesota, in February 1962. The association's original officers were Dr. C. O. Enge of St. James, president; and Dr. R. W. Rieke of Fairmont, secretary. The association served veterinarians in South Central and Southwestern Minnesota. Meetings were originally held six time a year. However, as attendance dropped, this group merged with the Southwest Minnesota Veterinary Medical Association.

EAST CENTRAL VETERINARY MEDICAL ASSOCIATION

The East Central Veterinary Medical Association was organized in 1965 with Dr. Leroy W. Thom of Cambridge serving as president and Dr. R. L. Hanson of Lindstrom serving as secretary. The membership includes veterinarians from Chisago, Isanti, Kanabec, Mille Lacs, Pine, and Sherburne Counties. Evening meetings are held at various locations four times a year.

HEART OF LAKES VETERINARY MEDICAL ASSOCIATION

The Heart of Lakes Veterinary Medical Association was founded at Perham in January 1984. Those responsible for organizing the association were Drs. W. M. Rose, W. E. Clauson, and Jeffrey Bryan of Perham. This association serves Northwestern Minnesota and meets four times a year in Perham.

JACK PINE VETERINARY ASSOCIATION

The Jack Pine Veterinary Association was organized in 1970 in Wadena with Dr. Warren Hartman of Wadena and Dr. James Schaefer of Staples serving as officers. Quarterly meetings were held in Wadena for a few years before the association ceased operation.

MCLEOD COUNTY VETERINARY MEDICAL ASSOCIATION

The McLeod County Veterinary Medical Association was formed on March 8, 1955, at the Garden Club in Hutchinson. As the name suggests, this association is composed of McLeod County veterinarians. The first officers of the association and other charter members are shown in Exhibit IV-12.

EXHIBIT IV-12

FIRST OFFICERS AND CHARTER MEMBERS OF MCLEOD COUNTY VETERINARY MEDICAL ASSOCIATION

President	Dr. M. R. Campbell, Winsted
1st Vice President	Dr. A. J. Thompson, Hutchinson
2nd Vice President	Dr. R. A. Thompson, Glencoe
Secretary/Treasurer	Dr. H. H. Fuglsang, Glencoe
Charter members	Dr. E. H. Braunsworth
	Dr. G. E. Jacobi
	Dr. Norman Fredrickson
	Dr. Fred Bathke
	Dr. H. H. Templin
	Dr. K. E. Griebe

The association holds eight evening dinner meetings with a scientific program each year. Additionally, this group has an annual Christmas party and, in June, a steak fry to which the spouses are invited.

METROPOLITAN ANIMAL HOSPITAL ASSOCIATION

While there had been an interest in forming an organization of small animal practitioners in Minneapolis and St. Paul, no concrete steps were taken until October 1952 when Dr. B. J. Porter contacted Drs. Ora B. Morgan, George W. Mather, Darrell Steele, George Hartle, Ernest Fitch, and Lyle Spakes about organizing an animal hospital association. These veterinarians indicated interest and a meeting was held on November 6, 1952, at the Covered Wagon Restaurant in Minneapolis. In addition to those veterinarians mentioned above, Drs. Griselda Hanlon, Maurice Palmer, Verdie Gysland, and Donald Clifford also attended the meeting. The group agreed that an organization named the Twin City Animal Hospital Association should be formed. The objectives of the new association included the promotion of a closer relationship between small animal practitioners in the Twin City area, the exchange of information, the development of educational programs, the drafting of a code of operating procedures, and the formulation of a range of approved charges for various types of veterinary services.

At the organizational meeting on December 18, 1952, the following officers were elected: Dr. Darrell Steele, president; Dr. George W. Mather, vice president; and Dr. Donald Clifford, secretary/treasurer.

On January 8, 1953, the name of the organization was changed to the Metropolitan Animal Hospital Association so as to encourage small animal practitioners outside of Minneapolis and St. Paul to join the association and attend the meetings.

Others who attended the early meetings included Drs. D. B. Palmer, Manuel Navarro, Fred Gehrman, Elmer Berg, Conway Rosell, Donald Low, Jay Sautter, John Henry, and Wesley Anderson.

During one of the early meetings, the association created the office of treasurer to collect the 50 cent per-meeting charge to cover the cost of postage and other expenses. Dr. Manuel Navarro was elected the association's first treasurer.

The Metropolitan Animal Hospital Association was incorporated on March 7, 1966. The incorporators included Drs. B. Robert Lewis, Thayer E. Porter, Richard H. McConnell, Thomas M. Willmus, and Donald Innes. The first officers of the newly incorporated association were Dr. B. Robert Lewis, president; Dr. Frank Barile, vice president; Dr. John Flynn, secretary; and Dr. Donald Innes, treasurer.

The Metropolitan Animal Hospital Association has been very active and has supported many projects affecting the veterinary profession. The MAHA, which periodically sponsors conferences with outside speakers, has a large membership that meets on a monthly basis (except during the summer months) at the Normandy Village in Minneapolis.

MINNESOTA ACADEMY OF EQUINE PRACTITIONERS

The Minnesota Academy of Equine Practitioners was organized at a meeting held on October 9, 1969, at the Chalet Bowl and Lounge in Plymouth. Dr. Wesley Schroeder had written to equine practitioners inviting them to a meeting for the purpose of considering the formation of an association. Those who attended the meeting included Drs. Victor Myers, F. W. Carlson and Robert Vander Pol. The original elected officers were Dr. W. G. Schroeder of Wayzata, president; Dr. Victor Meyers of St. Paul, vice president; and Dr. F. W. Carlson of Forest Lake, secretary/treasurer.

The academy's first spring meeting was held at Waconia with Dr. George M. Beeman of Littleton, Colorado, as the featured speaker. The academy has continued to hold spring meetings each year with an occasional fall meeting. The academy assists in arranging the equine section of the MVMA's annual meeting.

MINNESOTA ASSOCIATION OF BOVINE PRACTITIONERS

The Minnesota Association of Bovine Practitioners was organized in May 1976 at a continuing education program at the University of Minnesota's College of Veterinary Medicine. Drs. Stanley Held, James O. Hanson, and Robert Stone were active in the formation of the association. Dr. Held was elected president and has continued in that office through the present time. The association has held two or three informal meetings at the annual meetings of the Minnesota Veterinary Medical Association, but of late no meetings have been held. In the meantime, the organization has assisted in planning continuing education programs and the Preconditioning Program.

MINNESOTA VALLEY VETERINARY MEDICAL ASSOCIATION

The Minnesota Valley Veterinary Medical Association was formed at the Cat & Fiddle Club in New Ulm on February 1961. The first officers were Dr. C. L. Bohan of Madelia, president; Dr. John Eckstein of New Ulm, vice president; and Dr. C. R. Carlson of Gaylord, secretary/treasurer.

The association, which is one of the more active in the state, holds nine meetings a year and serves South Central Minnesota. The meetings are held alternately in New Ulm and St. Peter.

SOUTHERN MINNESOTA VETERINARY MEDICAL SOCIETY

The Southern Minnesota Veterinary Medical Society was organized through the efforts of Jay Hormel of the family that founded the George A. Hormel Packing Plant Family in Austin. Jay Hormel had a pet Chester White pig named Snowball. When winter came, she was kept in a horse stall in the stable with Hormel's fine horses. During the winter, Snowball had a litter of 11 pigs that were raised into healthy, vigorous pigs without problems. Jay Hormel was very proud of Snowball and her fine offspring.

The common practice at that time was to farrow pigs in the spring and in the fall. However, the highly successful farrowing of Snowball in the winter led Jay Hormel to believe that there really should be no ill effects in farrowing pigs every month of the year. If farmers would do this, it would solve the problem of an uneven supply of butcher hogs during the year at the Hormel Packing Plant. Hormel believed the best way to convince farmers that pigs could be farrowed every month of the year would be to establish a demonstration herd with year around farrowing.

The herd became Jay Hormel's pet project. He set about purchasing a herd of breeding swine that would be housed in a suitable building. In assembling the herds, it was necessary to purchase sows from several herds in order to obtain representative breeds and the desired number of animals.

All went well initially, and veterinarians were invited to see the operation with the hope they would encourage their clients to adopt year around farrowing. However, serious disease problems soon arose in the newborn and older pigs. The sows from different herds acted as carriers of diseases present on the farm from which they originated. The diseases were resistant to treatment and the project was threatened.

Drs. H. C. H. Kernkamp and Martin Roepke of the Veterinary Division of the University of Minnesota were sent to study the problem in the herd. Subsequently, Jay Hormel was instrumental in inviting veterinarians to meet at the Hormel Sales Cabin to discuss swine problems in 1943. This meeting led to the organization of the Southern Minnesota Veterinary Society. Dr. H. P. Hanson of Austin was elected the first president. Although there is no complete record of those persons who attended the initial meeting, the hall of the Hormel Sales Cabin was filled with veterinarians. Charter members included Drs. H. P. Hanson of Austin; L. A. Husby of Adams; P. H. Riede of Mabel; Karl Knoche of Austin; John Higbee of Albert Lea; W. F. Flanary of St. Charles; John N. Campbell of Fairmont; John P. Arnold and B. A. Zupp of Blooming Prairie; D. E. Trump of Owatonna; L. H. Phipps of Winnebago; E. S. Hobert of Blue Earth; J. L. Cavanaugh of Plainview; Carl Schlotthauer of Rochester; and H. M. Fisch of Spring Valley.

The George A. Hormel Co. continued to sponsor the organization by hosting a meeting every spring, sending out the invitations, and collecting the $2 dues that were used for postage and other expenses. The dinners served at the Hormel Sales Cabin featured generous portions of choice meat from the plant prepared by Jay Hormel's chef. Many veterinarians from Northern Iowa attended and, for a time, there was an effort to change the association's name to include a reference to Northern Iowa.

Wilson & Co. sponsored a few meetings in the fall of the year in Albert Lea, but these sessions never reached the popularity of those in Austin. After a few years, the meetings were dropped. In 1984, the Southern Minnesota Veterinary Medical Society ceased meeting altogether.

SOUTH CENTRAL MINNESOTA VETERINARY MEDICAL ASSOCIATION

The South Central Veterinary Medical Association was founded in New Richland on October 20, 1960. Veterinarians from Le Sueur, Blue Earth, Faribault, Freeborn, Mower, Dodge, Waseca, Rice, and Steele Counties attended the meetings. Dr. Roy C. Williams of New Richland was secretary for many years while the meetings were held in New Richland.

SOUTHEASTERN MINNESOTA VETERINARY MEDICAL ASSOCIATION

The Southeastern Minnesota Veterinary Medical Association was organized on August 2, 1956, at the Kahler Hotel in Rochester. The following veterinarians were present at the meeting: Drs. Bruce Hohn, Robert Leary, D. D. Hagen, John Anderson, Edmund Kohler, Warren Thurber, Alfred Carlson, Charles McPherson, W. H. Feldman, James Flanary, Robert Stader, and Paul Zollman. Dues were set at one dollar, and Dr. Zollman was elected the association's first secretary. With few exceptions, the association's meetings were held in Rochester. The association serviced members from Dodge, Goodhue, Fillmore, Houston, Mower, Olmsted, and Winona Counties.

SOUTHWESTERN MINNESOTA VETERINARY MEDICAL ASSOCIATION

The Southwestern Veterinary Medical Association was organized at Island in approximately 1950. Among those who helped organize the association were Drs. Alfred M. Anderson and M. J. Kontz, Luverne; P. C. Enge, Windom; R. A. Penkert, Hector; and J. A. Kempena, Edgerton. The association's meetings have been held at several locations including Slayton, Tracy, and Windom.

SUBURBAN VETERINARY MEDICAL ASSOCIATION

The Suburban Veterinary Medical Association was organized in the fall of 1960 in Chaska. The association's membership is composed of practitioners on the west side of the Twin Cities. Meetings are held monthly, except during the summer months. Dinners are held in conjunction with the meetings. Dues were initially set at $10 per year. The first members of the association are given in Exhibit IV-13.

EXHIBIT IV-13

FIRST MEMBERS OF SUBURBAN VETERINARY MEDICAL ASSOCIATION

Dr. W. D. Anderson of Rosemount
Dr. R. L. Conway of Watkins
Dr. D. W. Johnson of Maple Plain
Dr. L. W. Johnson of Maple Plain
Dr. George Koepke of Excelsior
Dr. A. J. Kunkel of St. Michael
Dr. D. F. Long of Lakeville
Dr. Donald Maas of Long Lake
Dr. R. G. Mackerwith of Annandale
Dr. D. A. Manthei of Norwood
Dr. R. G. Molnau of Waconia
Dr. P. L. Nelson of Minneapolis
Dr. Raymond Solac of St. Paul
Dr. A. C. Spannus of Waconia
Dr. Jack Stracke of Cokato
Dr. K. M. Tabberson of Cokato
Dr. R. T. Tibbits of Kimball
Dr. Leland Thal of Watertown
Dr. John Wright of Eden Prairie
Dr. D. W. Mittlestadt of Chaska

TWIN CITIES VETERINARY MEDICAL ASSOCIATION

The Twin Cities Veterinary Medical Association was organized in 1913. The following notice of the organization of the association appeared in the American Veterinary Review:

Vets living in and near the Twin Cities recently met and organized an association, to be known as the Twin City Veterinary Association. It is expected that a considerable number of vets practicing at railroad points within a convenient distance of the Twin Cities will take an active part with veterinarians from St. Paul, Minneapolis, South St. Paul and University Farm.

At the time this association was organized, there were 8 licensed graduate veterinarians in Minneapolis, 11 in St. Paul, 16 in South St. Paul, and 7 at the University Farm.

The following officers were elected at the organizational meeting: Dr. F. D. Ketchum, of South St. Paul, as president; Dr. L. Hay, of Faribault, as vice president; and Dr. Myron Reynolds, of University Farm, as secretary.

Meetings were discontinued during World War I, and did not resume until 1928. The main reason for the rebirth of the association was the fact the MVMA was hosting the annual meeting of the AVMA in Minneapolis. Meetings were discontinued for the second time during World War II. The association was revived again in 1945 with meetings taking place on a quarterly basis.

The growth of small animal practice and the decline in large animal practice in the Twin Cities area led to the formation of the Metropolitan Animal Hospital Association, which took many members away from the Twin Cities Veterinary Medical Association. The membership dwindled until only regulatory veterinarians and members of the College of Veterinary Medicine staff attended meetings. In about 1985, the association was disbanded.

WEST CENTRAL MINNESOTA VETERINARY MEDICAL ASSOCIATION

On June 30, 1935, twenty veterinarians (see Exhibit IV-14) met at Dr. O. H. Osborn's cottage on Lake Koronis in Paynesville to form a veterinary association. Dr. C. B. Estey was elected president; G. J. Paul vice president; W. T. Williams secretary; and Drs. R. W. Kiebel and J. R. Lupfer were appointed to the board of directors. The group decided to name this new organization the Central Minnesota Veterinary Medical Association. The name was later changed to the West Central Minnesota Veterinary Medical Association.

The association holds five meetings and a summer picnic each year. The meetings are held at the Minnewaske House between Glenwood and Starbuck.

EXHIBIT IV-14

CENTRAL MINNESOTA VETERINARY MEDICAL
ASSOCIATION FOUNDING VETERINARIANS

C. B. Estey, St. Cloud

J.C. McKee, Litchfield

H. G. Fleming, Alexandria

J.H. Newman, Little Falls

L. E. Frank, Hancock

O.H. Osborn, Paynesville

E. A. Hall, Little Falls

G.J. Paul, Melrose

Marion J. Jones, Milaca

C.L. Rackliffe, Delano

R. W. Kiebel, Monticello

H.L. Strandberg, Glenwood

M. C. Linneman, St. Joseph

Ed. Wanner, Willmar

J. R. Lupfer, Litchfield

W.T. Williams, Brooten

R. A. Merrill, Clara City

W.S. Wilson, Buffalo

Geo. McBroon, Atwater

G.F. Yager, Sauk Centre

WESTERN VETERINARY MEDICAL ASSOCIATION

The Western Veterinary Medical Association held its thirtieth anniversary party on April 21, 1983, at the Chalet Club, in Marshall. The association had its beginning in May 1953 when Dr. J. J. Kelly, of Marshall, sent cards to sixteen other veterinarians in Marshall and in the surrounding towns inviting them to a meeting at the Atlantic Hotel in Marshall. All of the sixteen veterinarians who were invited attended the meeting. The Western Veterinary Medical Association was organized at this meeting, and the members elected Dr. Donald M. Sook of Marshall as their first president.

Those present at the first meeting included Drs. J. J. Kelly, O. E. Dovre, and Donald M. Sook, of Marshall; Drs. E. K. Bicek and Donald B. Hicks, of Tracy; Drs. W. F. Ellgen and Lyle W. Klein, of Ivanhoe; Dr. D. B. Stewart, of Lake Benton; Dr. E. H. Allison, of Balaton; Dr. R. N. Reinertson, of Hendricks; Dr. E. J. Foley, of Wood Lake; Dr. M. P. Maher, of Vesta. Dr. B. F. Jahn, of Clarkfield, could not be a charter member because he graduated one month after the organizational meeting. He has nevertheless faithfully attended the association's meetings.

In the early years, the meetings were held at the Atlantic Hotel, in Marshall, with an occasional meeting at the Minnesota Club and Club 59, in Marshall, and the Mediterranean Club, in Tracy. In 1959, interest in the association lagged. However, it was revived through the efforts of a few members headed by Drs. Dovre and Hicks. The Chalet Club has been the regular meeting place since it was built in 1960. The regular meeting date is the third Thursday of each month.

CHAPTER V

Veterinary Education in Minnesota

The veterinary profession cannot continue, much less advance, without good educational programs. Veterinary colleges bring experts together to do research in their fields, present new ideas to advance the profession, and train the next generation of veterinarians. The demand for veterinarians is not great enough for each state to have a veterinary college. In Minnesota, a private college was created only to be destroyed by fire after a few years. The movement to create a college to train veterinarians in Minnesota nonetheless continued for many years thereafter. Eventually, a state supported veterinary college was established in the state.

EARLY VETERINARY EDUCATION IN MINNESOTA

The history of veterinary medical education in Minnesota is unique in that several attempts were made to establish colleges of veterinary medicine before the present College of Veterinary Medicine at the University of Minnesota was established in 1947.

In the late 1800s, there were only a few veterinary colleges in the United States, and most of these were located in the East. While some were connected with public universities or colleges, most veterinary colleges were proprietary institutions that were usually run for profit. As they were self-supporting, these colleges developed large numbers of clinical cases to generate income. The students helped take care of the cases as part of their training.

In 1881, Dr. C. C. Lyford founded the Northwestern Veterinary College in Minneapolis. Northwestern was located at 716 Third Avenue South in Minneapolis. Dr. Lyford had come to Minneapolis and established a practice in 1880. He was well educated, having received a degree in agriculture from the University of Illinois, and veterinary and medical degrees from McGill University in Montreal, Canada. In addition, Dr. Lyford had one year of post-graduate study at the Royal Veterinary College of London, England.

At the time, it was not uncommon for veterinarians to obtain medical degrees to gain respect and prestige in the community. In the planning and the early stages of the college, Dr. Lyford had the good fortune of making the acquaintance of a physician named Dr. F. Dunsmore. At the time, Dr. Dunsmore was planning the Minnesota Medical College in Minneapolis. They agreed that the veterinary students would attend classes in chemistry and physiology with the medical students. They further agreed that if any of the veterinary students wished to continue their education in the medical field and become a physician, they would have the privilege of completing the medical curriculum at the Minnesota Medical College.

The veterinary curriculum that was developed for the Northwestern Veterinary College extended over a three year period. The school year consisted of six months of instruction each year and a summer session following the second year.

Northwestern's faculty included H. J. Burnish, M.D., who taught chemistry and physiology; B. W. McLellan, V.S., who taught anatomy, pathology, and clinics; Richard Price, V.S. and M.D., who taught materia medica and therapeutics and clinics; and C. C. Lyford, B.S., V.S., and M.D., who taught surgery and clinics. Dr. Lyford served as the president of the college.

The first students who were accepted to the college when it opened in 1881 included J. J. Bradley, L. Graham, J. F. Lee, and R. C. Mason. Of these men, all but Graham graduated with a D.V.M. degree in 1885. Bradley and Mason also completed the medical curriculum and practiced as physicians. Mason began a veterinary practice in Winona, Minnesota.

In 1883, Dr. Lyford decided that none of the applicants met these high standards and admitted no students for that year. In 1886, Dr. Lyford again deemed that none of the applicants were considered worthy of admission. This rigorous admission process was unusual for proprietary veterinary colleges as they received no government support and were in great need of the tuition revenue and help that comes from students.

The high standards of admission to Northwestern Veterinary College and the reputation of Dr. Lyford inspired the editor of the American Veterinary Review to write, "[t]his country is large enough to support literally all institutions of this kind. Of the members of the faculty we are acquainted with but one, Dr. C. C. Lyford, V.S., and in the deserved repute obtained by this gentleman, may be found sufficient guarantee that the profession will never be disparaged by those whose diploma shall bear his name."

In 1884, Leo Briesacher, C. C. Burnham, and R. A. Van Nest were admitted as students to Northwestern. Briesacher dropped out in 1886, and Van Nest subsequently transferred to the American Veterinary College in New York City. Burnham graduated in 1887 and practiced at Stillwater, Minnesota.

In 1888, J. N. Gould was the only student admitted to Northwestern. He transferred to the Chicago Veterinary College, where he graduated in the same class with his father in 1893, and later practiced in Fairmont, Minnesota.

In 1889, fire destroyed the Northwestern Veterinary College, along with its the clinic and stable. Three of Dr. Lyford's fine trotting horses perished in the fire. Dr. Lyford's decision not to rebuild the college was unfortunate because Northwestern promised to become one of the leading proprietary colleges in the country.

FIRST ATTEMPT TO CREATE A VETERINARY COLLEGE AT THE UNIVERSITY OF MINNESOTA

The University of Minnesota catalog for 1888-89 listed "The Veterinary Curriculum" that contained a complete and comprehensive curriculum that would prepare students for the veterinary profession. The three-year course was open to students who either had completed two years in the School of Agriculture at the university or could demonstrate equivalent knowledge through an examination. The curriculum again appeared in the 1889-90 catalog with a few changes. The fact the veterinary curriculum was offered was unusual because there were no veterinarians on the staff of the university at this time. Indeed, there is no evidence that these courses actually were taught.

Professor Edward Porter of the College of Agriculture apparently was responsible for the development of the veterinary curriculum offered by the university. The idea for the veterinary curriculum may have been inspired by remarks made by Dr. R. White during a lecture on the university's Farm Campus in St. Paul. The lecture, which was entitled, "Diseases of the Fourth Stomach of Cattle," was part of a series of lectures arranged by Professor Porter to create interest and attract students to the College of Agriculture. At the close of the lecture, Dr. White, a veterinarian from South St. Paul, expressed the opinion that Minnesota should train its own veterinarians. A

Committee on Veterinary Science was soon appointed. While the minutes of the Board of Regents reflect the committee gave their report during the November 1888 meeting, contents of the report were not recorded.

During 1888, the Board of Regents decided to add a veterinarian to the university staff to teach courses on animal diseases. Dr. Michael Treacy, a native of New York City and a graduate of the Royal Veterinary College of London, was hired to fill the position. When Dr. Treacy appeared before the Board of Regents during their September 18, 1888, meeting, he informed them he was "moveable" and he would accept their original offer of $1,500 per annum to serve as veterinarian for the Experiment Station. However, Dr. Treacy resigned to join the army after working only two months. During the short time he was at the university, Dr. Treacy wrote an article entitled, "Tubercular Phthisis or Consumption in Animals," which was published as Station Bulletin No. 4.

Dr. Olaf Schwartzkoff, graduate of the Imperial Veterinary College in Berlin, Germany, was selected to succeed Dr. Treacy. Dr. Schwartzkoff began his duties in January 1889. The position was subsequently upgraded to Professor of Veterinary Services and Agricultural Experiment Station. The presence of the

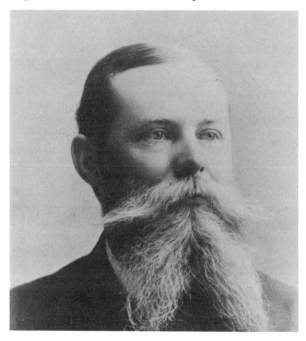

Dr. Olaf Schwartzkoff. courtesy University of Minnesota Archives.

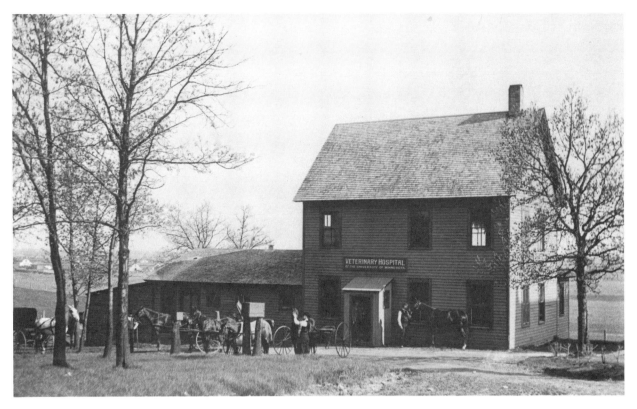

Veterinary Hospital, built in 1890 on St. Paul Campus.

"Veterinary Curriculum" in the university catalog and the demise of the Northwestern Veterinary College inspired Dr. Schwartzkoff to start a veterinary college at the University. With the approval of Professor Porter, Dr. Schwartzkoff made arrangements to teach the courses in the veterinary curriculum through the Departments of Botany, Zoology, and Chemistry in the College of Science, Literature and Arts. He made similar arrangements to teach veterinary courses in the Department of Physiology in the Medical School. He hired Dr. Frank Allen, a veterinary practitioner in St. Paul, to teach anatomy and Dr. S. H. Brimhall, a veterinarian with the state Board of Health, to teach materia medica on a part-time basis. Dr. Schwartzkoff himself planned to teach the courses in histology and veterinary hygiene.

The university needed a veterinary hospital to teach the veterinary clinics. At their August 20, 1889, meeting, the Board of Regents approved the following resolution: "That the Committee on Agriculture be authorized to make contract for the building of the veterinary hospital for $1200. Exclusive of painting and posts."[1]

At the May 6, 1891, meeting of the Board of Regents, President Cyrus Northrop stated: "Should the veterinary department grow into a

college by itself, doing for the Northwest what veterinary colleges in the East, especially Philadelphia, do for the whole country, the present hospital will prove too small." At this same meeting, the regents voted to increase Dr. Schwartzkoff's salary by $300.

During the summer of 1891, President Northrop took a leave of absence. While he was away, Dr. Schwartzkoff made arrangements for the teaching of the veterinary courses for the 1891-92 fiscal year. The new arrangements increased the expenses from $2,283.93 for the 1890-91 fiscal year to $6,085.24 for the 1891-92 fiscal year. When President Northrop returned and learned of the increase in the cost of the veterinary program, he was greatly disturbed and proposed that the regents abolish the program. President Northrop's proposal was discussed at the regents' May 3, 1892, meeting. Dr. Schwartzkoff, who was present at the meeting, gave "a statement as to the educational and financial conduct of the department." Details of the discussion that followed were not recorded. However, Dr. Schwartzkoff, who was educated in Germany and had served as an officer in the U.S. Army, was blunt, forceful, and a little arrogant in presenting his opinions. There is every reason to believe the discussion was heated. The minutes reflect "[a]fter further consideration it was voted that the request of Dr. Schwartzkoff to be relieved of his duties in

[1] The posts were for tying horses along the street in front of the building.

Curriculum with the School of Agriculture be granted [and] that the department of veterinary in the University be discontinued after the present year."

Twenty-one students enrolled in the veterinary curriculum during the two year period it had been offered by the University. Eleven of these students subsequently transferred to other veterinary colleges to obtain their veterinary degree. Charles E. Cotton of Prescott, Wisconsin, transferred to the University of Pennsylvania; J. R. Butters of Waverly, N. A. Christianson of Worthington, Thomas Falconer of Hendrix, and K. J. McKenzie of Northfield continued their studies at the Ontario Veterinary College; R. D. Eaton, F. A. Illstrop, J. A. Scott, and Jacob Sutzin, all students from Minneapolis, and J. N. Gould of Fairmont, each completed his degree work at the Chicago Veterinary College and later returned to practice veterinary medicine in Minnesota. The fate of the other ten students is not known.

CHANGE IN THE FOCUS OF VETERINARY MEDICINE

The university made several changes in the area of veterinary studies after Dr. Schwartzkoff left the university. Treatment of animals from nearby farms at the clinic was discontinued. The title of the veterinary curriculum was changed to "Veterinary Studies." Later, the curriculum was again renamed as "Anatomy, Physiology and Hygiene of Domestic Animals." The course work was tailored to meet the needs of students in the School of Agriculture who were planning careers as farmers or livestock husbandmen. The curriculum also grew to include instruction on the contribution of skeleton and muscle coverings to the conformation and soundness of the animal; the differences in digestive and reproductive systems between different species of animals; the physiology of milk production; and the digestion and assimilation of food. The course also included the cause and in some cases treatment of infectious and noninfectious diseases. Because it attempted to cover so many subjects, the curriculum was mostly a survey course with little depth in any particular subject.

Dr. Christofer Graham was selected to replace Dr. Schwartzkoff as the staff veterinarian at the university. As part of the university's change in focus, the position was downgraded from professor to instructor. Thus, Dr. Graham was officially appointed instructor of Veterinary Science in the School of Agriculture. He began his duties in October 1892. However, Dr. Graham, who had received his veterinary degree from the University of Pennsylvania in 1892, resigned his position with Minnesota after less than one year to return to medical school at Pennsylvania. He later became famous throughout the world as a staff member of the Mayo Clinic in Rochester.

DEVELOPMENT OF THE DIVISION OF VETERINARY MEDICINE

In 1893, Dr. Myron H. Reynolds was selected to fill the vacancy left by Dr. Graham. Dr. Reynolds had received his veterinary degree from Iowa State University in 1889 and had also earned both medical and pharmaceutical degrees. Oren C. Gregg, in charge of Agriculture Extension, first became aware of Dr. Reynolds in 1881 when he needed a veterinarian to give lectures for the Farmer's Institute. Gregg was referred to Dr. Reynolds, who was then practicing in southeastern Iowa and acting as an assistant to Dr. M. Stalker, the state veterinarian. Dr. Reynolds lectured at the Farmer's Institute for about two years before he was appointed staff veterinarian. When he started in the position on September 1, 1893, Dr. Reynolds received a salary of $1,000 per year. This was $800 less in salary than Dr. Schwartzkoff had been earning when he resigned, and $500 less than Dr. Treacy had been paid.

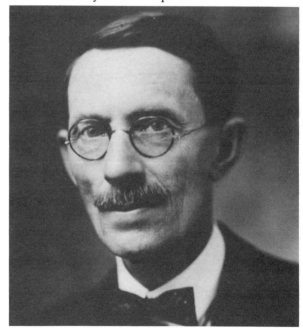

Dr. Myron H. Reynolds. Courtesy University of Minnesota Archives.

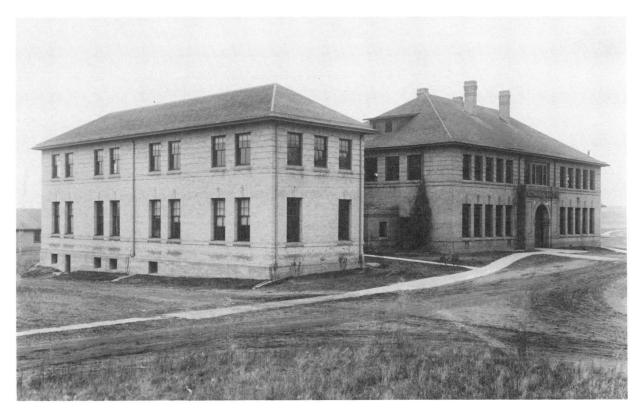

Veterinary Medicine Building (Old Anatomy), right building built in 1901, left building built in 1915.

Dr. Reynolds actively promoted animal disease control programs and the veterinary profession within Minnesota. He served on the state Board of Health (now the Department of Health) and the Live Stock Sanitary Board (now the Board of Animal Health). Dr. Reynolds also helped organize the Minnesota Veterinary Medical Association and served as its president in 1899-1900. He also served as secretary of the Board of Veterinary Examiners for several years. Dr. Reynolds was the only veterinarian on the university's staff until 1904 when Dr. C. C. Lipp was hired to assist him with his teaching responsibilities.

The volume of services and the research rendered by Dr. Reynolds and his staff eventually grew to the point where they needed more space. In 1901, the Veterinary Medicine Building was erected on the St. Paul Campus at a cost of $25,000. The first floor contained an operating room with amphitheater seating for 80 students, a pharmacy and instrument room, a box stall ward, a contagious disease room, and a dissecting room. The second floor included a large museum, a physiology laboratory, and a private office. In 1915, the east wing was added to the Veterinary Medicine Building at a cost of $25,000. Upon the establishment of the School of Veterinary Medicine in 1947, the Veterinary Medicine

Building was renamed "Old Anatomy." In 1992, the east wing of the building was torn down due to its deteriorating condition. The remainder of the building is in poor condition, and the second floor has been condemned as unsound and unsafe for use.

ANTI-HOG CHOLERA SERUM PLANT

Hog cholera was a deadly disease of swine that wiped out many hog herds. At first, the only means to control the disease was to quarantine infected herds. The subsequent development of anti-hog cholera serum helped prevent infection through early treatment of the disease. The anti-hog cholera serum was initially produced by State Laboratories. No commercial companies were willing to undertake production until a market was developed. In 1908, the College of Agriculture and the Board of Animal Health engaged in a joint venture to produce anti-hog cholera serum on the St. Paul Campus of the university. The Hyperimmune Shed, Bleeding Building, Scale Shed, and the Hog Cholera Virus Building were all built south of the Old Anatomy Building to produce the hog cholera products. The Swamp Fever Building was also built during this period. Dr. H. P. Hoskins was added to the university staff and assigned to run the Serum Plant. In 1916, Dr. Hoskins was replaced as manager of the Serum Plant by Dr. H. C. H. Kernkamp.

Dr. Kernkamp had previously worked in the Serum Plant during the summer of 1913 while he was a veterinary student at Ohio State University. He was appointed instructor in the Veterinary Division at the close of his senior year in 1914. At that time, Dr. Kernkamp unknowingly became the center of a dispute between Dr. Reynolds and Dr. Hoskins. Dr. Hoskins had hired Kernkamp and promised him a certain salary without first conferring with the division head, Dr. Reynolds. Dr. Kernkamp had started work before Dr. Reynolds learned of the salary arrangements. Dr. Reynolds came to Dr. Kernkamp and informed him there was not enough money in the budget to cover the cost of the salary that Dr. Hoskins had offered to Dr. Kernkamp. Dr. Reynolds stated he would have to lower Kernkamp's salary to balance the division's budget, but also promised to try to get him a raise the following year. Dr. Kernkamp, who really had no choice if he wished to keep the job, told Dr. Reynolds he was agreeable to the proposal. However, Dr. Hoskins resented what he considered to be Dr. Reynolds' interference with his position as director of the Serum Plant. This incident may have begun the ill feelings Dr. Hoskins had toward Dr. Reynolds.

Due to restrictions placed on state facilities by the legislature, commercial firms eventually produced the anti-hog cholera serum more economically than could state laboratories. By 1927, sales had dropped to such a low level that the Serum Plant was forced to close.

REORGANIZATION OF ST. PAUL CAMPUS

During the summer of 1916, the divisions of the University on the St. Paul Campus were reorganized. The Veterinary Division was renamed the Division of Veterinary Science, and included the following sections:.

I. Veterinary Sanitation, chaired by Professor Reynolds;

II. Veterinary Anatomy, temporarily chaired by Dr. C. C. Palmer;

III. Veterinary Physiology, chaired by Dr. C. C. Palmer;

IV. Veterinary Pathology, chaired by Assistant Professor Willard L. Boyd;

V. Veterinary Medicine and Surgery, chaired by Assistant Professor Willard L. Boyd;

VI. Veterinary Biochemical Products, chaired by Dr. H. C. H. Kernkamp.

TROUBLE IN THE VETERINARY DIVISION

Beginning in 1910, members of the veterinary profession in Minnesota grew concerned with the research performed by the Veterinary Division. They believed the research should focus more on problems in the livestock industry. They were also concerned that so many promising young researchers were leaving the university.

The concern had evolved to severe criticism by the early summer of 1916. During a farewell dinner for Drs. J. T. E. Dinwoodie and H. P. Hoskins, two well-respected veterinarians who had both resigned to accept positions elsewhere, both Dr. Dinwoodie and Dr. Hoskins stated they were sorry to leave Minnesota but they couldn't see any future for themselves at Minnesota.

As the result of these comments, the MVMA introduced a resolution during their summer meeting in Minneapolis on July 12, 1916, that cited the lack of research performed at the university and noted the departure of competent veterinarians because of conditions at the Experiment Station of the university. The resolution further stated the head of the Veterinary Division should be replaced with a person able and willing to take an active part in research and experimental work on animal diseases. The supporters of the resolution called for its immediate adoption. Notwithstanding the heated discussion that ensued, cooler heads prevailed in the end. The members voted to give Dr. Reynolds an opportunity to defend himself, and the business section of the program was recessed until the following morning to allow Dr. Reynolds time to prepare his defense.

On the following morning, Dr. Reynolds began his defense by stating that it was the "duty of the Veterinary Division to foster the animal industry by protecting it against infectious diseases and reducing the losses from other diseases, thus lessening the cost of production." He asserted research was an important vehicle to carry out this duty, and he had done his best to achieve these goals with the limited funds available and the division's heavy teaching commitments. Dr. Reynolds listed 22 publications, most of which were bulletins, and provided a resum_ of eight research publications prepared by the division. He also named an additional 17 research projects that were in progress at the time.

Dr. Reynolds also described his accomplishments outside the division that benefitted the livestock industry and the veterinary profession. These activities included helping to organize the Minnesota Veterinary Medical Association and the Board of Animal Health, and arranging cooperative efforts with livestock and agricultural industries. He also cited his service as secretary of the Board of Veterinary Examiners where he helped to organize the board's affairs and encouraged veterinarians to come to Minnesota.

Dr. Reynolds then reviewed his efforts to obtain research funds from the Department of Agriculture, and indicated that staff members who had left or were leaving the division were lured away by better paying jobs. Dr. Reynolds concluded his defense by submitting letters from officials in other states that praised the disease control programs in Minnesota.

When Dr. Reynolds had finished, Dr. Charles E. Cotton rose and praised Dr. Reynolds' loyalty to the profession. He then asked Dr. Hoskins to address the meeting. Dr. Hoskins confined his remarks to conditions at the university and avoided any comments relating personally to Dr. Reynolds. Dr. Hoskins stated he originally came to Minnesota to do research exclusively, but recent events had taken him away from research. He stressed that the pay of veterinarians on the St. Paul Campus was low when compared with other persons employed on the campus, and that research was the only accomplishment considered in setting individual staff members' salaries.

Dr. Reynolds asked Dr. Hoskins whether Reynolds, as chairman of the division, had lessened the amount or quality of Hoskins' research. He pressed Hoskins hard to say that Dr. Reynolds could not be blamed for the lack of research. Dr. Hoskins then responded by saying that he did not consider Dr. Reynolds had done any "real" research and, in fact, Dr. Reynolds was not "a research man." He continued by stating Dr. Reynolds had even said on occasion he was not interested in research. Dr. Hoskins concluded by

stating Dr. Reynolds was more interested and concerned with the Board of Animal Health than with conducting research.

In the discussion that followed, a motion was made for the Resolutions Committee to rewrite the proposed resolution. The committee was instructed to strike any wording that reflected on the present and past management of the division, and to urge a greater and better veterinary department in the future. There was a general feeling that Dr. Reynolds was not entirely at fault for the state of research in the division and he should not be castigated in this manner. The resolution was adopted as amended. Copies of the resolution were forwarded to the director of the Experiment Station, to the president of the university, and to each member of the Board of Regents. This marks the first and perhaps only time the Minnesota Veterinary Medical Association interfered in the internal affairs of the university.

DR. FITCH REPLACES DR. REYNOLDS

The Dean of Agriculture saw the need for a change in the leadership of the Veterinary Division before the matter came up at the MVMA meeting. He had been quietly conducting a search for a person with a greater commitment to research to head the division. He had offered the

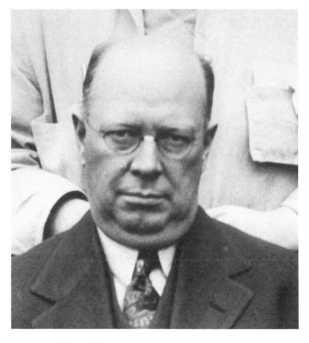

Dr. C.P. Fitch

position to Dr. John R. Mohler, who later became famous as chief of the Bureau of Animal Industry. Unfortunately, Dr. Mohler declined the offer.

The search for a new head of the Veterinary Division intensified following the MVMA meeting. On June 3, 1917, the Board of Regents voted to recommend the appointment of Dr. C. P. Fitch as Professor of Comparative Pathology and Bacteriology, and chairman of the Division of Veterinary Medicine. They also voted to designate Dr. Reynolds as Professor of Veterinary Medicine in charge of the Section of Veterinary Sanitation. Despite his demotion, Dr. Reynolds remained in the division and, to his credit, carried out his assignment in a commendatory manner until his death in 1929.

Dr. Clifford Penny Fitch, B.S., D.V.M., and D.Sc., was born on July 1, 1884, in Sauquit, New York. He received his veterinary degree from Cornell University in 1911. From 1911 to 1917, Dr. Fitch was a member of the faculty at Cornell University where he taught courses in bacteriology and parasitology, and managed the laboratory work conducted in conjunction with the New York Department of Agriculture. From 1915 to 1916, he was resident secretary of AVMA for the state of New York. Dr. Fitch was primarily known as a bacteriologist.

Dr. Fitch proved to be a good administrator who wasted little time making changes in the Veterinary Division. As the first order of business, he persuaded the Board of Regents to change his title to Professor of Animal Pathology and Animal Pathologist of the Experiment Station. He then set about to change the focus of the division to emphasize research by enlarging the staff and raising additional research funds.

Dr. Fitch set an example for the staff with his personal emphasis on research. He became involved in a cooperative research project with the U.S. Department of Agriculture on infectious abortion, or Bang's disease. Dr. Fitch served on the U.S. Livestock Sanitary Association Bang's Disease Committee from 1919-30. He also played a major role in standardizing the agglutination test, or tube and plate test, for brucellosis. At this time, the division conducted research projects in infertility and mastitis in cattle, swine diseases which included hog cholera, and poultry diseases.

Dr. Fitch was a tough but fair taskmaster. He was a very hard worker and he expected the same from the staff. On one occasion, Dr. Fenstermacher, a member of the staff, had been

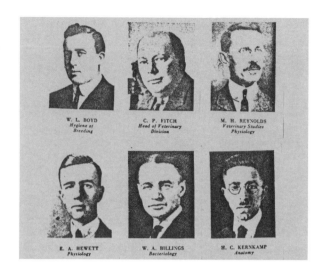

Veterinary faculty in 1922, from School of Agriculture publication.

out of town at an extension meeting the evening before giving a talk to a group of farmers. He returned quite late and overslept the next morning. Dr. Fitch, who was unaware he had been out representing the university the previous evening, was waiting for Dr. Fenstermacher when he reported to work in the middle of the next forenoon. Dr. Fenstermacher got out of his car and started walking toward the door of the building. There he saw Dr. Fitch standing by the door with his watch in his hand. Dr. Fenstermacher, who was not one to be pushed around, walked back to his car, drove off, and did not return until the following day.

Dr. Fitch had a significant ego. At the start of the brucellosis herd test program, it was necessary to instruct veterinarians on the technique of drawing blood from cattle for the test. Dr. Fitch demonstrated the technique at a meeting of veterinarians. A docile Guernsey cow was led into the room. A chair was then brought into the room and placed by the neck of the cow. Dr. Fitch, dressed in a white coat, walked in and sat down in the chair beside the cow. While the herdsman held the head of the cow, Dr. Fitch proceeded to draw a tube full of blood. The veterinarians had trouble controlling their amusement at the scene of Dr. Fitch sitting in a chair while drawing blood from the cow. It would be impossible to place a chair beside a cow in most dairy barns or barnyards. Even if one could place a chair beside a cow, it would be too easy for the cow to kick or strike the veterinarian.

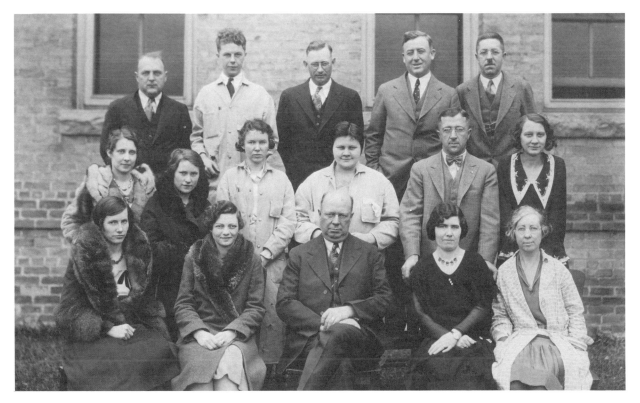

Veterinary staff in 1931, left to right; front row, Grace Whitmer, Francis Goldberg, Dr. C.P. Fitch, Rose Kenaley, Emma Miller, second row, Gladys Christenson, Jean Blocker Rollins, Eileen Davis, Hazel Hammersland, Dr. Ruel Fenstermacher, Lucille Bishop King, third row, Marvin Kent, W. Nilson, Dr. W.L. Boyd, Dr. H.C.H. Kernkamp.

Farmers would call on the Veterinary Division to request veterinarians to check their cows for pregnancy and to treat fertility problems. The procedure involved examining the ovaries, ovarian tubes, and uterus by rectal palpation. Dr. Willard L. Boyd, who was both a bacteriologist and an excellent fertility expert, was usually assigned to handle these problems. Although Dr. Boyd was usually well received by the farmers, Dr. Fitch decided that he, too, should go on these calls. During these calls, Dr. Fitch would palpate a cow first and make a very brief examination. On a nonpregnant cow, Dr. Fitch would say, "She has no chance, send her to market!" Dr. Boyd would follow and make his usual thorough examination. He would say he believed it was possible that with some treatment the cow could become pregnant again. Dr. Fitch would then say, "All right, we will give her another chance, but just one more chance." They would continue in the same manner in examining the other problem cows in the herd.

Dr. Fitch believed the staff needed a strong library to enhance the division's research capability. Although Dr. Reynolds had started the Veterinary Library, Dr. Fitch provided the impetus needed to create an excellent reference library. He modernized the scope of the library and purchased many books and periodicals, including important old reference volumes.

Dr. Fitch was widely respected throughout the country and was elected to many important offices. He served as secretary of the MVMA from 1918 until 1935, he was a member of the Board of Animal Health from 1922 to 1940, and he helped organize the Conference of Research Workers in Animal Diseases. He also served as president of the AVMA from 1933 to 1934. Dr. Fitch died suddenly on January 11, 1940, at the age of 56.

SECOND ATTEMPT TO ESTABLISH A VETERINARY COLLEGE AT THE UNIVERSITY

At the end of World War I, veterinarians in Minnesota anticipated a shortage of graduate veterinarians. Eight of the 14 proprietary veterinary colleges had closed between 1915 and 1920. While there were 10 state supported veterinary colleges in existence, these schools graduated only small classes and did not have the facilities to increase their class size.

During the 1920 annual meeting, the MVMA passed a resolution calling for the University of Minnesota to take whatever action necessary to establish a veterinary college. Copies of the resolution were sent to M. L. Burton, president of the university, and the Board of Regents. However, President Burton had just submitted his resignation as president and the Board of Regents was preoccupied with the process of selecting a successor. The board therefore delegated the question to a committee.

The closing of private veterinary schools was caused by the U.S. Army Surgeon General's refusal to approve entrance requirements at several of the private schools. The closing of the private schools decreased the opportunity to obtain a veterinary degree by 43 percent—a significant decrease as 90 percent of the veterinarians in Minnesota were graduates of private schools.

The committee assigned by the regents to review this situation determined the University Farm at the St. Paul Campus would be an ideal location for a veterinary school. The committee concluded, "[t]here already exists enough weak and poorly equipped veterinary colleges. Minnesota should not add to this number and be a party to turning out men who are not properly equipped to deal with the complex problems of animal disease. If there is to be a veterinary school in Minnesota, let it be such that its graduates can successfully cope with the present day problems which confront the animal breeder. This is an expensive undertaking and the cost must not be lost sight of when considering the advisability of a school."

On May 24, 1920, the Board of Regents referred the matter to the university's new president, Lotus D. Coffman. President Coffman apparently took no action as there is no further reference to the veterinary school in the minutes of the Board of Regents. The lack of support from the administration weakened the movement to establish a veterinary school in the university.

However, the lack of university support did not altogether stop efforts to create a veterinary school at the university. The MVMA, with the whole-hearted support of the Minnesota Livestock Breeders Association, went to the 1920 legislature to request authorization for funds to create a veterinary college at the University of Minnesota. Senator C. N. Orr of Ramsey County sponsored a bill, marked as Senate File 1621, for the creation of such a veterinary college. The bill moved through the legislature with little opposition until it was "pigeon-holed" in the Appropriations Committee. A hearing on the bill was scheduled to take place late one day at the end of the session. A large delegation from the veterinary and livestock associations came to

speak in support of the bill. At the time of the hearing, one of the members of the committee confronted the supporters of the bill and told them the bill would not be placed on the agenda as it was destined to be "pigeon-holed." The senator suggested the supporters of the bill pull up stakes and go home. This ended the second attempt to establish a veterinary college at the University of Minnesota.

DIVISION OF VETERINARY MEDICINE OFFERS GRADUATE DEGREES

In 1920, the Graduate School gave permission to offer the masters degree, or M.S., in the Division of Veterinary Medicine. The establishment of a graduate program greatly helped the veterinary division to increase the volume and quality of its research. The first graduate student in this program was Dr. Donald C. Beaver who had obtained a D.V.M. degree from Michigan State University. Dr. Beaver's thesis was entitled, "The Bacteriology and Pathology of Sterility in Cattle."

After Dr. Martin Roepke joined the staff in 1938, the division was granted permission to offer the Doctor of Philosophy Degree, or Ph.D., in Veterinary Medicine. The graduate program grew and was greatly enhanced through the cooperation of the University Medical School on the Minneapolis Campus. Graduate students in Veterinary Medicine were allowed to take courses and work in research laboratories at the Medical School. Medical School staff members served on graduate committees and as minor advisors. The assistance from the Medical School helped the Division of Veterinary Medicine become known as one of the better research centers in the United States. The quality of training graduate students received is reflected by the fact several graduates eventually became deans of veterinary colleges. Those who became deans and their schools include Drs. W.W. Armistead, Texas and Michigan State, Tennessee; Everett D. Besch, Louisiana; Robert H. Dunlop, Murdock, Australia, Minnesota; Donald Jasper, California; Ralph L. Kitchell, Kansas, Iowa; N. Ole Nielsen, Saskatchewan, Ontario; William R. Pritchard, California; George C. Shelton, Texas; and E.E. Wedman, Oregon.

DR. BOYD SUCCEEDS DR. FITCH

After Dr. Fitch died suddenly on January 11, 1940, Dr. Willard Lee Boyd was appointed

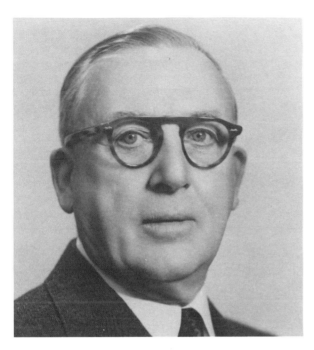

Dr. Willard L. Boyd

chief of the Veterinary Division. Dr. Boyd was born at Batavia, Iowa, on September 27, 1883. He graduated from the Kansas City Veterinary College in 1909 where he remained for two years following graduation as an instructor in veterinary pathology. In 1911, Dr. Boyd joined the faculty of the Division of Veterinary Medicine at the University. In 1918, he was appointed professor of Veterinary Medicine.

Dr. Boyd was an astute clinician who was widely known for his work on reproductive diseases and brucellosis. He was a good speaker and very popular among his fellow veterinarians. Dr. Boyd often appeared on scientific programs in other states. He was a mild mannered and congenial person who was a gentleman at all times.

Dr. Boyd was president of the MVMA in 1922-1923, and he later served as president of the AVMA in 1952-1953. He was active in the U.S. Animal Health Association and the Conference of Research Workers of America. Dr. Boyd served on the Board of Animal Health and the former Stallion Registration Board. He was also the official veterinarian at the Minnesota State Fair horse shows for many years.

Dr. Boyd believed in physical fitness and was a strong supporter of athletics. In the evenings, he exercised with walks in his neighborhood. He was a member of the University Senate Committee on Intercollegiate Athletics for more than 30 years, and he opened the gates at Memorial Stadium before football games for many years.

Under Dr. Boyd's direction, the Division of Veterinary Medicine continued to conduct high quality research and provide a great service to the veterinary profession and the livestock industry. The graduate program expanded substantially during his tenure as head of the division.

ESTABLISHMENT OF THE COLLEGE OF VETERINARY MEDICINE AT THE UNIVERSITY OF MINNESOTA

On April 28, 1947, the Minnesota legislature appropriated funds to establish a veterinary college at the university. The legislation was the result of a well-planned and extensive lobbying campaign by pre-veterinary students, members of the livestock industry, and members of many other interested groups.

Following World War II, there was a shortage of veterinarians, and surveys demonstrated the average age of veterinarians was on the rise. The value of livestock had risen dramatically by the end of World War II. Livestock owners had become increasingly hesitant to treat their animals with anyone other than a qualified veterinarian. All of these factors created public support for a veterinary college.

World War II veterans truly provided the momentum for a veterinary college. Veterans flooded colleges and universities after the war to pursue their education through the G.I. Bill. Many of these veterans took pre-veterinary courses to meet the entrance requirements of veterinary colleges. These pre-veterinary students overwhelmed the veterinary colleges when they applied for admission. The veterinary colleges had more qualified students applying for admission than they could accommodate. For example, Colorado State University had 450 in-state residents applying for admission to its veterinary college. This was ten times the number the college could admit.

To further intensify problems faced by Minnesota veterans, colleges gave priority to admission of in-state applicants. Pre-veterinary students in Minnesota had virtually no chance of gaining admission to veterinary colleges in other states. In the midst of this situation, a meeting of Minnesota pre-veterinary students was called by Ithel Schipper and Glen Nelson during the winter of 1945-1946. The Pre-Veterinary Club, or Pre-Vet

Establishing Of U Veterinary School Urged By Farmers

By ALFRED D. STEDMAN

An effort to include establishment of a school for veterinary medicine in current plans for expansion of the Minnesota College of Agriculture is gaining state-wide support among farmers and farmers' sons, many of them veterans of World War II, who are pre-veterinary students, it was revealed Thursday.

A shortage of veterinarians is injuring the state's livestock industry, which is Minnesota's main source of farm income, and refusal of veterinary colleges outside of Minnesota to accept students from this state is theatening to make the present scarcity of veterinarians permanent and chronic, supporters of the proposal contend.

Some contrary opinion that the shortage is being exaggerated has come to light. But numerous letters urging establishment of a veterinary school at University Farm have been received by J. S. Jones, president of the Minnesota Farm Bureau federation and member of the board of regents of the University of Minnesota.

The Pre-Veterinary club of University of Minnesota students has taken up the movement and is appealing actively for public support of the plan.

"With admittance to veterinary colleges throughout the United States restricted to residents only, Minnesota pre-veterinary students are unable to gain entrance to any of the 10 recognized veterinary colleges," Robert Bossing, president of the club, has written the Pioneer Press in a statement of the case for establishing the school. The condition, he asserts, will continue until at least 1949, so the shortage of veterinarians and the effects of such shortage promise to be prolonged many years unless quickly remedied.

Seventy students at the University now are registered in pre-veterinary medicine, Bossing says, and 20 others have transferred to other fields because of restricted facilities for the veterinary training they want.

Bossing's letter continues:

"Minnesota, one of the leading agricultural states, has only 403 veterinarians today; one for every 489 farms, one for every 21,714 head of livestock, and one for every 72,047 units of poultry. The average age of these veterinarians is 51 years. The livestock income for the past year was $666,229,000; 74.4 per cent of the entire agricultural income of the state of Minnesota came from livestock. The local practitioner is too busy caring for emergency cases in his community to aid in disease prevention. The disease prevention program, if fully carried out, will save the Minnesota farmer thousands of dollars each year. It is evident that this industry should be protected to the fullest extent.

"Due to the lack of graduates in the field of veterinary medicine, because of restricted educational facilities, the profession lacks competition among its own men to such an extent that it is 15 years behind other professions in research. Much research is needed in the diseases of animals transmissible to man.

"Large numbers of veternarians were graduated in the 1911-1920 era. The number of veterinarians in the United States in 1920 was 13,466; in 1931, 12,240; in 1942, 12,500, and at the present time approximately 13,500 to 14,000. From these figures it will be noted that the veterinarian population is not increasing sufficiently to meet present and future needs.

"The establishment of a veterinary college in Minnesota seems to be the only solution to the problem. Other states cannot be expected to train veterinarians for Minnesota.

"The University of Minnesota owns a greater number of livestock than any other university in the country, and there is ample land available on the farm campus for construction of a veterinary school."

From St. Paul Pioneer Press, Nov. 29, 1946

Club, was formed at this meeting. The mission of the Pre-Vet Club was to establish a veterinary college at the University of Minnesota. Mr. Robert Bossing was elected president of the Pre-Vet Club.

The Pre-Vet Club sought the advice and support from several persons including members of the veterinary staff at the university. J. Senaca Jones, who was secretary of the Farm Bureau and a regent of the university, was especially supportive of the club's efforts. Dr. W. E. Peterson of Dairy Husbandry in the College of Agriculture also provided the club members with valuable advice and support. The students collected data on the size and value of the livestock and poultry population in Minnesota, the number and age of veterinarians providing veterinary services in the state, the number and location of veterinary colleges, and the number of students enrolled in each college. Dr. Ruel Fenstermacher, who was the head of the Diagnostic Laboratory and an officer in the Minnesota Veterinary Medical Association, rendered great assistance in helping the students gather this information.

Once this information was gathered, pre-veterinary students sought permission to attend and speak at meetings of livestock organizations, poultry organizations, creamery associations, Farm Bureau, Farmer's Union, Grange, commercial and service clubs, war veteran organizations, and any other organizations that could provide important support to the Pre-Vet Club's efforts to create a veterinary college. During the meetings, the students would relate the information they had collected to demonstrate the need to train more veterinarians. They also told these groups of the great difficulties they had, as Minnesota residents, in gaining admission to out-of-state veterinary colleges. The agricultural press, metropolitan press, and many of the newspapers throughout Minnesota soon gave wide publicity to the students' cause. The students also contacted and received important support from the Minnesota Veterinary Medical Association and the Board of Animal Health.

During the 1946 annual meeting, the Minnesota Veterinary Medical Association passed the following resolution:

Resolved that the Minnesota Veterinary Medical Association favor the establishment of a school of veterinary medicine at the University of Minnesota, said school to be of the highest standards and must meet the requirements for accreditation as set

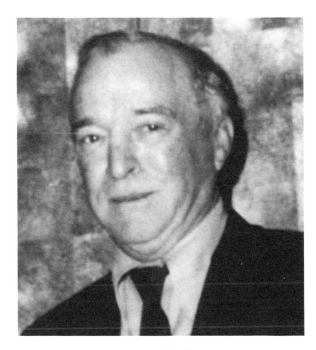

Representative August Mueller.

forth by the committee on colleges of the American Veterinary Medical Association.

Copies of the MVMA's resolution were sent to the members of the state legislature and the Board of Regents.

By the summer of 1946, the campaign had reached the point where members of the Pre-Vet Club began to urge legislators to introduce legislation to establish a veterinary college. Representative August Mueller, a farmer from Sibley County, and Senator Ancher Nelsen, a farmer from McLeod County and later a member of the U.S. Congress, agreed to sponsor the legislation. Both of these men were experienced and able legislators who were well respected by their colleagues.

On February 7, 1947, Representatives August Mueller, Aubrey W. Dirham, L. B. Erdahl, John J. Kinzer, and Rueben Tweten introduced House File 420. Section 1 of the bill read: "There is hereby appropriated out of any monies in the state treasury not otherwise appropriated to the University of Minnesota, the sum of $50,000.00 for the establishment of a School of Veterinary Medicine at the University of Minnesota." The bill, which became known as the "Veterinary Bill," was referred to the Committee on Dairy Products and Livestock for hearings.

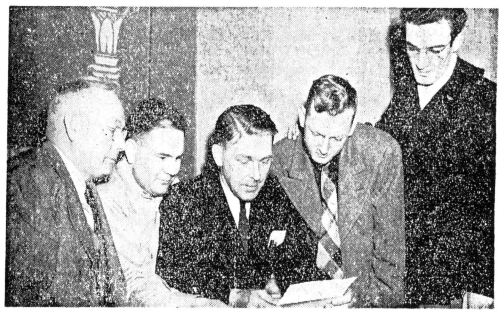

WOULD-BE VETERINARIANS—University of Minnesota students interested in studying veterinary medicine appeared at a Senate finance committee hearing Tuesday in behalf of a proposed bill to establish a veterinary college in the state. Discussing the measure with Sen. D. M. Crey, left, of Wells are, left to right, Ithel Schipper of Wayzata, Sen. Ancher Nelson of Hutchinson, Bruce Hohn of 1614 Hewitt ave., St. Paul, and Walter Mackey of Silver Lake.—PIONEER PRESS PHOTO.

Senators Told Need Of Veterinary School

Minnesota's dairy and livestock industry faces a serious crisis unless action is taken now for establishment of a school of veterinary medicine at the University of Minnesota, the Senate finance committee was told Tuesday.

More than 30 persons— would-be veterinarians now attending the University of Minnesota, leaders in various farm groups and members of the Senate—appeared before the committee in support of a bill to appropriate $600,000 to start a veterinary school.

Sponsors of the measure are Sens. Ancher Nelson of Hutchinson, William Dietz of Montgomery, and D. M. Carey of Wells. Carey is a veterinarian.

"This action seems to us to be an absolute must," said W. S. Moscrip of Lake Elmo, who appeared as a representative of the livestock sanitary board. "We must act now if we are to have proper livestock disease control."

Sen. Carey called enactment of the bill "the best move the state could make at this time."

Sen. Nelson explained that there are only 409 veterinarians in the state now, 300 of whom are practicing in rural areas, and that the average age of the practicing veterinarians is 51.

Ithel Schipper, president of the Pre-veterinary Medical club at the university, said there are about 150 men at University Farm who have had pre-veterinary training but are unable to continue their studies because schools offering such courses already are over-crowded.

Ninety-five per cent of the group are World War II veterans, he said.

Others appeared included Henry Derenthal, president of the Minnesota Livestock Breeders association; Clarence Palmby of Mankato, president of the Blue Earth County Farm Bureau; M. W. Thompson, representing the St. Paul Association of Commerce, and Sens. Werner Wuertz of Austin, Milford Davis of Reading, and C. E. Johnson of Almelund.

From St. Paul Pioneer Press, March 19, 1947.

Individuals who appeared at the hearings and urged the adoption of the Veterinary Bill included Dr. Ralph L. West, secretary of the Board of Animal Health; Colonel E. B. Miller, commander of the Minnesota branch of the American Legion; J. Seneca Jones, secretary of the Farm Bureau; Messrs. Alfred Stedman, Randall Hobart, and Russell Aslesen, editors of the agricultural sections of the metropolitan newspapers; and Pre-Vet Club members Robert Bossing and Ithel Schipper.

In the meantime, the Board of Regents authorized "President Morrill to take the case of a veterinary college to the legislature in the strongest terms." In his presentation to the legislature, President Morrill stated the need for a veterinary college in Minnesota was uncontestable. Furthermore, President Morrill argued it would be folly to establish such a college unless it was well funded and fully accredited. At the same time, he stressed that a veterinary college should not be established at the expense of other critical needs of the university.

Notwithstanding its public support for the legislation, behind the scenes the university administration sought to discourage the establishment of a veterinary college. They emphasized the great cost of the proposed veterinary college and argued that, in balance, the university had other needs that were more important than establishing this new college. When the university presented its formal budget request to the legislature, it did not include proposed funding for a veterinary college.

The lack of meaningful support for a veterinary college by the university administration was a source of great annoyance to rural legislators. In the past, the rural legislators had been concerned by the university administration's apparent lack of consideration for the needs of the St. Paul Campus. The administration's limited support for a veterinary college only added to these legislators' frustration. Consequently, a bill was introduced by Senator Oscar Swenson of Nicollet County to separate the Department of Agriculture on the St. Paul Campus from the Minneapolis Campus of the university. The proposed legislation caught the university by surprise and caused the administration some uneasy moments. Although it did not pass, the proposed legislation caused the university administration to pay more attention to the St. Paul Campus.

The Veterinary Bill received favorable consideration from the Committee on Dairy Products and Livestock. The proposed legislation was then referred to the Appropriations Committee where representatives questioned whether $50,000 would be enough to create a veterinary college. A subcommittee was formed to investigate the probable cost of establishing an acceptable veterinary college. The subcommittee held hearings and recommended the amount be increased to include $150,000 for staffing and $450,000 for permanent equipment and temporary buildings, for a total appropriation of $600,000. On March 4, 1947, the subcommittee re-referred the bill to the Appropriations Committee with a favorable recommendation.

Once the Veterinary Bill seemed to be moving smoothly toward passage in the House, Senators Ancher Nelson, William L. Dietz, and D. M. Carey, himself a veterinarian, introduced a similar version in the Senate. Senate File 877 was referred to the Senate Committee on Dairy Products and Livestock where hearings were promptly scheduled. For the most part, the same persons who appeared in the House hearings also participated in the Senate hearings. However, the proposed legislation had a more difficult time in the Senate where the central roadblock involved the question of where the state would get the money to pay for this new veterinary college. The Veterinary Bill was subsequently tabled where it seemed certain to die in committee.

On March 12, 1947, Alfred Stedman of *The St. Paul Pioneer Press* wrote, "[t]he veterinary bill is up against such hard going that some of the sponsors openly admitted its chances for enactment at this session was [sic] not good." When the students of the Pre-Vet Club read the newspaper reports, they raced to the Capitol and asked to be recognized before the legislature. When their request was refused, the 70 members of the Pre-Vet Club called a special meeting on the evening of March 12, 1947, at the Student Center on the campus. Approximately 25 legislators, several regents, several members of the veterinary staff, and members of the MVMA, Board of Animal Health, news media, radio stations, and university administration attended the meeting. Dr. C. II. Bailey, dean of the St. Paul Campus, was invited to the meeting but declined to attend due to another commitment.

The meeting was lively and sometimes heated, and included discussion of the importance of the veterinary service to the livestock industry; whether the teaching faculty could be recruited from the present veterinary staff; whether the state should assume the financial obligations created by the veterinary college; and the difficulties qualified students faced in admission to veterinary colleges.   During the meeting, Dr. Boyd indicated that, if the legislature enacted legislation to create a veterinary college, classes could begin that fall.

The next morning, the Dairy Products and Livestock Committee referred the bill to the Committee on Finance recommending the passage of the bill into law.

Soon after the meeting took place, one of the student leaders, Glen Nelson, found a note in his post office box from Dr. Boyd asking him to see Dean Bailey as soon as possible. Dean Bailey subsequently let Nelson know in no uncertain terms he was upset by the Pre-Vet Club's audacity to invite legislators to the meeting on the St. Paul Campus. Due to the cost of a veterinary school in balance with other items of higher priority needed on the St. Paul Campus, Dr. Bailey strongly recommended discontinuing the pressure to create a veterinary school.

In the meantime, Senator Nelson asked Glen Nelson to contact and arrange for Dr. Boyd to come to the Capitol and give an estimate on the cost to create a veterinary college. The following day, President Morrill, Dean Bailey, and Dr. Boyd appeared before the committee and estimated the creation of a veterinary college would cost approximately $600,000.[2]

When the Veterinary Bill was tabled by the Appropriations Committee, Alfred Stedman, a writer for *The St. Paul Pioneer Press* who had continued to keep a close watch on the proceedings at the legislature, waved a warning flag signaling the bill was in trouble.

The following people appeared at a hearing of a subcommittee of the Appropriations Committee to urge serious consideration of the bill: Messrs. W. S. Moscrip and Henry Derenthal,

prominent livestock breeders; Messrs. George Woodward and Clarence Palmby of the Minnesota Farm Bureau Federation; Mr. E. W. Thompson of the St. Paul Association of Commerce; Senators D. M. Carey, Milford Davis, C. E. Johnson, and Ancher Nelson; and pre-veterinary student, Ithel Schipper.

Although the subcommittee of the Appropriations Committee approved the creation of the college, members of the subcommittee had failed to include the $600,000 agreed upon to fund the creation of the veterinary college. Representatives August Mueller and Joe Daun recognized the error and sought to have the appropriations inserted in the bill. The bill was finally amended to include the $600,000 appropriation.

At this point, the university administration began to believe the bill had a good chance to pass and they suggested the school of veterinary medicine should open the following year in 1948. The pre-veterinary students who were attending college under the GI Bill were alarmed by this suggestion because they would lose their GI benefits if their college education was interrupted for a year. Thus, Senator Ancher Nelson added an amendment to the bill to require that the first class of students had to be accepted in the fall quarter of 1947. The bill, with the amendments, passed without opposition. Thus, after a long struggle and many disappointments, the third attempt finally succeeded in establishing a veterinary college at the University of Minnesota.

THE BEGINNING OF THE VETERINARY COLLEGE AT THE UNIVERSITY OF MINNESOTA

Following the passage of the Veterinary Bill, the university initially was not aware of the amendment to the bill directing the university to accept the first class in the upcoming fall quarter. The university began to leisurely plan for classes beginning in 1948, and identified certain problems that would have to be resolved before the college could actually open. When the university finally realized the first class had to be accepted for the fall quarter, there were only 110 working days left before the quarter was scheduled to begin and shock waves raced through the university administration.

President Morrill nonetheless delayed preparation of the veterinary school until he was assured the inclusion of the veterinary college in the university budget was legal. He quickly

[2]   The figure of $600,000 given to the committee seemed low in light of an earlier estimate of $1,000,000 offered by President Morrill. The February 15, 1947, issue of the Minnesota Daily stated: "President Morrill will ask the state legislature for an additional $1,000,000 for each of the 1947-1948 biennium for the establishment of a new veterinary school at the University. . . . The school outlined by President Morrill, would need $1,000,000 for each of the next two bienniums to get started and $375,000 thereafter for maintenance."

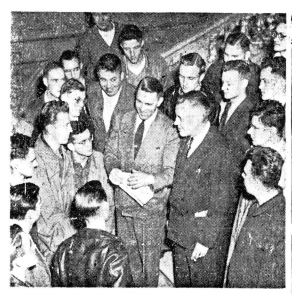

BOOSTS VETERINARY SCHOOL—Sens. Ancher Nelsen of Hutchinson, left, and Val Imm of Mankato on the steps to the Senate with Minnesota agricultural students boosting the veterinary school project before Senate finance committee approval Friday —PIONEER PRESS PHOTO.

PRIORITY ASSURED AGAIN—

Student Pleas Win Veterinary School Aid

By ALFRED D. STEDMAN

With Minnesota agricultural students flocking to its support at the Capitol, the project for a new veterinary school at University Farm won a critical round Friday in its long and hard fight for approval by the State Legislature.

The pleas of the Minnesota students, most of them GI's, for a chance to get a veterinary education got a definite and positive "yes" answer from the Senate finance committee.

After the students had hurried to the Senate in alarm over a report by this writer that the project had suffered a stinging defeat at the hands of a Senate finance subcommittee the day before, the entire finance committee voted to recommend priority along with other projects to a $600,000 appropriation to get the veterinary school

Earlier the students had given their own personal experience stories of how they had traveled hither and yon around the country to every one of the 11 existing veterinary colleges in the United States with appeals for admission, and how they had found these others full of resident students, had heard their own appeals turned down, and had been given no possibility of gaining admission anywhere until some time in the dim distant future.

The Senate finance committee adopted a motion by Sen. Val Imm of Mankato, chairman of the subcommittee in question, to give priority to the veterinary school project along

(Please Turn to Page 2, Col. 3)

with others in the 20-million-dollar construction program.

Sen. Imm presented the motion after Sen. Ancher Nelsen of Hutchinson, pressing his fight in the main committee for the veterinary project, declared it in his judgment "the most vital need in the state as far as agriculture is concerned."

At least 50 college students went to the Capitol or telephoned in behalf of the veterinary school project. Most impressive were their personal stories of futile efforts to get veterinary education while the state's 800 million dollar livestock industry is crying for veterinary service and the public is suffering from a spread of undulant fever because of the lack.

The fact was, however, that Sen. Imm's subcommittee earlier, instead of rejecting the $600,000 veterinary school project outright, as this writer had reported, had favored it but had not given it a place among the projects for which it had recommended priority. It was this desired priority which the entire Finance committee voted Friday afternoon.

WOUNDED VET SPEAKS

"I want a veterinary education so I can go into farm practice but can't get in anywhere," said Emmet Boyer, disabled veteran of Eveleth, injured by a buzz bomb at Mannheim, and whose height of 6

getting all the way in the Pioneer Press photograph.

"I tried to get into Colorado A&M college," said Glen Nelson, army veteran of Brainerd. "My wife and I got a place to live there. But the dean told me that 450 Colorado veterans were waiting for admission, that Colorado would have to take its first non-resident students from adjoining states, and that I might just as well give up trying to get in there for many years to come."

"I drove down to Ames," asserted Warner Christeson of Clinton, Minn., a war veteran and a farmer who wants to be a veterinarian and can't unless Minnesota provides a way.

"I tried Iowa state, too, and it didn't do any good," said Norman Fredrickson of Hanska.

TELLS OF NEED

"So did I and if I can't get a veterinary education at Minnesota I'll have to quit, because that's the one big thing that interests me," asserted Walter Mackey of Silver Lake, who has been three years preparing for such a course.

"I saw half the lamb crop and 25 per cent of the ewes lost on my uncle's farm near Duluth due to nodular disease, and no veterinarian could be had to help," declared Bruce Hohn of Duluth, sophomore at the college and an army veteran.

"And I went to Texas and Georgia and Alabama trying to get a veterinary course and not one of them would let in a non-resident. I traveled by train and spent quite a lot of money and time, but without results," related William Bowers of Gradstone.

"I saw my father's horses get sleeping sickness and one of them die when he couldn't get a veterinarian for four days," asserted Delvin Zinter of Minneapolis.

And so on down the line went the testimonials of attempts to get into Ohio State, Kansas A. C., Cornell, and other veterinary colleges without results.

From St. Paul Pioneer Press, April 12, 1947.

called a meeting of the veterinary staff and announced the organization and chain of command on the St. Paul Campus. All of the administrative units on the St. Paul Campus were placed under the Department of Agriculture with C. H. Bailey, Ph.D., as dean and director. Under Dean Bailey, Henry Schmitz, Ph.D., served as dean of the College of Agriculture, Forestry, Home Economics and Veterinary Medicine; W. L. Boyd, D.V.M., was appointed director of the School of Veterinary Medicine; and Harold Macy, Ph.D., was appointed director of the Agricultural Experiment Station.

President Morrill assured the veterinary staff his office would see to it the university met its obligation to students entering the college on September 29, 1947. As the meeting adjourned, President Morrill added, "We'll open in September if we have to begin in a tent." President Morrill kept his word. He and his office provided complete support in the opening of the School of Veterinary Medicine.

At the time the Veterinary Bill passed, the staff of the Division of Veterinary Medicine consisted of the following individuals

Dr. Willard L. Boyd, professor and chief
Dr. Martin H. Roepke, professor
Dr. Howard C. H. Kernkamp, professor
Dr. Benjamin D. Pomeroy, associate professor
Dr. Ruel Fenstermacher, associate professor
Dr. Alvin F. Sellers, instructor
Dr. John R. Collier, assistant veterinarian
Dr. Jay H. Sautter, research fellow
Dr. Donald E. Jasper, research fellow
Margaret K. Grady, laboratory technologist
Florence Jones, laboratory technologist
Fern B. Frost, laboratory technologist
Adelaide Holland, laboratory technologist[3]
Wilma T. Tomlinson, junior librarian
Rose M. Kenaley, secretary[4]
Loraine L. Peterson, clerk stenographer
Lawrence Jergenson, herdsman
William T. Kehr, assistant herdsman
Arden Ostergaard, assistant herdsman
Magdalene West, laboratory attendant

[3]   Staff member on loan from Bureau of Animal Industry

[4]   Rose Kenaley joined the staff as secretary in 1931 and remained for 30 years. She clipped newspaper articles about veterinary medicine over that period of time. These clippings were an important source of information in preparing this book.

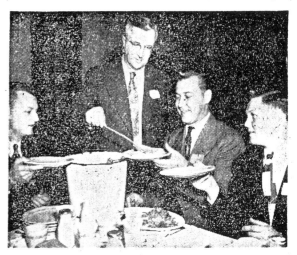

PROFESSOR BECOMES CHEF — Dr. Reuel Fenstermacher, ladle in hand, dishes food he cooked for the University veterinary dinner Monday night in the Farm Union. Students waiting their turn are, left to right, Bruce Hohn, 1614 Hewitt ave., St. Paul; Glen Nelson, Brainerd; Paul Cox, 908 Vista ave., St. Paul.

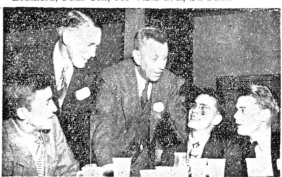

NEW STUDENTS MEET SPONSORS—Dinner in appreciation for new University veterinary school founding finds new students meeting guests. Left to right are, Con Russell, Stillwater; Sen. Ancher Nelson; J. S. Jones, secretary of Minnesota Farm Bureau; Paul Bailey, Marshall; Robert Bakke, Minneapolis.

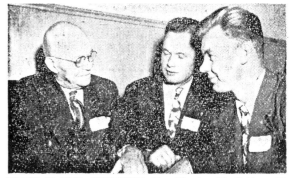

FIRST U VET STUDENT—Dr. Charles E. Cotton, 79 years old, of Minneapolis, tells new students, John E. Fogarty, Belle Plain, and Stanley Jepson, Renville, about veterinary study in 1888-89.

From St. Paul Pioneer Press, September 30, 1947.

In midsummer, two graduate students, Dr. Ralph L. Kitchell and Dr. Francis A. Spurrell, were added to the staff.

The Division of Veterinary Medicine's total budget for the 1946-1947 fiscal year was $66,273, which reflected $59,477 for salaries and $6,796 for supplies, expenses, and equipment. Twenty-four students were admitted in the first class. The beginning curriculum and instructors included, respectively:

Gross Anatomy was taught by Instructors H. C. H. Kernkamp, Ralph L. Kitchell, and Francis A. Spurrell;

Microscopic Anatomy and Embryology were taught by Instructors Ralph L. Kitchell and Jay H. Sautter;

Bacteriology was taught by M. H. Roepke and B. S. Pomeroy; and

Physiological Chemistry was taught by Instructor David Glick of the Medical School.

To ease the immediate space and equipment concerns, Physiological Chemistry was taught in the Medical School, and the Genetics and Nutrition courses were taught in the College of Agriculture. Three rooms in Old Anatomy were remodeled as classrooms and labs to teach Gross Anatomy and Microscopic Anatomy and Embryology. Additionally, the library in the building was enlarged. The Department of Buildings and Grounds on the St. Paul Campus responded to the challenge and, in the short time available, the building was essentially ready by the start of the first class on September 29, 1947.

While Old Anatomy was remodeled, the academic and Civil Service staff were busy preparing teaching aids for the first class. Drs. Kernkamp, Sautter, Kitchell, and Spurrell, with assistance from the Civil Service staff, worked feverishly to get these items ready for the first class. There was a pressing need for 50 sets of slides for the Microscopic Anatomy and Embryology course. Bone sets were needed to teach the Gross Anatomy course.[5/] Frantic calls were made to other departments in the university to obtain microscopes for the opening day of classes. Many of these microscopes came from storage rooms and were of ancient vintage.

Dr. Willard Boyd's leadership played an important role in the preparation for the first class. He was a source of encouragement and help to the staff in their efforts to prepare for the opening of the school. Through his good relations with members of other departments of the University, Dr. Boyd obtained their cooperation in teaching some of the courses, and thus eased some of the strain and stress on the veterinary staff.

FIRST CLASS ENTERS SCHOOL OF VETERINARY MEDICINE

September 29, 1947, was "blast off day" for teaching the art and science of veterinary medicine at the professional level at the University of Minnesota. On the morning of that date, 24 young men, armed with notebooks and pencils, were formally inducted into the study program that would prepare them for careers in veterinary medicine. The members of the first class included Archibald Alexander, Minneapolis; Wesley Anderson, Aneta, North Dakota; Robert Bossing, Minneapolis; Goodwin Branstad, Grantsburg, Wisconsin; John Busch, Morris; Paul Cox, St. Paul; Vern Dahl, Arlington; John Fogarty, Belle Plaine; William Gladisch, Gaylord; Donald Hicks, Tracy; Bruce Hohn, St. Paul; Robert Leary, New Ulm; Paul Lundgren, Minneapolis; Walter Mackey, Cokato; Glen Nelson, Brainerd; Vern Olson, South Haven; Kenneth Palmer, Forest Lake; Robert Pyle, Minneapolis; Lester Redder, Canby; Conway Rosell, Stillwater; Ithel Schipper, Wayzata; David Stanley, Breckenridge; and James Stewart, Minneapolis. Twenty of these men were World War II veterans. Only six members of this class had been members of the Pre-Vet Club. Other members of the Pre-Vet Club were accepted in later classes.

[5/] Horse bones were obtained from a horse slaughtering plant; cattle bones from a packing plant; and dog bones from a dog pound. The bones were cleaned of flesh by cooking them in two 55-gallon drums. The drums were set up west of the Round Room (part of the Old Anatomy Building) and heated by steam that ran from steam lines in the Round Room. The hoses were immersed in the water in the drums, and sodium hydroxide was added to assist the process. The bones were placed in baskets and immersed in the drums. After the initial cooking, the bones were removed from the hot water and cleaned as much as possible. Then the bones were cooked again. This process was repeated until there was no soft tissue left on the bones. The last step of this process was to whiten the bones by placing them in chlorine solution.

When the school opened, experienced veterinary teachers were in short supply. There had been limited training during World War II. Additionally, several new veterinary colleges were starting and there was great competition for the few available experienced teachers. The School of Veterinary Medicine at the University of Minnesota had not received additional funds to enter the market and compete for the experienced teachers.

The administration on the St. Paul Campus decided that a limited number of experienced staff would be hired to teach in areas in which the present staff were not qualified to teach. Drs. Henry Griffiths and Allen Hemingway were experienced teachers who were hired by the university to join the faculty. Dr. Griffiths had taught parasitology at several veterinary colleges and Dr. Hemingway had taught physiology in the Medical School at the university. Dr. John Campbell, a successful practitioner in Fairmont, Minnesota, was hired to develop and direct the veterinary teaching hospital. Dr. Robert Merrill, a well-known practitioner in Clara City, Minnesota, was later hired to develop the ambulatory clinic.

However, the administration on the St. Paul Campus believed teachers they trained would be as good, if not better, than any outside staff they could hire. They also believed this approach provided a better opportunity to evaluate prospective staff members to determine if they would blend well with the other staff members. Finally, graduate students received far less salary than an experienced teacher. Thus, long term staff needs were intended to be filled from the ranks of the university's graduate students.

The new School of Veterinary Medicine wished to accept patients to develop teaching material for the students in the clinical stage of the curriculum. However, there was no suitable space available for handling and keeping clinical cases. The new veterinary clinic was eventually completed in 1950. In the meantime, clinics were held in three barns for research animals located across the street from the Old Anatomy Building. The hospitalized dog cases were kept in cages along with horses in "Unit I." Cattle were housed in "Unit II" with the overflow going into the main barn, "Unit III." Surgery was performed in the Round Room of Old Anatomy.

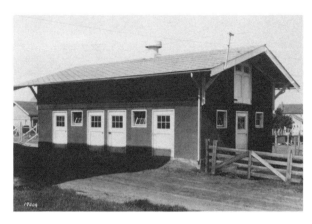

Unit I, Unit II was similar in design, except for the location of the doors. Courtesy University of Minnesota Archives.

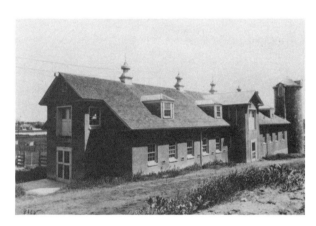

Unit III

TEACHING STAFF AND PROGRAM, FALL QUARTER 1950

The first class entered their senior year in the Fall Quarter of 1950. Exhibit V-1 lists the academic and Civil Service staff that had been assembled by that time to teach the four year curriculum.

EXHIBIT V-1

SCHOOL OF VETERINARY MEDICINE STAFF, FALL 1950

Willard L. Boyd	Professor and Chief
John N. Campbell	Professor
Ruel Fenstermacher	Professor
Allen Hemingway	Professor
H. C. H. Kernkamp	Professor
Benjamin S. Pomeroy	Professor
Martin H. Roepke	Professor
Henry J. Griffiths	Associate Professor

(Exhibit V-i Continued)

Robert A. Merrill	Associate Professor
Jay H. Sautter	Associate Professor
Alvin F. Sellers	Associate Professor
Alvin F. Weber	Assistant Professor
John P. Arnold	Instructor
David E. Bartlett	Instructor
Reid B. England	Instructor
Thomas M. Christison	Instructor
Jean C. Flint	Instructor
William J. Hadlow	Instructor
John F. Henry, Jr.	Instructor
Harvey H. Hoyt	Instructor
Ralph L. Kitchell	Instructor
Donald G. Low	Instructor
William A. Malmquist	Instructor
George W. Mather	Instructor
Jack E. Moulton	Instructor
Thomas E. O'Dell	Instructor
William R. Pritchard	Instructor
Clarence M. Stowe	Instructor
Calvin C. Turbes	Instructor
James E. Williams	Research Fellow
Ambrose Lein	Principle Clerk
Rose M. Kenaley	Secretary
Dorthea Brightman	Secretary
Donna M. Klett	Clerk-Typist
Mary Baker	Junior Librarian
Fern Frost	Laboratory Technologist
Toby Lea Gitis	Laboratory Technologist
Margaret Grady	Laboratory Technologist
Wilma C. Hayes	Laboratory Technologist
Florence Jones	Laboratory Technologist
Mary Grace Phillips	Laboratory Technologist
Agnes M. Opstad	Laboratory Technologist
Remi J. Brooke	Laboratory Technician
Judith Leah Shapiro	Laboratory Technician
Melvin E. Nelson	Senior Laboratory Attendant
Kenji Horita	Principal Laboratory Attendant
Arden Ostergaard	Principal Laboratory Attendant
Verner A. Severson	Principal Laboratory Attendant
Thomas Van Koersel	Laboratory Attendant
William T. Kehr	Herdsman
Millard Jensen	Assistant Herdsman[a]

[a] a/Many of the Civil Service personnel did not assist in the teaching program but instead limited their work to research projects. The staff of other departments that taught courses to the veterinary students are not listed above.

Among the senior staff members, Dr. Boyd focused on administration and planning, Dr. Campbell developed the teaching hospital, Dr. Fenstermacher was in charge of the Diagnosis Laboratory, Dr. Merrill provided full time supervision of the ambulatory clinic, and Dr. Roepke, a biochemist, served as the school's secretary, administered the graduate program, and oversaw many of the research projects. Because these staff members had little time to devote to teaching, Drs. Griffiths, Hemingway, Kernkamp, Pomeroy, and Weber, and later Drs. Sautter and Sellers, were the senior staff who had the most extensive involvement in the four year teaching program. Only two members of the senior staff, Drs. Griffiths and Hemingway, and one graduate student, John Arnold, had previous experience teaching professional level veterinary courses. However, most of the graduate students who taught in the college were recent graduates who were familiar with the content of the veterinary courses in the 1940s.

The veterinary staff made up for their lack of experience with enthusiasm and hard work. The graduate students took many of their courses on the Minneapolis Campus. This often caused difficulties in meeting class schedules. Graduate students rushed from teaching a class on the St. Paul Campus to catch the intercampus street car that took them to a class on the Minneapolis Campus. At the completion of the class on the Minneapolis Campus, these students would have to scurry back to the St. Paul Campus to teach another class. Graduate students found it difficult to keep ahead of the veterinary students with lecture preparation, and some graduate students were accused of lecturing from the notes they had taken in their course at the Medical School.

In this early period, the academic and Civil Service staff were a small, closely knit group. They became well acquainted with each other, knew where each other worked or officed, and were aware of each other's duties and how each other was doing. Everyone also knew who was taking graduate work and what courses they were taking. Everybody knew of the ongoing research projects and the progress of those projects. If a person needed help, others in this community tried to assist him. This collegial and encouraging environment was due to Dr. Boyd, who was a kind and outgoing person. He wanted the staff to be like a large family, and he took great pains to

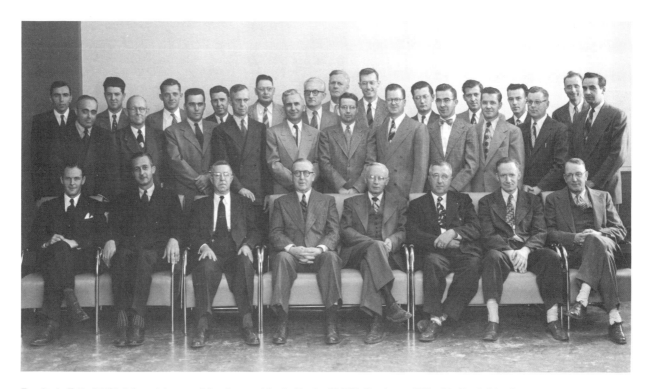

Faculty in Fall of 1950, left to right; seated, Jay Sautter, Martin Roepke, H.C.H. Kernkamp, Willard L. Boyd, John Campbell, Ruel Fenstermacher, B.S. Pomeroy, Robert Merrill, standing, Peter Obstopochek, George Mather, John Henry, Jean Flint, Paul Hammond, Francis Spurrell, Reid England, Allan Hemmingway, David Bartlett, Thomas Christison, Alex Korsunsky, Ted Setterquist, Henry Griffiths, Richard Brown, Ralph Kitchell, Clarence M. Stowe, Thomas O'Dell, Harvey Hoyt, James Williams, Donald Low, Winston Malmquist, Alvin sellers, William Hess.

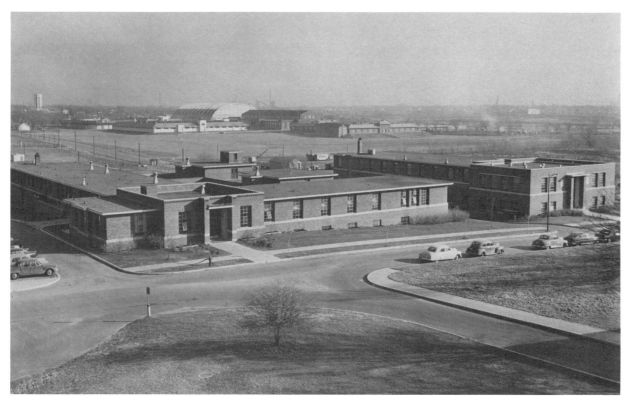

New Veterinary Clinic, dedicated in 1950. Courtesy University of Minnesota Archives.

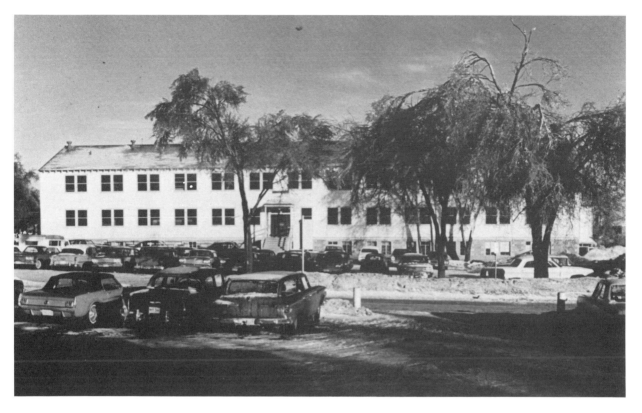

TEH (Temporary East of Haecker) World War II Army Barrack Building moved in to provide teaching facilities for second year students.

avoid hurting any person's feelings and to make everybody feel wanted.

DEDICATION OF THE VETERINARY CLINIC

On October 25, 1950, the new Veterinary Clinic was dedicated in an impressive ceremony held in Coffey Hall Auditorium. President of the university James Morrill presided, Vice President Malcom Willey made the dedication, and President Emeritus Walter Coffey gave the invocation. The featured speaker was Dr. W. A. Hagen, dean of the New York State Veterinary College at Cornell University. His presentation was entitled, "Veterinary Medical Education — Its Evolution and Its Present Status."

Following the dedication, an open house was held at the new Veterinary Clinic. Staff members were present to guide visitors through the facilities and displays of equipment. When Dr. Hagen arrived a day before the dedication, he was given a V.I.P. tour of the veterinary facilities. (In such tours, the good points were emphasized and the poorer areas were bypassed.) Later that evening, Dr. Hagen returned to the Veterinary Clinic alone and gained admittance. He went through every drawer and cabinet in the clinic. Dr. Hagen looked at every piece of equipment and all of the supplies the new veterinary school

had acquired for the clinic. There is little doubt Dr. Hagen relayed his findings to the members of the AVMA Council on Education who, as the accrediting body, were scheduled to inspect the new school in a few months.

The new Veterinary Clinic consisted of two floors and was built on the side of a hill. The upper-street level floor housed the Small Animal Clinic, the director's office, a business office, staff offices, clinical laboratory, and a classroom. The building also contained sleeping rooms for students assigned to after-hours duty. The lower floor of the new building contained the Large Animal Clinic, staff offices, a conference room, a drug and supply room, a garage, and a research room. The building also contained student and staff locker rooms for men. No locker rooms or other facilities then existed for women students or staff.

As director of the clinic, Dr. Campbell supervised the clinical teaching program. He assigned the teaching duties to clinical staff and managed the clinic's business operation. Dr. Campbell delegated the supervision of the daily operations of the Small Animal Clinic to Dr. Mather. Drs. Pritchard, Hoyt, and Arnold served at different times in the same capacity in the large animal clinic. Dr. Robert Merrill operated the

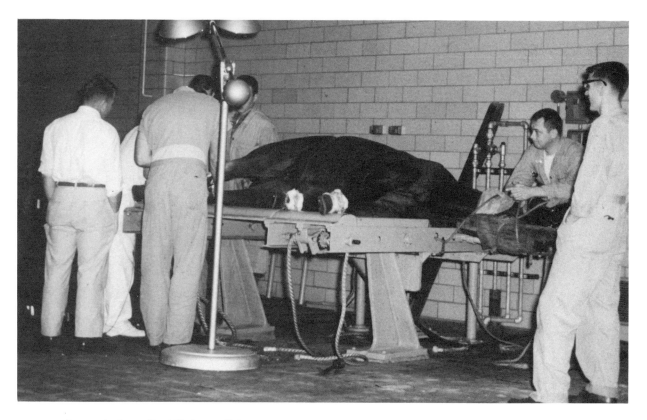

Large animal operating table in new clinic.

ambulatory clinic under the supervision of Dr. Campbell.

Much of the equipment in the School of Veterinary Medicine was World War II surplus that had been stored in a large warehouse at the Rosemount Experiment Station. Practically all the chairs, desks, tables, and lockers in the Temporary East of Haecker (T.E.H.) and the Veterinary Clinic were war surplus painted in the army olive-drab color. Most of the other supplies at the new school were also war surplus painted in the same olive-drab color. Students were furnished with army surplus coveralls, boots, and Turkish towels.

The clinic was essentially closed on Saturdays and Sundays. No classes were scheduled on Saturdays and, although they were officially responsible for the care of their hospitalized patients on weekends, senior students were frequently excused from these duties by senior staff members. One staff member was regularly assigned to weekend duty for the Small Animal Clinic and one was assigned for the Large Animal Clinic. They were usually not notified a student had been excused, and when students did not show up before noon the staff member would have to care for the patient. In addition, staff members had to answer the telephone on the weekend. The staff member on large animal duty

also had to take the weekend ambulatory calls.

During the school year, students were assigned to the pharmacies as part of the rotation system. Dr. Stowe and Dr. Hammond of the pharmacology staff were alternately assigned to supervise the students in the pharmacy where solutions were prepared and drug mixtures were compounded. The students also cleaned instruments, prepared and sterilized surgical packs, and sterilized solutions.

When the school started no particular staff member was designated as surgeon in the Small Animal Clinic. However, Drs. Mather and England generally performed the more difficult procedures. In the Large Animal Clinic, Drs. Pritchard, Hoyt, and Low were assigned the medical cases, Dr. Arnold was responsible for the surgical cases, and Drs. Bartlett and Spurrell were assigned the obstetrical cases. Dr. Spurrell also served as radiologist for both clinics.

Students were not required to take clinics during the summer months. However, the clinics could not afford to operate only nine months a year without losing clients. Thus, the clinic was open as usual throughout the summer vacation months. There were problems in staffing the clinics over the summer because staff members took vacations and graduate courses during those months. In the Small Animal Clinic, the diversity

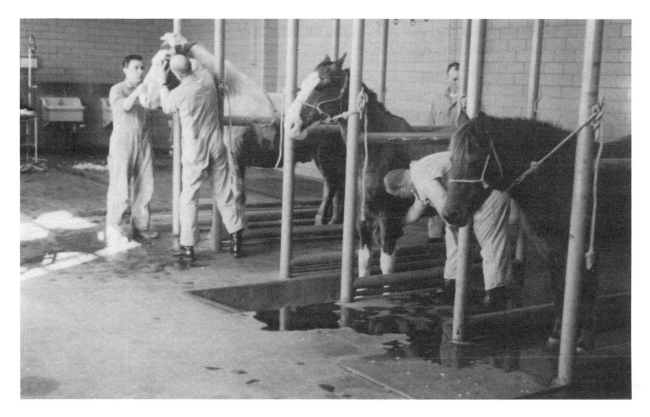

Horse stocks built for draft horses in new clinic, casting mat in background.

of the staff minimized the scope of these problems. In comparison, there were only two clinicians assigned to handle the Large Animal Clinic. Drs. Hoyt and Arnold both had to work mornings, and they would alternate taking their vacation time during the afternoons. Because of patient commitments, they often were not able to leave the clinic until after 2:00 p.m. in the afternoon of their vacation day.

The new Veterinary Clinic Building was designed by architects who were not familiar with the needs and uses of an animal clinic. For example, the design did not include ventilation capable of providing intake of fresh air for animals or for the removal of urine and fecal odors. The air in the small animal cage rooms was always stale, and odors would linger in the hallways. In the Small Animal Clinic, the doorway provided the only ventilation for the drug and supply room located at the foot of the stairs. The situation was unbearable during the summer, thus making the room a poor place to store drugs. The cattle ward was difficult to walk through in the morning because of the odors. Some years later, staff members discovered the ventilation fan for the area was running backwards. But even after this error was corrected, the ward was still an extremely uncomfortable place to work.

Animals had difficulty walking in the large animal treatment area and halls. The surface was smooth and hard, and animals could not get traction on the floor. The conditions were made even worse when the floor was wet. Horses would fall on their knees, strike their mouth on the floor, and often break off their front teeth. Cattle would lose control of their hind legs and "spraddle" on the floor. These incidents were difficult to explain to the owners of the injured animals. The floor was covered with the same type of surface used in packing plants. However, designers did not recognize that animals do not walk on the floors in packing plants. They are placed in chutes or hung on tracks. Workers who walk on the floor in packing plans wear rubber boots. The administration finally recognized the problem and spent $1,500 to paint a rubber surface on the floor. Unfortunately, the rubber coating would wash off when the floors were cleaned. Eventually, a machine with chain flails was used to beat the floor and roughen the surface.

When weather permitted, restraining horses and cattle in a recumbent position, or "casting," was done on the grass in the courtyard. During the winter months or in inclement weather, the animals were placed on a large animal operating table. A tanbark casting area later was constructed. The area consisted of a ring approx-

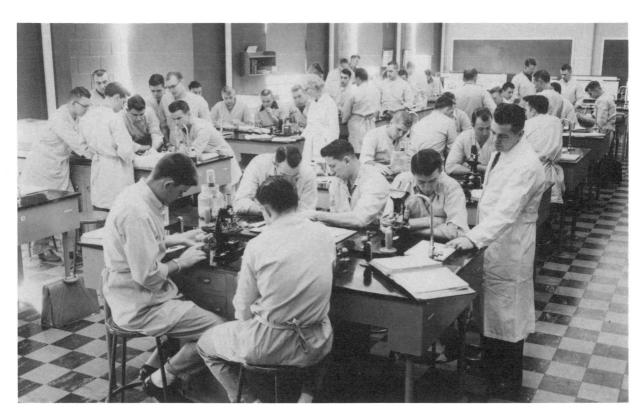

Bacteriology Laboratory.

imately 20 feet in diameter with sandbags around the outer edge. The inside of the ring was covered with an 8-inch layer of tanbark that made a soft landing for the animal. Although an attempt was made to keep the tanbark damp, the animal that was being "cast" or thrown on the tanbark would usually stir up a cloud of dust. The dust would cover both the animal and the persons doing the casting. This arrangement was not very conductive to antiseptic surgery.

Eventually, the Goodrich Tire Company, which had recognized the commercial demand for a rubber padded casting mat, installed the first mat of this kind at the School of Veterinary Medicine. Goodrich sent several high ranking company officials to supervise the installation. These representatives strutted around in their white shirts giving directions for the installation of the mat. At noon, when the company officials left to have lunch with senior staff, the Goodrich employee who came with them to install the mat went to work. During the morning, "Joe" had appeared to comply with their orders and suggestions but had actually done nothing of substance. As soon as they left for lunch, he sprang into action and had the mat installed by the time his "superiors" had returned. The high-ranking company representatives, who believed "Joe" had followed their instructions, were very pleased with the installation.

The X-ray equipment installed in the new clinic was considered the most powerful in any veterinary college in the country. The reputation of the power of the X-ray machine is reflected in an incident involving J. C. Penney, founder of J. C. Penney Co. Mr. Penney had a farm in Missouri where he kept a show herd of Aberdeen Angus cattle. He was particularly proud of his prize winning bull. However, one of Penney's competitors accused the Penny farm of tampering with this bull in order to win in a show and inferred the handlers had injected a "filler" under the skin to fill a defect on the back of the bull.[6] Penney, who was incensed by the accusation, was told a radiograph would demonstrate whether an injection had been made and that the only machine capable of radiographing the back of his bull was at the University of Minnesota. He immediately ordered his herdsman to load the bull in a trailer and take it to the School of Veterinary Medicine. The radiographs showed no evidence of any oil or other foreign substance in the subcutaneous tissue. Having vindicated Mr. Penney, the happy but tired herdsman returned to Missouri with the bull.

[6]   Some animals with otherwise good conformation would have depressions along the spine in the back. Unscrupulous showmen would inject a filler under the skin, usually mineral oil, to make the back level and look smooth.

ACCREDITATION

Students must graduate from an accredited veterinary school or college to qualify to sit for state licensing examinations. The Council on Education of the American Veterinary Medical Association periodically visits institutions to determine whether they meet the standards for accreditation. They report their findings and make a recommendation to the Executive Board of the American Veterinary Medical Association. That board ultimately decides whether an institution will be accredited and, if accredited, whether it will receive full or probationary accreditation.

One of the major challenges faced by the School of Veterinary Medicine was to become accredited. Members of the Council on Education scheduled their initial inspection on March 1 and 2, 1951, in order that, if accreditation was granted, the school's first graduates would be able to sit for state licensing examinations. The Council members made a thorough inspection of the physical plant, including laboratories, clinics, and equipment, and reviewed teaching aids and the library. They interviewed staff members at all levels and conferred with President Morrill and other administrative officials of the university.

The council placed the School of Veterinary Medicine on public probation, which is the lowest level of probationary accreditation. Public probation meant the school had one or more major deficiencies. The council's primary criticism was the school "was not a major administrative unit in the University but was subordinate to the Dean of the Department of Agriculture." The Executive Board of the AVMA supported the council's criticism in this regard by voting to withdraw public probation in April 1952 unless substantial changes in the college's administration did not occur.

The debate was eventually taken to the meeting of the AVMA House of Delegates where there was disagreement over AVMA's "essentials of an acceptable veterinary college." The relevant AVMA provision read as follows:

A school or college of veterinary medicine should find its most advantageous environment if it is a part of an accredited institution of higher learning. In the best interests of both the institution and the veterinary medical school, the latter requires the same recognition and autonomy as other professional schools. A veterinary medical school may be fully accredited only when it is operated as a major administrative division of the parent institution and under the direction of a dean who is a veterinarian.

The majority of the members of the Council on Education and Executive Board believed the position of the School of Veterinary Medicine in the University of Minnesota did not meet the criteria set forth by the AVMA. After debate, the House of Delegates voted to support the action taken by the council and the board by requiring the administrative head of Minnesota's School of Veterinary Medicine to be directly responsible to the president of the university.

In contrast, the university believed there was precedent for maintaining the School of Veterinary Medicine within the College of Agriculture, Forestry, and Home Economics. After all, the Schools of Nursing and Public Health were academic units within the Medical School, and each was headed by a director while the Medical School was headed by a dean. This same structure applied to the School of Journalism, which was a smaller unit within the College of Science, Literature, and Arts. The academic units of Forestry and Home Economics in the College of Agriculture had become schools and were headed by the dean of the College of Agriculture. Thus, the fact the School of Veterinary Medicine was headed by a director who was a veterinarian and reported to the dean of the College of Agriculture was consistent with the manner in which other units in the university were designed and administered.[7]

ADMINISTRATIVE CHANGES

Dr. Willard L. Boyd retired as director of the School of Veterinary Medicine on June 30, 1952, approximately three months before his 68th birthday. His long service to the university was unusual as the university regulations required staff in administrative positions to "step down" at age 65. Because the school was in a critical stage of development and no successor had been found, the Board of Regents approved a request that Dr. Boyd remain in the post. Dr. Boyd agreed to remain until he reached age 68. However, Dr. Boyd decided to retire just prior to that time as he was president-elect of the American Veterinary Medical Association and would become president

[7] President Morrill was also concerned that, if the School of Veterinary Medicine became a college, the Schools of Forestry and Home Economics would demand that they, too, be elevated to the college status.

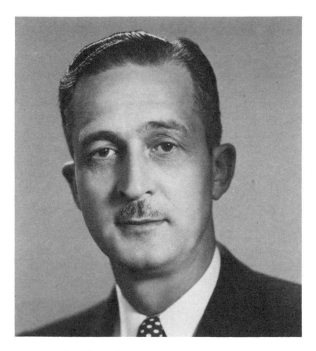

Dr. Martin Roepke.

in August 1952. Dr. Boyd wished to have sufficient time to attend the various meetings and events that were the function of the office.

DR. MARTIN ROEPKE APPOINTED ACTING DIRECTOR

When Dr. Boyd retired, Dr. Martin Roepke, a biochemist, was appointed to serve as acting director of the School of Veterinary Medicine. He was familiar with the way the school had been operated as he had previously served as the school's secretary and had administered most of the graduate and research programs of the school. However, Dr. Roepke did not have a veterinary degree and the Council on Education of the American Veterinary Medical Association looked upon his appointment as an act of defiance by the university. The veterinary profession was further irritated by the fact the search committee appointed by Dean Bailey to recommend candidates to become the new director did not include any veterinarians. The absence of veterinarians on the committee prompted Dr. Carl Schlotthauer of the Mayo Clinic, father of Drs. John and Charles Schlotthauer, to write to Dr. C. W. Mayo of the Mayo Clinic who was a member of the Board of Regents. As the result of this letter, Drs. Harvey Hoyt and George Mather, members of the school's staff, were added to the search committee.

DEAN BAILEY RETIRES

Dr. Bailey, Dean of the College of Agriculture, Forestry, Home Economics, and Veterinary Medicine, retired on December 31, 1952. He was famous world-wide as a cereal chemist and had received many honors for his contributions to the cereal industry. However, as an administrator, Dean Bailey was interested in detail and, based on a review of his written communications, seemed more concerned with spelling and punctuation than the substance of the message. His attention to detail was described as clouding his vision in the development of the St. Paul Campus. Dean Bailey desired to impress the university administration and the legislature with the efficient and economical operation of the St. Paul Campus. Dean Bailey was not regarded as a friend of veterinary medicine. He lacked an understanding of the manner in which veterinary medicine should be taught at the professional level. He did not seem to understand graduates must pass an examination to become licensed to practice, and he resented the involvement of an outside agency such as the Council on Education that established requirements to accredit a school of veterinary medicine.

Dean Bailey's resignation was preceded by the resignation of Dean Henry Schmitz. Dean Schmitz was the "other dean" on the St. Paul Campus who reported directly to Dean Bailey. The resignation of both deans gave President Morrill the opportunity to revamp the administration on the St. Paul Campus. He promptly reported the resignations to the Council on Education of the American Veterinary Medical Association. He also informed the council that the name of the Department of Agriculture would be changed to the "Institute of Agriculture." The Council on Education hoped these changes would also include an administrative restructuring so the head of the School of Veterinary Medicine would report directly to the President of the University and thus remove the last major obstacle to full accreditation.

The St. Paul Campus administration was eventually reorganized as follows:

Harold Macy, dean of the Institute of Agriculture

R. J. Sloan, director of Agricultural Experiment Station

A. A. Dowell, director of Resident Instruction

Paul E. Miller, director of Agricultural Extension

T. M. Fenske, assistant to dean of institute and assistant dean in charge of School of Veterinary Medicine

The administration hoped the Council on Education would determine these changes met the AVMA's criteria on administration. Although the council regarded the reorganization as a move in the right direction, the university still did not meet the AVMA's requirements.

DEAN MACY MOVES TO SAVE THE SCHOOL OF VETERINARY MEDICINE

One of the major problems Dr. Macy inherited when he became dean of the Institute of Agriculture was the School of Veterinary Medicine. Little progress had been made in the effort to find a replacement for Dr. Boyd. Dr. Roepke, as a nonveterinarian, had received little support as the acting director from the veterinary profession in Minnesota. The school was, of course, having problems receiving accreditation by the AVMA. Students were concerned they would not be able to take licensing examinations. Younger staff members worried the school would fail. These problems and this apprehension lowered morale of the student body and faculty alike.

The administration made little effort to retain the graduate students on the faculty after they finished their degrees. Junior staff members came to believe the administration had decided many of the professional courses could be taught entirely by graduate students. This situation, combined with the university's apparent lack of effort to correct the accreditation situation and the fact the school was headed by a nonveterinarian, greatly frustrated the junior staff. New veterinary schools throughout the country soon realized that the University of Minnesota was a fertile ground for staff recruitment.

Dean Henry Schmitz, second in command on the St. Paul Campus, recognized the problem and tried to prevent the departure of junior staff members. He called individuals to his office and promised that things were bound to improve under Dean Macy. These staff members wondered how much credence to give Dean

Schmitz's predictions since he had submitted his resignation and would not be present to help improve the school in the future.

Soon after taking office, Dean Macy met with some of the junior faculty who had received offers from other veterinary schools. Sitting at his desk, he looked the young staff members in the eye and promised to stake his reputation as dean on making the School of Veterinary Medicine one of the best schools in the country. Dean Macy was taken at his word and the young staff members turned down the offers to teach at other institutions.

KERNKAMP APPOINTED ACTING ASSISTANT DEAN

In June 1953, Dr. Roepke requested to be relieved of his duties as acting director. Dr. Roepke was an important member of the staff and an exceptional research worker. Unfortunately, as a nonveterinarian, he had been placed in an untenable position as acting director.

Dr. H. C. H. Kernkamp was appointed acting assistant dean of the School of Veterinary Medicine in June 1953. Dean Macy also appointed an administrative committee made up of Drs. Ralph L. Kitchell and William R. Pritchard to assist Dr. Kernkamp. When Dr. Pritchard left the university, Dr. Harvey H. Hoyt took his place on the administrative committee.

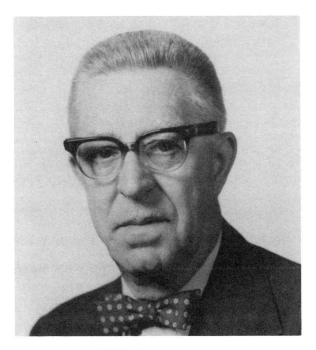

Dr. H.C.H. Kernkamp.

Dean Macy asked the staff of the School of Veterinary Medicine to propose a table of organization. At the time, the school was informally organized along discipline lines with a staff member designated with responsibility for each discipline. These included veterinary anatomy; veterinary physiology; veterinary pathology; veterinary parasitology; veterinary bacteriology; and veterinary medicine, which included all of the clinical areas that made up roughly the last two years of the curriculum. Pharmacology and physiological chemistry were taught in the Medical School.

In response to Dean Macy's request, the staff developed the following divisions in the table of organization:

Veterinary Anatomy, headed by Dr. Ralph L. Kitchell

Veterinary Physiology and Pharmacology, headed by Dr. Alvin F. Sellers

Veterinary Pathology and Parasitology, headed by Dr. Jay Sautter

Veterinary Bacteriology, headed by Dr. B. S. Pomeroy

Veterinary Obstetrics, vacant

Veterinary Medicine and Clinics, headed by Dr. John N. Campbell

Veterinary Surgery and Radiology, headed by Dr. John P. Arnold

The table of organization was approved and the persons listed as heads were appointed to their respective positions.[8]

DR. THORP BECOMES DIRECTOR

Dean Macy intensified the search for a successor to Dr. Boyd. The entire faculty had the opportunity to propose and interview candidates. This process was in stark contrast with the previous search for a director conducted by Dean Bailey where there was little contact between the faculty and the candidates. Dr. W. T. S. Thorp, who was one of the last candidates to visit the campus, was eventually selected and appointed assistant dean and director of the School of Veterinary Medicine effective July 1, 1954.

[8]   Graduate students were appointed "acting heads."

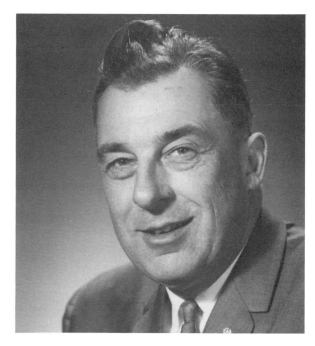

Dr. W.T.S. Thorp. Courtesy University of Minnesota Archives.

Dr. Thorp was born in Edmonton, Canada, on April 4, 1914. He received his D.V.M in 1935 and his M.S. in 1937 from Michigan State University. He had served on the faculty of Pennsylvania State University until he joined the staff of the National Institutes of Health in 1948. At the time of his appointment at Minnesota, Dr. Thorp was chief of the section on comparative pathology and hematology, and was commissioned Veterinary Director of the National Institutes of Health, U.S. Public Health Service, in Bethesda, Maryland. His rank at the institute was equivalent to that of colonel in the U.S. Army.

Dr. Thorp's first challenge was to resolve the school's problems with accreditation. Members of the AVMA Council on Education had visited the School of Veterinary Medicine on April 5-7, 1954. The council's report, which was sent to the university on June 2, 1954, stated the deficiencies identified therein had to be corrected by May 1955 or public probation would be withdrawn.

Notwithstanding improvements that had been made, the council's report contained strong criticism of the school's administrative organization. The report also identified the following deficiencies: meat and milk hygiene courses were the weakest of any veterinary school; the Ambulatory Clinic did not have enough cases and provided no

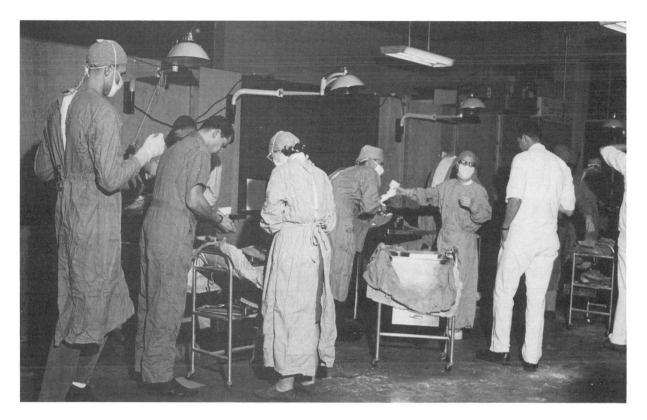

Small Animal Surgery Laboratory.

service on Saturdays and Sundays; the school needed more staff; the director of clinics should be more involved in teaching; and the report questioned the Department of Veterinary Science.

The visiting team was quite displeased with the progress made by the School of Veterinary Medicine since the 1951 accreditation inspection. One of the members expressed privately, "Minnesota started with the best nucleus of a faculty of any of the new schools and has made the least progress."

Many staff members believed at least some of the criticism was due to the failure of the visiting inspection team to obtain sufficient input from the faculty. Some of the faculty members were not available for interviews by the members of the council. This, of course, did not help the school's cause as some of the inspection team regarded their absence as a snub.

Dr. Thorp wasted no time in getting to work on correcting the deficiencies and criticism of the Council on Education. In an October 4, 1954, letter to Dr. R. A. Rabrassier, chairman of the council, Dr. Thorp promised to make the following changes effective July 1, 1955:

1. Department of Veterinary Science would be eliminated;

2. Division of Veterinary Diagnostic Laboratories would be established with Dr. Fenstermacher as head, and Dr. Donald Barnes would be added to the division's staff;

3. Division of Veterinary Bacteriology would be renamed Division of Veterinary Bacteriology and Public Health;

4. Dr. Henry Griffiths would be appointed assistant director of School of Veterinary Medicine and professor of parasitology;

5. The school would hire four additional staff members; and

6. The school's facilities would expand, including appropriations of $8,000 to replace small animal cages and $6,000,000 for an addition to Veterinary Science Building.

Dr. Thorp went to the Minnesota legislature to obtain funds for more buildings and facilities. When funds were initially appropriated to construct the original Veterinary Science Building, a member of the university's administration had stated that "this (appropriation) would more or less finish the major building programs of the School." Dr. Thorp began a campaign to overcome this statement and to make known the needs of the school to the legislators and the people of Minnesota. He contacted members of the legislature and university administration, and he spoke to farm organizations, commercial clubs, members of the veterinary profession, the general public, and the media throughout the state. He revealed that the School of Veterinary Medicine had the poorest research facilities of any school in the country. At the annual meeting of the Minnesota Veterinary Medical Association in February 1957, Dr. Thorp informed members the school needed $3,000,000 to $3,500,000 to provide the necessary teaching, research and service buildings.

Dr. Thorp's efforts to obtain more buildings, facilities, and staff for the School of Veterinary Medicine received the full support of Dean Macy and President Morrill. Once the school was created, President Morrill was committed to making it a success. When Dr. Thorp requested more support for the School of Veterinary Medicine, President Morrill was very helpful and recommended all of these requests to the Board of Regents.

Dr. Thorp's efforts were aided by many people including legislators such as Senator John Olson and Representative Delbert Anderson. In 1957, the legislature appropriated $600,000 for a Diagnostic Laboratory (which was completed in 1960) and an additional $600,000 for the first addition to the Veterinary Science Building (which was completed in 1958). In 1961, the legislature appropriated $616,000 to build another addition to the Veterinary Clinic Building. This appropriation was matched by $500,000 from Title I funds. In 1967, the legislature appropriated $720,000 to add the Diagnostic and Research Laboratory to the Diagnostic Laboratory. In 1967, the legislature appropriated $171,000 for Phase I planning of a building that would be shared by Animal Husbandry and Veterinary Medicine, and $522,182 to cover a deficiency in the funds for the addition to the Veterinary Clinic. In 1971, $121,000 was appropriated to develop construction plans for an addition to the Veterinary Clinic (Phase II). Finally, the legislature appropriated $10,000,000 for the construction of the Phase I Building.

SCHOOL OF VETERINARY MEDICINE BECOMES A COLLEGE

Dean Macy lived up to his promise to support efforts to make the School of Veterinary Medicine one of the best veterinary schools in the country. Dean Macy decided the time had come to elevate the School of Veterinary Medicine to the status of a college. President Morrill agreed and made this recommendation to the Board of Regents. On May 10, 1957, the regents voted that "the School of Veterinary Medicine, now a unit of the Institute of Agriculture, be given full and separate status as a college for professional training and research in veterinary medicine, that the administrative head of the College be a dean responsible to the president of the University in respect to administration and budget and that W. T. S. Thorp be designated Dean." With the elevation of the school to a college, the former divisions of the school became departments in the college effective July 1, 1957. See Exhibit V-2 for a listing of faculty and staff in 1960-61.

These changes raised questions as to the relation of the College of Veterinary Medicine to the Institute of Agriculture in regard to space, services, and research on the St. Paul Campus. The respective deans of the Institute of Agriculture and College of Veterinary Medicine eventually agreed on terms for location of buildings, services provided by the cashier's office, admissions and records services, and operation of the farm shop. Finally, academic employees of the College of Veterinary Medicine remained eligible for research funds from the Agricultural Experiment Station.

The elevation of the School of Veterinary Medicine to the College of Veterinary Medicine wherein the dean reported directly to the presi-

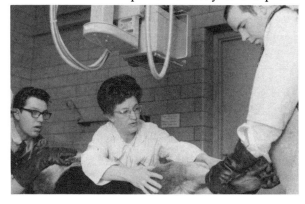

Dr. Bee Hanlon positioning a dog for hip dysplasia radiograph.

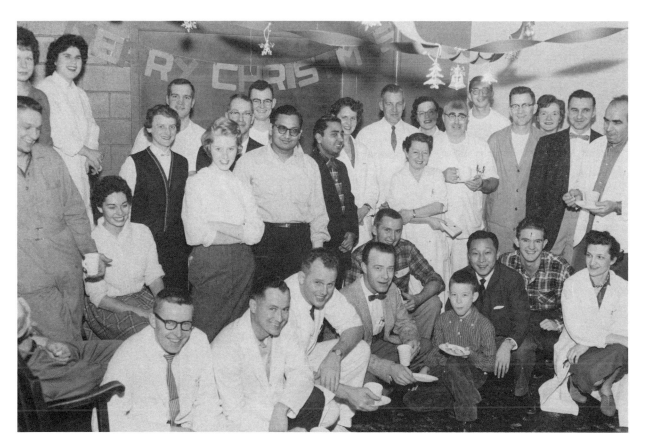

1961 Veterinary Clinic Christmas Party, left to right, kneeling, Dr. Dale Sorensen, Dr. Wm. Cates, Dr. Ira Gourley, Dr. Donald Low, Dr. LaRue Johnson, Ronnie Low, Dr. Cheong Chang Kook, Lauren Madden, Dr. Bee Hanlon, seated, Alice Stuber, standing, Lawrence Sirinek, Carol Bergeland, Denise Verbrugghen, Donna DenBoer, Dr. Ronald Engel, Bertha Cowan, Dr. John Arnold, Dr. Donald Simes, Dr. Rajendra Singh, Dr. I.H. Siddique, Katherine Smith, Dr. Harvey Hoyt, Fern Bates, Barbara Nelson, Dr. George Mather, Dr. Richard Herschler, Arden Ostergaard, Shirley Anderson, Dr. Vic Perman, Dr. Raimunds Zemjanis.

dent met the administrative requirements previously imposed by the AVMA's Council on Education. Thereafter, much to the relief of all concerned, full accreditation was granted by the AVMA.

Research continued to be an important part of the programs of the College of Veterinary Medicine. The first new research projects in the college included a grant from the U.S. Air Force to study the regulation of temperature control, and a commercial grant to study trichlorethelylene extracted soybean meal.

Dr. Thorp worked hard to increase the number of research grants and other sources of funding for the College of Veterinary Medicine. His contacts in the National Institutes of Health and other federal agencies were invaluable in this regard. The first major research project obtained by the college from a government agency was a grant to Dr. Francis A. Spurrell from the Wright Air Development Center, at Wright-Patterson Air Force Base in Ohio, to determine the effects of irradiation on large animals. Burros were used in the project, which spanned from July 1, 1958, to January 1, 1962. The total budget for the project was $225,000. Dr. Spurrell also obtained a large grant to study hip dysplasia in dogs.

Other large projects in the early days of the college involved the porphyria project and later the bovine leukemia project that was supported by National Institute of Cancer funds and had an initial budget of $300,000. In 1960, the Agricultural Experiment Station funded the purchase of an electron microscope unit used in research under the supervision of Dr. A. F. Weber.

EXHIBIT V-2

COLLEGE OF VETERINARY MEDICINE FACULTY AND STAFF 1960-61 ADMINISTRATION

William T. S. Thorp	Dean and Professor
Ralph L. Kitchell	Assistant Dean and Professor
Margaret T. Alm	Office Supervisor
Rose M. Kenaley	Principal Secretary
Sandra V. Petricka	Secretary
Judith Widersk	Senior Account Clerk
Rosemary Finnegan	Senior Clerk-Typist

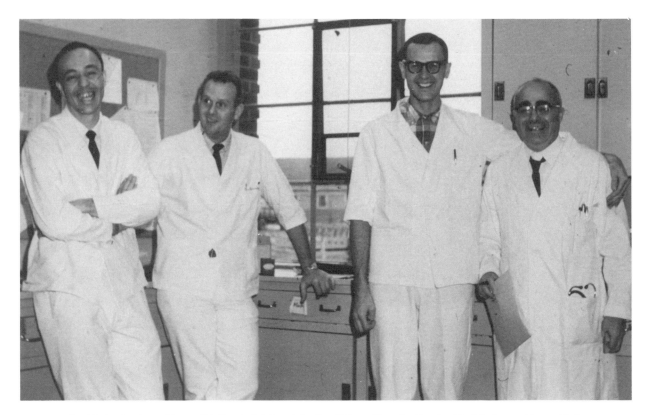

Dr. Mather has just told one of his "stories", left to right, Drs. Delmar Finco, Ira Gourley, Neal Anderson, George Mather.

| Janice C. Hystad | Senior Clerk-Typist |
| Karel DeWerff | Secretary |

DEPARTMENT OF VETERINARY ANATOMY

Ralph L. Kitchell	Professor and head
Alvin F. Weber	Professor
Melvin W. Stromberg	Associate Professor
Al W. Stinson	Instructor
Mary G. Phillips	Junior Scientist
Southwell C. Edgell	Laboratory Attendant

DEPARTMENT OF VETERINARY BACTERIOLOGY AND PUBLIC HEALTH

Benjamin S. Pomeroy	Professor and head
Robert K. Anderson	Professor
Robert K. Lindorfer	Associate Professor
Keith Loken	Assistant Professor
Calvert Larson	Instructor
Margaret Grady	Junior Scientist
Valborg Anderson	Senior Laboratory Attendant

DEPARTMENT OF VETERINARY PATHOLOGY AND PARASITOLOGY

Jay H. Sautter	Professor and head
Henry J. Griffiths	Professor
William J. Bemrick	Assistant Professor
N. Ole Nielsen	Instructor

Victor Perman	Instructor
John C. Schlotthauer	Instructor
Donald A. Willigan	Instructor
Roger A. Ball	Research Fellow
Wilma C. Hayes	Laboratory Technologist
Barbara J. Nelson	Student Technologist Supervisor
Denise Verbrugghen	Student Technologist Supervisor

DEPARTMENT OF VETERINARY PHYSIOLOGY AND PHARMACOLOGY

Clarence M. Stowe	Professor and head
Alvin F. Sellers	Professor
Archie L. Good	Associate Professor
Paul B. Hammond	Associate Professor
Emmett N. Bergman	Assistant Professor
Robert Dunlop	Instructor
Angelika A. Jegers	Junior Scientist
Leonard D. Walter	Principal Laboratory Attendant

DEPARTMENT OF VETERINARY MEDICINE AND CLINICS

Harvey H. Hoyt	Professor and head
John N. Campbell	Professor
George W. Mather	Professor
Dale K. Sorensen	Professor
Donald G. Low	Associate Professor
Robert A. Merrill	Associate Professor
William F. Brown	Instructor
Stanley E. Held	Instructor
Donald W. Johnson	Instructor
William E. Moore	Instructor
Fred W. Gehrman	Clinical Instructor
Arden Ostergaard	Principal Laboratory Attendant
Millard P. Jensen	Principal Laboratory Animal Attendant
Gustave Wendland	Stores Clerk
Lillian R. Fields	Laboratory Animal Attendant
Carol A. Bergeland	Senior Secretary
Janice Anderson	Senior Clerk-Typist
Alice Stuber	Senior Clerk-Typist
Bertha M. Cowan	Clerk Typist

DEPARTMENT OF VETERINARY SURGERY AND RADIOLOGY

John P. Arnold	Professor and head
Francis A. Spurrell	Associate Professor
Edward A. Usenik	Associate Professor
Donald H. Clifford	Assistant Professor

MAPLE PLAIN AMBULATORY CLINIC

As the suburbs of the Twin Cities grew, farmland was taken over for housing developments. The number of farm animals near the veterinary school decreased and there were fewer animals and less variety of cases seen by the students on Ambulatory Clinic. In an effort to bolster training opportunities in the Ambulatory Clinic, the college took over Dr. Fred Gehrman's farm practice in Wayzata, Minnesota.

On July 1, 1956, the college leased Dr. Gehrman's house and land with the option to buy. Dr. Gehrman and his staff stayed on to provide assistance in telephone and radio communication, and in consultation under the terms of the lease. The practice was located in Maple Plain, a small farming community about 20 miles west of Minneapolis.

Dr. Donald W. Johnson was placed in charge of the Maple Plain Ambulatory Service. Students who were rotated through the service would room in the upstairs of the house. At first, Dr. Johnson and his wife lived in the downstairs of the house. As the practice grew, Dr. Stanley Held was added to the staff. When he left, Dr. LaRue Johnson took his place, and later Dr. Marlin Baker joined the staff.

The venture proved to be very successful and, in December 1958, the university purchased the property from Dr. Gehrman. In 1959, a garage, an office, and a small treatment area were built to establish a regular and more efficient veterinary practice.

Over time, more people moved into the community, and some of the large farms were replaced by housing developments and hobby farms. The number of veterinary calls dropped as the number of animals decreased. Drs. Donald, Johnson, and Baker — all of whom had a large following among the animal owners in the area — subsequently left the college. The veterinarians who replaced them were never able to establish the same sort of relationship with the clientele. In July 1971, the facilities were sold to a private practitioner and the college ended the Maple Plain Ambulatory Clinic venture.

The teaching program of the Maple Plain Ambulatory Clinic was transferred to the St. Paul Campus and a herd health program was instituted to fill the void. The college also started an extern program with students spending time with practitioners. See Exhibit V-3 for the faculty and staff in 1970-71.

EXHIBIT V-3

COLLEGE OF VETERINARY MEDICINE FACULTY AND STAFF 1970-71 ADMINISTRATION

William T. S. Thorp	Dean and Professor
Robert K. Anderson	Associate Dean and Professor
Jane H. Van Avery	Senior Executive Secretary
Marilyn Rasmussen	Principal Account Clerk
Betty L. Covington	Senior Account Clerk
Carol Lynn Seefeld	Senior Clerk Typist
Judith Faye Roper	Secretary
Pamel Michie	Account Clerk

SPECIAL SERVICES

Wendell J. DeBoer	Assistant to the Dean
Myron Henry Nelson	Administrative Fellow

Hannis L. Stoddard	Professor and Director of International Programs
James O. Hanson	Associate Professor and Project Leader of Veterinarian Extension
Raymond B. Solac	Assistant Professor and Extension Veterinarian
Joan H. Lilleodden	Principal Secretary
Jeanette Dexheimer	Senior Secretary
Dandra Sue Sather	Clerk Typist

DEPARTMENT OF VETERINARY ANATOMY

Alvin F. Weber	Professor and head
Thomas F. Fletcher	Associate Professor
Caroline Czarnecki	Assistant Professor
Everett H. Heath	Assistant Professor
J. C. Vanden Berge	Assistant Professor
Robert F. Hammer	Instructor
William D. Martin	Instructor
Barbara Dickinson	Teaching Assistant
Richard L. Leino	Assistant Scientist
Southwell C. Edgell	Junior Scientist
Nancy N. Bjorndahl	Senior Laboratory Technician
Karen Gloege	Senior Secretary

DEPARTMENT OF VETERINARY MICROBIOLOGY AND PUBLIC HEALTH

Benjamin S. Pomeroy	Professor, head and Associate Dean
Robert K. Anderson	Associate Dean and Professor
Robert Lindorfer	Professor
Stanley L. Diesch	Associate Professor
Keith L. Loken	Associate Professor
Richard E. Shope, Jr.	Associate Professor
James Andree Libby	Assistant Professor
S. K. Maheswaran	Instructor
Robert A. Robinson	Instructor
Margaret Grady	Assistant Scientist
Kathryn Gilbert	Senior Laboratory Attendant
Nettie E. Anderson	Laboratory Attendant
Rosemary Finnegan	Principal Secretary
Marie Joy Cano	Senior Clerk Typist

DEPARTMENT OF VETERINARY MEDICINE

Dale K. Sorensen	Professor and head
Donald G. Low	Professor, head of Veterinary Hospital, and Associate Dean
Donald W. Johnson	Professor

George W. Mather	Professor
LaRue Johnson	Associate Professor
John F. Anderson	Assistant Professor
Vaughn L. Larson	Assistant Professor
Carl A. Osborne	Assistant Professor
Ralph J. Farnsworth	Instructor
Ronald E. Werdin	Instructor
Shelia Jo Olson	Laboratory Animal Technician
June Marie Swope	Senior Clerk Typist

DEPARTMENT OF VETERINARY DIAGNOSTIC LABORATORIES

John M. Higbee	Professor and Head
Donald M. Barnes	Associate Professor
Martin Bergeland	Associate Professor
Glen Harold Nelson	Associate Professor
Fern Yvonne Bates	Associate Scientist
Mildred R. Hakomaki	Junior Scientist
J. K. Steffenhagen	Junior Scientist
Magdalena Tainter	Senior Laboratory Technician
Richard J. Roback	Senior Laboratory Animal Technician
Frank Henry Parker	Laboratory Animal Technician
Barbara I. Lucast	Laboratory Technician
Delphine M. Yurick	Laboratory Technician
Ella K. Kuch	Laboratory Attendant
M. B. Christensen	Senior Secretary
Barbara J. Anderson	Senior Clerk Typist

DEPARTMENT OF VETERINARY OBSTETRICS

Raimunds Zemjanis	Professor and head
Francis A. Spurrell	Professor
Melvyn Fahning	Associate Professor
Richard M. Schultz	Associate Professor
Robert A. Wescott	Clinical Assistant Professor
Charles D. Gibson	Instructor and Extension Veterinarian in Animal Reproduction
William Kehr	Herdsman
George Williamson	Laboratory Animal Technician
Diane C. Halstenson	Senior Secretary

DEPARTMENT OF VETERINARY PATHOLOGY AND PARASITOLOGY

Henry J. Griffiths	Professor and head
Victor Perman	Professor
Jay H. Sautter	Professor
William J. Bemerick	Associate Professor
Kenneth H. Johnson	Associate Professor

Harold John Kurtz	Associate Professor
John Schlotthauer	Assistant Professor
Jerry B. Stevens	Assistant Professor
C. A. Christensen	Junior Scientist
Wilma C. Hayes	Junior Scientist
Beverly J. Johnson	Senior Laboratory Technician
William M. Reed	Laboratory Animal Technician
Betty Rosalie Rud	Senior Secretary
Barbara L. Roseen	Senior Clerk Typist

DEPARTMENT OF VETERINARY PHYSIOLOGY AND PHARMACOLOGY

Clarence M. Stowe	Professor and head
Harold E. Dzuik	Professor
Archie Leroy Good	Professor
Paul B. Hammond	Professor
Everett C. Short, Jr.	Associate Professor
Gary E. Duke	Assistant Professor
Grace W. Gray	Assistant Professor
Edward P. Jankus	Assistant Professor
Garth Miller	Assistant Professor
John P. Sullivan	Assistant Professor
Angelika Jegers	Associate Scientist
Carl W. Edborg	Principal Laboratory Attendant
Lorraine Tomkins	Principal Laboratory Attendant
Judith A. Brown	Senior Secretary

DEPARTMENT OF VETERINARY SURGERY AND RADIOLOGY

John P. Arnold	Professor and head
Donald Piermattei	Professor
Edward Usenik	Professor
Griselda W. Hanlon	Associate Professor
Victor S. Myers, Jr.	Associate Professor
Carl Roger Jessen	Assistant Professor
John Cowell Ellery	Instructor
Eberhard Rosin	Instructor
Lawrence Oberste	Herdsman
Ernest Waytashek	Principal Laboratory Animal Attendant
Linda J. Johnston	Laboratory Animal Technician
M. J. Christison	Senior Secretary

ADMINISTRATIVE PROBLEMS IN THE COLLEGE

Dr. Thorp had worked extremely hard to attain full accreditation and elevate the school to the rank of a College of Veterinary Medicine. The staff grew, additional research grants were obtained, the graduate program expanded through National Institutes of Health (NIH) Training Grants, and an international program was developed. The class size grew through NIH grants and new facilities were built and equipped. At the same time, Dr. Thorp developed an excellent relationship with veterinarians and legislators throughout the state.

Dr. Thorp's success at Minnesota attracted national attention. He was appointed to many committees and offices of national professional associations. The responsibilities of the positions took Dr. Thorp away from the college more and more, and he began to lose touch with events at the college.

During this time, student unrest and demonstrations were prevalent on the university's Minneapolis Campus. While the students on the St. Paul Campus did not demonstrate, students in the College of Veterinary Medicine had become more assertive, questioned the authority of faculty members, and challenged the content of courses. Students and faculty alike began to question decisions made by the university administration.

In November 1970, some members of the faculty circulated a petition demanding a change in the administration of the College of Veterinary Medicine. The petition was presented to Vice President of Academic Affairs William G. Shepherd, who ordered the formation of a committee to investigate the charges and complaints lodged against Dean Thorp. After completing the investigation, the committee concluded that, regardless of whether the accusations were true, the dissatisfaction in the college was so extensive that Dean Thorp could no longer function effectively as dean. On March 24, 1971, President Malcolm Moos and Dr. Thorp agreed on a transition plan for the administration of the College of Veterinary Medicine.

DR. DALE E. SORENSEN APPOINTED ACTING DEAN

Effective January 1, 1972, Dr. Sorensen was appointed acting dean of the College of Veterinary Medicine to replace Dr. Thorp. Dr. Sorensen was born on July 21, 1924, in Centuria, Wisconsin. He obtained his D.V.M. from Kansas State University in 1953, and he had received his M.S. in 1950 and Ph.D. in 1953 from the University of Wisconsin. Prior to his appointment, Dr.

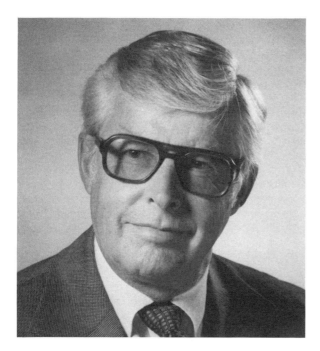

Dr. Dale K. Sorensen.

Sorenson had been professor and head of the Department of Veterinary Medicine.

Some people were not pleased with Dr. Sorenson's appointment as acting dean and were suspicious of his actions. The faculty had been divided during the final months of Dr. Thorp's regime. Deep animosity had developed and the divided faculty was not in a mood to put aside their differences to work together for the good of the college.

In the meantime, construction plans for the Phase II building program had to be finalized in order to request construction funds from the 1973 legislature.[9/] Phase II involved construction of a new small animal hospital (which became the Lewis Hospital for Companion Animals), administrative and faculty office suites, remodeling of the large animal hospital, and remodeling of the Veterinary Science Building. The college had to mobilize public and legislative support for the building projects.

A search committee for a new dean was appointed with Dr. Wesley Spink, professor emeritus of the Medical School, serving as chairman. Dr. Spink was an authority on brucellosis, or undulant fever, in humans and, therefore, was

familiar with brucellosis in animals. He had worked with veterinarians and was supportive of the College of Veterinary Medicine. The committee interviewed several candidates who also presented lectures at the college.

DR. SIDNEY A. EWING APPOINTED DEAN

Dr. Sidney Allen Ewing was appointed dean during the fall of 1972. He was born on December 1, 1934, on the campus of Emery University, Atlanta, Georgia. Before his appointment on December 1, 1972, Dr. Ewing had been head of the Department of Veterinary Parasitology, Microbiology, and Public Health in the College of Veterinary Medicine at Oklahoma State University. He had earned his B.S.A. and D.V.M. from the University of Georgia, his M.S. from the University of Wisconsin, and his Ph.D. from Oklahoma State University. Dr. Ewing had also held teaching and research positions at the University of Wisconsin, Kansas State University, and Mississippi State University.

Following the announcement of his appointment, Dr. Ewing made several trips to Minnesota in preparation for his new position. He recognized he was assuming deanship of a college that had various divisions among the faculty and where faculty and staff alike were apprehensive about the new administration.

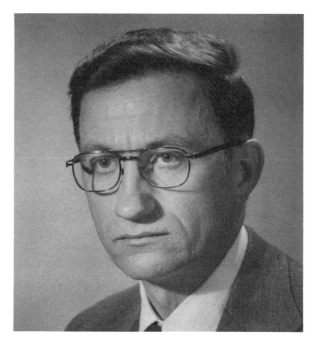

Dr. Sidney A. Ewing.

[9/] The 1971 legislature had appropriated $120,000 for preliminary planning of Phase II facilities.

The Council on Education of the AVMA had criticized the college, stating "faculty coordination seems to be lacking. The designated management structure appears to have a limited role in leadership and is in need of strengthening. ... There may be excessive departmentalization and a need would appear for creating a more effective management structure."

Dr. Ewing quickly appointed a committee to make recommendations on the organization and administration of the college. The committee was chaired by Dr. Carl Jessen and included Drs. Kenneth Johnson, Keith Loken, and Kirk Gelatt. After consulting with faculty and staff, the committee recommended streamlining the administrative structure.

The following spring, Dean Ewing announced that effective July 1, 1973, the existing nine departments would be merged into two departments — Veterinary Biology and Veterinary Clinical Sciences — and the collegiate administration would be reorganized into three programmatic areas: veterinary medical services; professional and undergraduate education; and veterinary research and graduate education. The objective behind these changes was to emphasize programmatic areas rather than academic disciplines, and thus both enhance the exchange of ideas between faculty and multiply interdisciplinary projects.

After soliciting faculty opinion on existing staff members who might be suited for the administrative positions, Dr. Ewing made the following appointments:

Veterinary Biology, Chair — Dr. Harold Dzuik

Veterinary Clinical Sciences, Chair — Dr. Dale K. Sorensen

Veterinary Medical Services, Associate Dean — Dr. Timothy Brasmer

Veterinary Professional and Undergraduate Education, Associate Dean — Dr. Everett C. Short

Veterinary Research and Graduate Education, Associate Dean — Dr. Benjamin S. Pomeroy

The Department of Veterinary Clinical Sciences created eight divisions to carry out its teaching and service commitments: (1) Large Animal Medicine; (2) Large Animal Surgery; (3) Small Animal Medicine; (4) Small Animal Surgery; (5) Theriogenology; (6) Radiology; (7) Specialties; and (8) Continuing Education and Extension.

The Department of Veterinary Biology was organized and administered by electing coordinators for each course who would provide leadership in teaching the courses.

Soon after announcing the reorganization, Dean Ewing was surprised with a "gift" presented by a faculty member of the Theriogenology Division at a collegiate banquet. The "gift" was a freeze-dried bull's penis. The presentation was made with fanfare and levity in the otherwise solemn setting. Dr. Richard Schultz read a "poem" that was open to interpretation and invited Dean Ewing to respond. Dean Ewing accepted the "gift" and, while displaying it to the audience, commented that he recognized the complexity of its function as a structure designed for delivery. The observation won him a round of applause.

COLLEGE CONSTITUTION

In the fall of 1970, the Department of Veterinary Physiology and Pharmacology drafted a constitution to define the administration and faculty's respective roles in conducting department affairs. The constitution was forwarded to Dean Thorp on October 3, 1970. The Department of Veterinary Pathology and Parasitology subsequently developed its own constitution. On November 10, 1970, Dean Thorp called a special faculty meeting to consider the need for a college, rather than departmental, constitution. The faculty voted to establish a constitutional committee that included the following faculty members: Drs. William Bemrich, Paul Hammond, Robert Lindorfer, Caroline Czarnecki, Victor Myers, and Vaughn Larson. Drs. William Benrick and Hammond served as co-chairs of the committee. When Dr. Hammond left the university, Dr. Everett Short took his place as co-chair.

The committee developed a constitution that defined the powers and duties of the college's dean, department heads, and faculty. The constitution also defined the organization and duties of the faculty, student, civil service, and administrative councils, and outlined the composition and responsibilities of all of the college's standing committees. Dr. Ewing provided his comments on a draft of the constitution and, after extensive rewriting, review, and revision, the constitution and bylaws of the College of Veterinary Medicine were approved by the Board of Regents in February 1973.

ADMINISTRATIVE CHANGES

After two years, the strong tradition of academic-centered department administrations at the University of Minnesota caused the faculty to become dissatisfied with the two department structure of the College of Veterinary Medicine. The faculty felt it was difficult for department chairs to become familiar enough with all of the areas covered in their respective departments to adequately represent faculty concerns to the dean. The faculty was also concerned that the decision making process had become too centralized. In response to faculty calls to change the departmental structure, Dean Ewing reorganized the college, effective July 1, 1976, as follows:
Veterinary Biology, Chair — Dr. Harold Dzuik

Veterinary Pathobiology, Chair — Dr. Kenneth Johnson

Large Animal Clinical Sciences, Chair — Dr. Dale K. Sorensen

Small Animal Clinical Sciences, Chair — Dr. Carl A. Osborne

Research and Graduate Education, Associate Dean — Dr. Raimunds Zemjanis[10]

To even the number of faculty between the two clinical departments, Radiology and Clinical Specialties were merged into Small Animal Clinical Sciences, and Public Health and Continuing Education and Extension opted to be placed within the Large Animal Clinical Sciences.

CONTINUED PROBLEMS WITH ACCREDITATION

In October 1974, the AVMA Council on Education visited the College of Veterinary Medicine. The following spring, the council informed the university the status of the college

would be reduced from full accreditation to probationary accreditation effective late September 1975. The council recommended: (1) increased clinical case material for in-hospital instruction of food animal and equine medicine and surgery; (2) development of additional field service in the area of food animal and equine practice, and greater student exposure to patients during the four years of instruction; (3) development of a program for instruction in laboratory animal medicine; and (4) increased faculty and opportunities for their professional development. The council scheduled its next visit for 1978.

The council's demotion of the college's accreditation status gave renewed credence to the college's earlier requests for additional resources. The university administration became more receptive to requests from the College of Veterinary Medicine. For example, the university facilitated the creation of a free ambulatory service for sick cattle within a 50-mile radius of the Veterinary Clinic. The service, which began on a trial basis, was successful in increasing the number of patients at the clinic. In 1978, the service was expanded to include a radius of 100 miles for sick animals referred by a veterinarian. The service was available five days a week. The college also entered into a special arrangement to treat sick animals from the stockyards at South St. Paul. Additionally, the college's internship program was strengthened to improve the instructional program with greater patient contact with students. The herd health program was also expanded to give the students more experience in this field. Students traveled to Cannon Falls to study with Dr. John F. Anderson, who had several private herds on herd health programs.

The college also carried out a curriculum study. Under the direction of Dr. Everett Short, the Curriculum Committee developed a new curriculum that was subsequently adopted by the faculty. The new curriculum went into effect for the fall quarter of 1978. As part of the new curriculum, all lecture/laboratory courses were presented in the first three years of the veterinary medical program. The four quarters comprising the fourth year consisted of 36 weeks of core clinical assignments, four weeks of elective assignments, and three weeks of vacation.

Dean Ewing believed increasing the food and equine medicine coursework and surgery, along with other adjustments to the curriculum, had succeeded in correcting the deficiencies iden-

[10]   Dr. Zemjanis replaced Dr. Benjamin S. Pomeroy, who had accepted the responsibility of Director of Alumni and Public Affairs.

tified by the council. With the agreement of the Administrative Council, Dean Ewing requested the Council on Education to reevaluate Minnesota's veterinary medical program before originally scheduled. Members of the Council on Education agreed to move their visit up a year earlier in the spring of 1978. In the fall of 1978, the council granted the College of Veterinary Medicine full accreditation.

DEAN EWING RESIGNS

By 1978, Dean Ewing had served six years as dean. While he had sustained teaching and research activity in his scientific discipline, parasitology, he wished to return to scientific research full time. He decided to resign as dean soon after he learned the college would be granted full accreditation. Dean Ewing subsequently returned to the Veterinary College at Oklahoma State University as head of the Department of Veterinary Parasitology, Microbiology, and Public Health.

At the July 7, 1978, meeting of the Board of Regents, University President Peter Magrath reported Dean Ewing had announced his resignation as dean of the College of Veterinary Medicine effective December 31, 1978. Vice President Henry Koffler formed a search committee to fill the position.

The College of Veterinary Medicine underwent several important changes during Dean Ewing's tenure. The college operated in accordance with a constitution that prescribed the roles of the administration and faculty, fixed terms of appointment of administrators, established administrative reviews, held regular faculty meetings, and established standing committees with defined organization and responsibilities. The college operated through a close association between administration and faculty. The college was reorganized twice, and had been reduced from full accreditation to probationary accreditation, and then returned to full accreditation. The curriculum was revised to increase opportunities for clinical training. The physical plant was significantly expanded to include new facilities for instruction of the basic sciences. Funds were secured to complete the extensive renovation of the Veterinary Science Building and the construction of a new teaching hospital. Although actual construction of the Lewis Teaching Hospital was completed after he had returned to Oklahoma, Dean Ewing returned to St. Paul to attend the formal dedication.

BUILDING NEEDS — RECIPROCITY

The College of Veterinary Medicine became a regional center for veterinary education. Since its establishment in 1947, the college had accepted students from the Wisconsin, North Dakota, South Dakota, and Nebraska. In 1972, Acting Dean Sorensen initiated discussions with these states concerning the cost of instructing these out-of-state students. In 1973, Minnesota finalized arrangements with North Dakota and Nebraska. The college agreed to annually accept up to four qualified students from North Dakota and up to 20 qualified students from Nebraska in return for payment of a negotiated level of instructional costs.

Negotiations with Wisconsin proved more complex as Wisconsin sought admission of a larger number of students. In 1970, the Board of Regents approved a long-range plan to accept 60 to 120 students per year. However, the facilities would have to be obtained to accommodate these students. Discussions were held with University of Wisconsin administrators and legislators to negotiate a contract that was tentatively approved by both universities. The University of Minnesota proposed to admit 16 to 18 students from Wisconsin until the number in the class reached 80. At that point, the number of Wisconsin students would increase to 25 percent of the entering class. This agreement was never finalized or implemented.

In 1973, Governor Wendell Anderson of Minnesota and Governor Patrick Lucey of Wisconsin met and negotiated a reciprocity agreement for unlimited student exchange in higher education. Under the agreement, the University of Minnesota would admit 18 qualified Wisconsin residents each year to the College of Veterinary Medicine. The reciprocity agreement also allowed residents of each state to attend the other's public university and only pay resident tuition.

The cost of instruction to veterinary students is much greater than tuition. Thus, Minnesota taxpayers were paying much of the cost to educate Wisconsin residents. This situation inspired additional negotiations and, in 1976, the states were near agreement. Wisconsin requested 35 places in the entering class with a marginal cost method to determine the net educational costs. Wisconsin residents would pay resident tuition rates, and Wisconsin would participate in admission and curriculum policies. The agreement was contingent on appropriations from the Minnesota legislature to increase the college's facilities. Powerful legislators and interest groups, as well as many Minnesota veterinarians, were opposed to expanding the enrollment to accommodate Wisconsin residents. In 1977 and 1978, the legislature refused to appropriate the funds for more facilities. In 1978, the legislature instructed the college to present plans to accommodate only 80 Wisconsin students. In 1979, the university requested and received $12,500,000 from the legislature for additional facilities based on this reduced figure.

In the meantime, groups in Wisconsin promoted the creation of a veterinary college in Wisconsin. In 1976, the Wisconsin legislature passed a bill to establish a veterinary college in Wisconsin. The establishment of the college was delayed for a time to watch developments in Minnesota.

In 1975, a southwestern Minnesota legislator introduced a bill to move the College of Veterinary Medicine to Southwest University at Marshall. The Marshall campus was having trouble attracting students and, according to the legislator, the campus had $50,000,000 worth of unused buildings. He argued the move would bring more students to the campus and solve the facility needs of the College of Veterinary Medicine. Although the bill caused concern among the faculty, the legislation died in the legislature from lack of support.

DR. BENJAMIN S. POMEROY APPOINTED ACTING DEAN

Dr. B. S. Pomeroy was appointed acting dean of the College of Veterinary Medicine effective January 1, 1979. Dr. Pomeroy was born on April 24, 1911, in St. Paul. He was a 1933 graduate of Iowa State University, received his M.S. from Cornell University, and received his Ph.D. in 1944 from the University of Minnesota. He was known and honored world-wide for his work on poultry diseases. He was also very active in the professional organizations, including service as secretary-treasurer of the Minnesota Veterinary Medical Association from 1950 to 1975. Dr. Pomeroy was also well-known in political circles and lobbied hard for College of Veterinary Medicine requests to the legislature.

During his term as acting dean, Dr. Pomeroy improved the college relations with veterinarians throughout Minnesota, the livestock and poultry industry, and the legislature. In par-

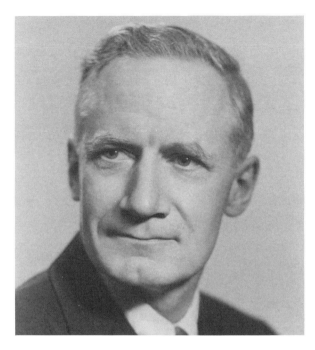

Dr. B.S. Pomeroy.

ticular, he played an important role in obtaining $13,600,000 from the legislature to complete Phase II of the construction plan. Dr. Pomeroy served until December 31, 1980, when Dr. Dunlop was appointed dean.

DR. ROBERT DUNLOP APPOINTED DEAN

Dr. Dunlop became dean effective January 1, 1980. He was born in London, England, where he received his early education. In 1949, he came to Canada and, in 1956, he graduated from Ontario Veterinary College. He obtained his Ph.D. from the University of Minnesota in 1961. Dr. Dunlop then returned to England where he served as pathologist and directed the Wickham Laboratories. In 1962, he accepted a position at Cornell Veterinary College to teach pharmacology. In 1965, he became head of the Department of Physiological Sciences in the Western College of Veterinary Medicine at the University of Saskatoon, Canada. He went to Uganda, Africa, in 1971 to help the British and Canadian governments develop a veterinary school. The project was terminated prematurely due to political pressure in the country. He then went to Malaysia to assist that nation's college of veterinary medicine and to evaluate a cattle program. Late in 1973, he became dean of the Murdock Veterinary School in Western Australia.

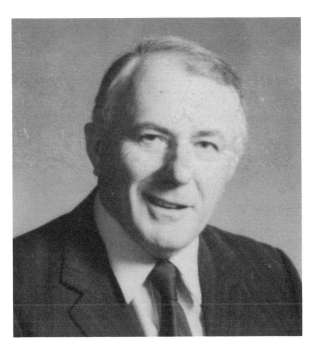

Dr. Robert Dunlop.

Upon becoming dean, Dr. Dunlop found the College of Veterinary Medicine had changed in many ways during the 19 years since he had been a graduate student. Both the physical plant and the staff had greatly expanded. The staff was less unified then when he had been a graduate student. Although Dean Ewing had eased tension between staff factions, there remained distrust and friction in the faculty ranks.

Members of the staff of the Diagnostic Laboratory had been greatly disturbed when their department was placed within another department. The head of the Diagnostic Department had resigned and practitioners had criticized the arrangement. Dr. Dunlop restored the laboratory to department status in an effort to ease the concerns of laboratory staff.

The vice president of the university, Kenneth Keller, developed the Commitment to Focus Plan to raise the standard of excellence in the university. The plan was subsequently approved by the Board of Regents. When he became president of the university, Dr. Keller brought in a new vice president of academic affairs to implement the plan. Each department of the college was asked to redirect fifteen percent of its funds from the maintenance and operations budget. Ten percent was to be channeled to high priority programs and five percent directed to programs on a noncontinuing basis. This arrangement greatly disadvantaged professional schools like the College of Veterinary Medicine where it is necessary to cover many disciplines in order to provide the proper professional education.

The new vice president of academic affairs instituted a new system to measure the effectiveness of colleges and departments based on the number of credit hours taught by each staff member; the amount of research funding brought in by each staff member; and the number of Ph.D. candidates who were graduated per staff member. The College of Veterinary Medicine fared poorly in this type of evaluation. The criteria did not consider the large volume of service work expected of the staff and the relatively small number of students enrolled in the college. The college was advised to reduce its staff size and facilities to fit in the budget calculated by the evaluation system.

A committee was appointed to recommend ways for the university to raise the standard of excellence. However, the committee's recommendations required substantial funding. As the legislature was not likely to appropriate more money, these funds had to be found within the university. The committee considered the closing of several colleges and elimination of certain departments. The committee recommended the closing of the College of Veterinary Medicine, Dental School, School of Public Health, and Department of Mortuary Science.

The recommendation to close the College of Veterinary Medicine alarmed veterinarians throughout the state. The Minnesota Veterinary Medical Association, livestock and poultry organizations, and owners of pet animals came to the support of the college. The reputation and standing of the college suffered nationally because of the wide publicity the recommendation was given in the media. However, the recommendations were eventually rejected by the Board of Regents.

FELINE HEALTH CENTER

There was a belief among cat fanciers, cat breeders, and practitioners who treated cats that insufficient attention had been given to research in cat diseases. Thus, the Feline Health Center was organized in 1981 to promote feline health research. The Feline Health Center used a cooperative approach wherein feline owners and practitioners were encouraged to make their problems known to the center. Faculty members interested

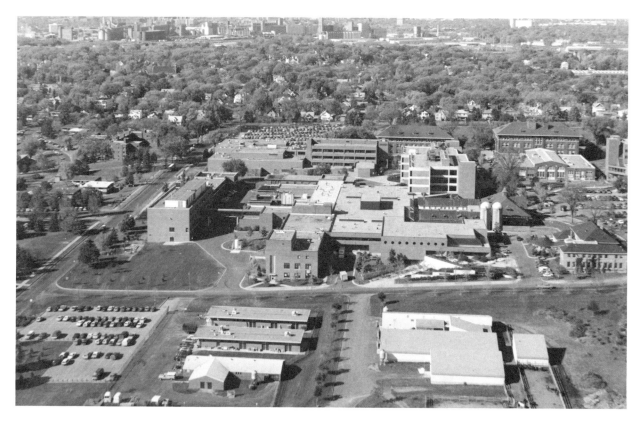

College of Veterinary Medicine, c. 1988.

in feline health from different areas of the College of Veterinary Medicine cooperated in the use of facilities, equipment, and supplies, and worked together to conduct research.

The center has conducted research on feline urinary diseases, mammary cancer, reproduction, anemia, and diabetes. The most dramatic research findings occurred in the area of feline diabetes where the center discovered a new hormone. The results of this research have been applied to human diabetes as well as diabetes in cats.

Drs. Kenneth H. Johnson and Carl A. Osborne serve as co-directors of the Feline Health Center. The remaining members of the steering committee include Drs. David Hayden, Shirley D. Johnston, and Vic Perman of the College of Veterinary Medicine. Dr. Mike McMenomy, a feline practitioner, and Patricia Jacobberger, a cat fancier and breeder, have also been appointed to the committee to represent practitioners and cat breeders.

SWINE CENTER

The University of Minnesota Swine Center is an interdisciplinary program that was established in 1982 by the College of Veterinary Medicine, College of Agriculture, Agricultural

Experiment Station, and Agricultural Extension. Participants in the program include the faculty of the Departments of Animal Science, Agricultural Engineering and Agricultural and Applied Economics in the College of Agriculture, as well as from Large Animal Clinical Sciences, Veterinary Biology, Veterinary Pathobiology and Veterinary Diagnostic Laboratory Departments in the College of Veterinary Medicine.

The purpose of the center is to promote and enhance interdisciplinary swine research and to provide efficient lines of communication between university personnel, pork producers, and businesses with swine interests. The center seeks to develop a database to measure the effectiveness of swine programs and attract additional faculty members. Finally, the center works to generate private funds to accomplish projects that cannot be supported through traditional funding sources.

The center's research programs have included studying the environment for swine, reproductive efficiency, reproductive diseases, nutrition, genetics, cell culture, pseudorabies, and enteric diseases. The Swine Center has also developed a computerized program known as "Pig Champ." The program follows the history of all of the individual pigs in a herd and includes farrowing, weaning, growth and sales. The data collected have been used to reveal factors that may limit production.[11/]

.   Dr. Al Leman of the College of Veterinary Medicine, was largely responsible for the establishment of the Swine Center and served as its first director. Dr. Leman was succeeded as director by Professor Ron Moser of Animal Science. Dr. Gary D. Dial subsequently became director, and he was eventually succeeded by Dr. John Fetrow. Genetic engineering is a new concept in the college. However, it has been developed to the point that two faculty members devote their time to this area.

AVIAN HEALTH CHAIR CREATED

The poultry industry led by Lloyd Peterson of the Turkey Growers Association raised two million dollars to establish a chair in avian health. The Board of Regents accepted the funds on January 11, 1985, and the chair was named the Benjamin S. Pomeroy Chair of Avian Health in recognition of Dr. Pomeroy's 45 years of teaching, research, and service to the poultry industry. Dr. Jagdev Sharma was appointed to fill the chair effective in July 1988.

DEAN DUNLOP RESIGNS

Dr. Dunlop announced his resignation on April 26, 1988, effective August 1, 1988. Although he had planned to resign earlier, Dr. Dunlop had delayed his plans to resign until the threat of closing the college had passed. After the Board of Regents rejected the recommendation, Dr. Dunlop decided the time had come for him to return to teaching and research.

DR. DAVID THAWLEY APPOINTED INTERIM DEAN

Dr. David G. Thawley was appointed interim dean of the College of Veterinary Medicine effective August 1, 1988. In 1990, he became the dean of the college. Dr. Thawley received his D.V.M. from the Massey University Palmerston North, New Zealand in 1969. In 1974, he received his Ph.D. from his University of Guelph, in Guelph, Ontario, Canada. He came to the University of Minnesota in 1986 from the College of Veterinary Medicine at the University of Missouri, where he had been professor of veterinary microbiology, director of research, and

[11/]   Later a comparable program known as "Dairy Champ" was developed. The same principles were applied to poultry.

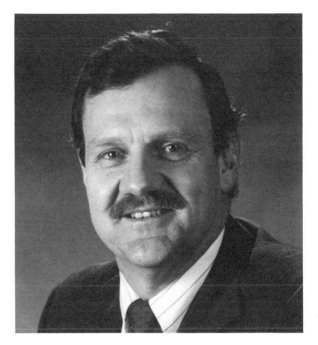

Dr. David Thawley.

assistant director of the Missouri Agricultural Experiment Station. Prior to his appointment, he had been chairperson of the Department of Large Animal Clinical Sciences at the college.

Upon his appointment, Dr. Thawley undertook an extensive long-range strategic planning program for the college. The college participated in the Pew National Veterinary Educational Program to develop a plan to meet the challenges for veterinary medicine in the 1990s. The college developed a five-year strategic plan that included extensive changes to the curriculum.

Additionally, the Department of Animal Science has become affiliated with the College of Veterinary Medicine. Staff members had been working together on an individual basis. However, this affiliation allows staff members in animal science and veterinary medicine to coordinate much more extensive teaching, research, and extension programs.

DEPARTMENT OF DIAGNOSTIC INVESTIGATION

The Department of Diagnostic Investigation is the Minnesota Board of Animal Health's official laboratory for diagnostic work on animal and poultry diseases. The laboratory is supported through special appropriations from the legislature.

The laboratory began in a rather quiet and unobtrusive manner. Veterinarians on the St. Paul Campus of the university began diagnosing animal diseases for the public when Dr. M. H. Reynolds joined the staff in 1893. When the Board of Animal Health was created in 1903, the animal disease laboratory work was conducted at the state Board of Health laboratory. After a short time, the two boards met to work out terms for providing the state Board of Health with reimbursement for the cost of this service. When they were unable to agree, the Board of Animal Health began searching for alternative laboratory services. Dr. Reynolds, who was a member of the Board and on the staff of the Agricultural Experiment Station, proposed the Board move its animal laboratory facilities and equipment to the St. Paul Campus. Dr. Reynolds saw this arrangement as a way for the College of Agriculture to obtain specimens for educational and research purposes. The Board of Animal Health adopted the proposal in June 1904.

The Board hired Dr. W. L. Beebe, a veterinarian, to do the bacteriological work. In 1905, the Board wrote to veterinarians throughout the state instructing them to send specimens to Dr. Beebe at the Experiment Station, in St. Anthony Park, in care of Ballard's Express, St. Paul, Minnesota. (The company is now known as Ballard Moving and Storage Co., Inc.)

The Board later arranged to have a laboratory installed in the basement of the Old Capitol Building. In 1912, Dr. Beebe resigned to establish a private laboratory. The Board of Animal Health offered the position to Dr. Willard L. Boyd at a salary of $1,600 per year. At the time, Dr. Boyd was a member of the staff at the university and declined the offer.

Failing to hire Dr. Boyd, the Board of Animal Health contacted Dean W. F. Wood of the College of Agriculture to negotiate an arrangement for continued laboratory services. On July 12, 1912, the Board and Dean Wood reached an agreement wherein the laboratory equipment would be moved to the St. Paul Campus. The Board agreed to pay the laboratory assistant's salary for six months of the year. The university agreed to furnish the supplies needed, and Dr. Boyd was assigned to conduct the laboratory diagnostic work for the Board of Animal Health.

Although Dr. Boyd was in charge of the general laboratory work, other members of the veterinary staff provided assistance in their specialty areas. The laboratory's work increased over the years. When Dr. Fitch replaced Dr. Reynolds as head of the Division of Veterinary Medicine in 1917, the operation of the laboratory was placed under the university's direction and became known as the Livestock Sanitary Board Laboratory.[12]

In October of 1926, the College of Agriculture notified the Board of Animal Health the amount of work requested of the laboratory had increased so greatly that it would be impossible to continue without more funding. The college requested $7,500 to operate that year and $6,000 to operate the following year. The Board of Animal Health included this request for additional funds in its legislative request. Although Governor Theodore Christenson deleted the request for extra funds from the Board's legislative request, he promised to convince the University to provide the extra funds. However, the university determined it could not continue to provide the service with the available funds.

On September 26, 1927, a meeting was held to consider the problem. The university was represented by President L. D. Coffman, Dean W. C. Coffey, and Dr. C. P. Fitch. The Board of Animal Health was represented by Colonel C. H. Marsh, W. S. Moscrip, and Dr. C. E. Cotton. Everyone in attendance agreed the service should continue to be provided if at all possible. To cover the immediate biennium, the Board of Animal Health committed to find within the limits of its budget sufficient funds to defray half of the costs of routine service for the next two years. The university agreed to supply the remaining funds.

On November 21, 1926, Dr. Cotton, the executive secretary of the Board of Animal Health, wrote to President L. D. Coffman stating that they were able to raise $2,000 annually, or $166.66 per month, for the next two years to operate the laboratory. The university matched this amount and the laboratory continued in operation. However, both parties agreed to make an urgent appeal to the 1929 legislature. Their combined efforts were successful. The 1929 legislature appropriated $7,500 per year for the next biennium and funded the salary of a technician for pullorum testing.

In the meantime, the laboratory had become known as the Veterinary Diagnostic Laboratory. Dr. Ruel Fenstermacher joined the

---

[12] Unofficially, Dr. Kernkamp was in charge of the laboratory from about 1926 to 1928.

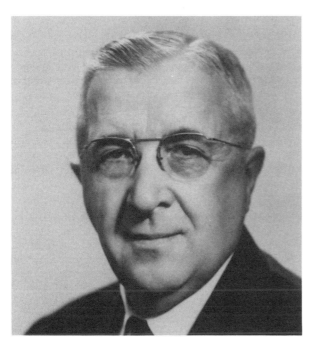

Dr. Ruel Fenstermacher.

staff as Director of the Veterinary Diagnostic Laboratory on January 1, 1928. Dr. Fenstermacher was a 1917 graduate of Ohio State University. After being discharged from the Veterinary Corps in 1919, he began work with the Board of Animal Health. He was assistant secretary of the Board at the time he was appointed director of the laboratory. Dr. Fenstermacher was especially interested in diseases of wild animals with a particular emphasis on moose and deer disease. Under his direction, laboratory services to the animal and poultry industries increased dramatically.

In the beginning, the laboratory was located in what is now known as the Old Anatomy Building. Poultry was necropsied in a room opposite the outside entrance to the east wing of the building. For necropsy, animals were taken down the hall from the main entrance of the building. Occasionally, some animals were posted in the round room and later taken to the autopsy room of the Serum Building. Dr. Boyd handled the laboratory work involving cattle, Dr. Kernkamp handled the swine, and Dr. Pomeroy handled the poultry.

On November 19, 1943, a fire started in a large walk-in incubator on the second floor of the Old Anatomy Building and spread to the attic. The fire destroyed much of the laboratory equipment, part of the library, and the older records of

the Minnesota Veterinary Medical Association that were stored in the attic. Laboratory equipment was in short supply and difficult to replace due to the demands of World War II. As a result, the Diagnostic Laboratory was moved to the Serum Building. This building had previously been used in the anti-hog cholera serum and virus production operation located on the campus.

As the services provided by the Diagnostic Laboratory grew, the laboratory needed to improve its facilities. In 1948, the laboratory moved into the first floor and part of the second floor of the Temporary East of the Haecker Building, or "T.E.H."

Under a cooperative agreement with the Bureau of Animal Industry, the federal state Brucellosis Laboratory became associated with the Diagnostic Laboratory. A cooperative arrangement was made with the state Department of Health on diseases such as rabies that affect both animals and humans.

The laboratory staff gradually increased over the years. Remi Brooke served faithfully as a laboratory technician beginning in 1949. Dr. Robert Leary assisted in the laboratory for a short time after he graduated in 1951. In 1953, Dr. Charles Gale joined the staff while he also took graduate work. Dr. Donald Barnes came in 1955 and also took graduate work. Dr. Earl Thompson worked in the laboratory for a short time after graduating in 1955.

Upon the creation of the School of Veterinary Medicine, the Diagnostic Laboratory was placed in the Department of Veterinary Science. When the AVMA Council on Education questioned the arrangement, Dr. Thorp cut the college's ties with the Diagnostic Laboratory and created the Division of Veterinary Diagnostic Laboratory, thus allowing Dr. Fenstermacher to participate in division head administrative meetings.

In 1957, Dr. John Higbee was recruited to fill a new staff position in the laboratory in response to requests from veterinarians throughout the state to have a staff member with practice experience. Dr. Higbee graduated from Iowa State University in 1939 and had a successful practice in Albert Lea, Minnesota. In addition to Dr. Higbee, Dr. Martin Bergeland and Dr. Harley Moon were also hired in 1959 and 1960, respectively.

The move to T.E.H. gave the Diagnostic Laboratory more space. However, by the late

1950s, the laboratory had outgrown these facilities due to increased demand for its services. The 1957 legislature appropriated funds to construct a new building that was completed in 1961. In a short day, Drs. Martin Bergeland, Clifford Ling, Harley Moon, and Ned Olson moved all of the equipment into the new building using the veterinary medicine truck. The building was dedicated in 1961. Sadly, Dr. Fenstermacher died before the dedication.

Dr. John Higbee was subsequently appointed head of the Department of Diagnostic Laboratories. Dr. Glen Nelson joined the staff in 1961 and Dr. Barnes returned from a research project in Montana the following year. Dr. Moon left the staff in 1965 and Dr. Bergeland left in 1970. Drs. Ronald Werdin, Dr. Harold Kurtz, and Dr. George Ruth subsequently joined the staff in 1971, 1972, and 1976, respectively.

In October 1973, to balance the budget and provide necessary services, the Diagnostic Laboratory began charging a fee for processing the animals and specimens.

In 1973, when Dean Sidney A. Ewing reorganized the college administration, the Diagnostic Laboratory was placed under the direction of Dr. Timothy M. Brasmer, associate dean of Veterinary Services, and the staff was placed in the Department of Veterinary Pathobiology. This arrangement caused some difficulties as the Diagnostic Laboratory was the official laboratory of the Board of Animal Health and was supported by a special legislative appropriation.

Except for a short period, Dr. John Higbee was head of the Diagnostic Laboratory until 1980. He died the following year. Dr. Harold Kurtz served as acting head on two occasions. Dr. George Ruth served as head of the laboratory from January 1, 1979, to June 30, 1979.

Dean Robert Dunlop restored the department status of the Diagnostic Laboratory effective July 1, 1982. On August 1, 1983, Dr. Martin Bergeland returned as chairman of the new Department of Diagnostic Investigation and director of the Veterinary Diagnostic Laboratory.

The 1971 legislature appropriated funds to build additional facilities for the Veterinary Teaching Hospital and the Diagnostic Laboratory. The new additions provided the laboratory with more space on the upper level of the building.

The laboratory has been involved in teaching undergraduate veterinary students since the first class became seniors in 1950-1951. Students were rotated through the laboratory to gain experience in necropsy. Graduate students have also spent time in the laboratory for experience and study of disease problems. The arrangement was unusual as the Diagnostic Laboratory provided the staff but had no curriculum listed in the records. However, the department eventually developed five graduate courses that are listed in the university catalog.

The eradication of diseases such as hog cholera and the appearance of important and new diseases have resulted in the need for different and more complicated laboratory equipment, as well as the need for increased space. Staff expertise has been added in virology, toxicology, and electron microscopy. Additional staff members who have been hired to provide this expertise included Dr. Sager in 1982, Dr. Lawrence Felice in 1984, Dr. James Collins in 1986, and Dr. Daniel Shaw in 1987. In addition, in 1984, the official laboratory of the Minnesota Racing Commission was placed in the Diagnostic Laboratory.

Laboratory accessions have increased from 3,450 in 1961 to 43,421 in 1991. The increase in the number of accessions has required an increase from 13 staff members in 1961 to 64 staff members in 1991.

To provide larger facilities that were badly needed, the legislature appropriated funds to build a new building with 18,850 square feet of laboratory and office space. The new building, which cost $7,900,000, was dedicated on October 6, 1992.

VETERINARY CONTINUING EDUCATION

The first veterinarian in Agricultural Extension was Dr. William A. Billings who joined the staff in 1918. Dr. Billings had worked in the Diagnostic Laboratory until October 1, 1922, when he was transferred to the Division of Agricultural Extension. He was classified as extension specialist in veterinary practice with no change in collegiate rank or salary.

While working in the Diagnostic Laboratory, Dr. Billings performed many post mortem examinations on turkeys that had died of blackhead disease. Chickens were recognized as carriers of organisms that caused the disease. At the time, the custom was to raise chickens and turkeys together on farms. Chicken flocks were small and turkeys were allowed to roam about the farm. Turkey hens acted like wild turkeys in secreting their nests, and would take great pains, such as taking a circuitous route, to prevent their nests from being found. If they suspected they were being followed, the turkeys would go to another area to throw off whoever was following them. When their eggs had hatched, the turkey hens would take care to keep the young poults away from the farm buildings. As the young turkeys became larger and needed more food, the hen would bring them to the farm yard where they ate with the chickens. The poults would subsequently catch blackhead disease from the chickens. The death loss was high, and blackhead disease soon threatened to wipe out the turkey industry in the Midwest.

Dr. Billings and Professor C. A. Smith devised a method of raising turkeys away from chickens. To demonstrate the feasibility of the method, Dr. Billings convinced some farm women to hatch turkey eggs in an incubator and raise the poults in confinement away from chickens. When this method proved successful, Dr. Billings publicized the method through a bulletin entitled, *Talking Turkey*. Over one million copies of this bulletin were distributed.

When the 1923 legislature passed an act directing the University of Minnesota to conduct hog cholera vaccination schools for farmers, Dr. Billings was assigned to conduct these schools. Dr. Billings became very unpopular among veterinarians in the large hog-raising area in Minnesota because, by training laymen to vaccinate hogs, he was taking away part of these veterinarians' practice.

Dr. Billings was otherwise a popular speaker at poultry meetings throughout Minnesota. He was colorful and had a caustic wit. He would tell stories of people who thought they had "disinfected" their chicken house by sweeping out the chickens and dusting off a few cobwebs. In fact, this was how most people believed a chicken house was disinfected. Having got the attention of the audience with this story, he would then proceed to tell them how to properly disinfect a chicken house. Dr. Billings also had a turkey dressing recipe that became very popular. He spent much time promoting the recipe in his later years at the university. Dr. Billings died in 1970.

Dr. Raymond Solac became the second veterinarian on the extension staff in 1957. He had graduated from Michigan State University in 1950 and practiced for a time in Eyota, Minnesota.

In 1953, he became a district veterinarian for the Board of Animal Health and was later placed in charge of all district veterinarians.

When he joined the extension staff, Dr. Solac was assigned an office in the College of Veterinary Medicine. This marked a new trend of locating extension personnel in areas they represented. This brought extension veterinarians in closer contact with other university veterinarians and helped keep them abreast of the latest developments in veterinary medicine.

Dr. Solac participated in the scabies and hog cholera eradication programs. His primary interest in extension was poultry with an emphasis on geese and waterfowl. Dr. Solac retired in 1984.

Dr. James O. Hanson joined the extension staff in 1967. When he was appointed director of continuing education and project leader of Veterinary Medicine. This marked an increased emphasis on continuing education for veterinarians. Dr. Hanson had a dual appointment requiring him to devote 60 percent of his time in the College of Veterinary Medicine and 40 percent in Agricultural Extension. This allocation of time and responsibility was subsequently changed to an equal division between their duties.[13] Dr. Hanson had graduated from the Minnesota College of Veterinary Medicine in 1953 and had practiced at St. Peter, Minnesota, before he joined the extension staff.

Dr. James A. Libby joined the staff as extension veterinarian of Meat Hygiene and Public Health in 1968. Dr. Libby had graduated from the College of Veterinary Medicine in 1959. He had practiced after graduation before joining the federal Meat Inspection Service of the Department of Agriculture. He took part in the Meat Inspection Service program at Ohio State University where he obtained his M.S. and taught in the veterinary medicine college. He was subsequently assigned to teach at the U.S. Department of Agriculture Meat Hygiene School in Chicago, Illinois. Dr. Libby both taught Meat Hygiene and performed extension work at the College of Veterinary Medicine. He resigned in 1973 to start a small animal practice in Bloomington.

[13] The joint appointments enabled extension to obtain more specialized personnel and the services of those engaged in teaching, research, and service. The growth of the professional staff was accompanied by an increase in the Civil Service support staff, which grew from a shared secretary to 2.3 full-time employees.

Dr. James O. Hanson retired on June 30, 1991. At the time that Dr. Hanson came to the university extension, veterinarians on the staff frequently spoke at livestock and poultry meetings and other farm groups, and prepared leaflets and bulletins. While they had some interaction with veterinarians, the staff's main focus was the dissemination of information to lay groups.

Since Dr. Hanson's arrival, the number of continuing education courses for veterinarians has increased to more than 30 per year. The presentation format has evolved from straight lectures to include workshops or participation courses.

Dr. Robert Dunlop succeeded Dr. Hanson as director on a temporary basis until Dr. Charles Casey was appointed as director effective September 1, 1992. Dr. Casey had graduated from the College of Veterinary Medicine in 1963. He served in the U.S. Army Veterinary Corps from 1963 to 1965. Dr. Casey practiced in West Concord, Minnesota, for more than 25 years after being discharged from the service, and he served as a member and chair of the Board of Regents of the University of Minnesota for twelve years.

INTERNATIONAL PROGRAMS

In 1954, the University of Minnesota signed the Minnesota FAO[14/] Cooperative Agreement for Rehabilitation of Seoul National University, also known as the International Cooperative Agreement Minnesota Project. This program was administered by the U.S. Department of State. When the program was started, former Minnesota Governor Harold Stassen was special assistant to President Eisenhower and is given credit for the fact the University of Minnesota received the first contract of this type after World War II.

The College of Agriculture and other colleges of the university had early involvement in the project. Animal diseases were a serious problem in Korea. The Korean veterinary profession needed assistance and the College of Veterinary Medicine was asked to help. In 1957, faculty members of the Veterinary College of Seoul National University began coming to Minnesota to study and observe teaching methods at the College of Veterinary Medicine. That same year, Professor Emeritus Willard L. Boyd went to Korea to study that country's needs in veterinary medicine. In 1960, Dr. John P. Arnold was sent to

Korea to coordinate activities and assist the faculty at Seoul National University. Under the agreement, 12 faculty members of the Veterinary College of Seoul National University spent various periods of time at the College of Veterinary Medicine at the University of Minnesota. Many of these faculty members earned advanced degrees from the University of Minnesota.

Dr. Hannis Stoddard joined the staff of the College of Veterinary Medicine in 1970 as professor and director of International Programs. When Dr. Stoddard left the university, Dr. Dale Sorensen assumed responsibility for the international programs.

In 1980, the College of Veterinary Medicine became a participant in the program to assist the Institute Agronomique at Veterinarie Hassan II in Morocco through the U.S. Agency for International Development. The major emphasis of this program has been on Ph.D. level training and development of the veterinary faculty in Morocco. The College of Veterinary Medicine and the College of Agriculture have played important roles in developing veterinary research and education in Morocco. Several College of Veterinary Medicine faculty members have gone to Morocco to provide expertise in special areas. Dr. Donald Johnson, professor in the Department of Large Animal Clinical Sciences, has served as Team Leader in Rabat, Morocco.

In November 1983, the dean of the College of Veterinary Medicine and the dean of the Republic Faculty of Veterinary Medicine in Montevideo, Uruguay, signed a memorandum of understanding to conduct a technical exchange in teaching and research. The agreement was entitled the Minnesota Uruguay Partners of the Americas Program. Dr. Stanley Diesch, professor of Large Animal Clinical Sciences, has served as chairman of this project and several faculty members from the College of Veterinary Medicine have traveled to Uruguay to assist in the project. In 1984, the American Express Company Partners Award was presented to the Minnesota-Uruguay Partners in Veterinary Medicine for Outstanding Achievement in Program Development.

In addition to involvement in these projects, members of the faculty of the College of Veterinary Medicine have taken numerous assignments in foreign countries for various agencies of the Department of State while others have been employed for various periods of time by other nations or private industry in foreign coun-

4/   "FOA" stood for Foreign Operations Agreement.

tries. Additionally, the scope of training graduate students from foreign countries in the College of Veterinary Medicine is evident by the fact that 58 percent of the 1987 graduate students were from foreign countries.

ANIMAL HOUSING UNITS AND VETERINARY FARM

Large animals such as horses and cattle used for research were housed in the three barns that had been labeled as Units I, II, and III, as well in the area now occupied by the first animal research building. The "Units" were built in about 1920. Teaching animals were also housed in these buildings after the College of Veterinary Medicine was established. For a long time, the teaching animals were used in an informal and uncontrolled manner. However, in 1953, the college decided to assign one person to coordinate the use of these animals. Dr. Lester Larson was placed in charge of the teaching animals and the barns. When Dr. Larson left the university in 1958, Dr. Edward Usenik assumed these responsibilities. In 1960, Dr. Wallace Wass was given charge of the animals and these barns, as well as the veterinary farm at Rosemount. When Dr. Wass left the university, the position passed between Drs. Usenik and John P. Arnold, and was eventually delegated to Dr. William Olson. In 1980, Mr. Lester Westendorp was assigned responsibilities for these duties and Dr. Olson continued to provide services in an advisory capacity. Over the years, responsibility for the housing of all the teaching animals has been placed under the direction of Mr. Westendorp.

The veterinary farm at Rosemount is located on land formerly owned and used by the Gopher Ordnance Works. During World War II, the U.S. Government took over farm land near Rosemount and built an ordnance plant to produce ammunition. However, the war ended just as production had started. In July 1946, the university began negotiations with federal agencies to acquire the land known as the Gopher Ordnance Works. In the fall of 1947, the Farm Credit Administration turned over 4,684 acres of land to the university. In 1948, the War Assets Administration turned over 3,325 acres of land to the university, including nearly 300 buildings complete with fixtures, machinery, and other contents. The total amount of land received by the university was 8,019 acres. The government provided the land at no cost but with the express stipulation that the university must use the property

continuously for 25 years. In 1958, the College of Veterinary Medicine was assigned 133.5 acres of the land ceded to the university by the government. Ultimately, the college would receive a total of 260 acres of this land.

The veterinary farm, or the Rosemount Research Center, had been a farm before the Government acquired the property, and the original buildings were still standing on the land. These buildings included a house, dairy barn, laboratory building, and several small buildings or sheds. The college intended to use the farm for housing teaching and research animals and for growth support feeds. Indeed, much of the alfalfa hay feed used in the college still comes from the veterinary farm at Rosemount.

A buffer zone was set up around the farm to prevent the introduction of pathogens, or disease producing agents, that would ruin the research projects by causing disease among research animals and birds. No other domestic animals or birds were permitted within a mile radius of the farm. This buffer zone was especially important when the only fowl pathogen free turkey flock in the state was maintained on the farm. Research on diseases of large animals included respiratory diseases as well as porphyria and leukemia. Research on canine hip dysplasia also took place on the farm.

For years, the farm was operated by Lawrence Oberste. For many years, the farm was the site of the senior picnic, which featured roast pigs and turkeys and later included mutton. Drs. Perman and Hardy supervised the roasting of the pigs, turkeys, and sheep, which always began shortly after midnight.

RAPTOR CENTER

The Raptor Center was organized in 1972 to serve the following objectives: (1) provide care for ill or injured wild raptors and release rehabilitated raptors into wild populations; and (2) gather scientific information about raptors.

The Raptor Center arose out of a research project supervised by Dr. Gary Duke that was intended to study the efficiency of the digestive system in meat-eating birds. The meat-eating birds were compared with grain-eating turkeys. Dr. Duke, who decided to use owls as the research bird, contacted officials with the Department of Natural Resources (DNR) and asked them to provide him with injured owls they found along the road or were brought to the DNR for assistance.

Dr. Duke, an avian physiologist, hoped that he could obtain five or six owls for use in the research project. However, much to his surprise, the DNR brought him 30 owls in response to his request. The care of this many birds presented several problems. However, Dr. Duke never considered destroying the extra birds. He instead resolved to care for their injuries or illnesses. Fortunately, there was a veterinary student named Patrick Redig who offered to help Dr. Duke care of the birds. The combined efforts of these two men to save these owls eventually led to the development of the Raptor Center.

In caring for the injured owls, Dr. Duke and Patrick Redig determined that some of the owls could be healed and returned to the wild. Gradually, they developed successful methods of anesthetizing, treating injuries, and rehabilitating raptors to allow them to return to their native habitat.

News of their success in repairing and healing injured raptors spread, and they received more and more raptor patients. Veterinary students and others who learned of the project volunteered to help the budding Raptor Center. From 1972 to 1974, 280 birds were saved, and 120 of these were set free in the wild. Two rooms were obtained in the basement of Temporary East of Haecker to house the raptor birds. One room housed the research birds and the other room housed the patients. In addition, because of the lack of space and because some of the birds needed 24 hour care, Dr. Duke and Patrick Redig took many of the birds home with them.

In the beginning, the care of the injured or ill raptor birds was done on a shoestring operation. Funds to take care of raptors were practically nonexistent. A few donations were received for essential equipment, and some supplies and equipment had been left over from other research projects. The funding situation changed dramatically following a meeting Duke and Redig had with the director of a local humane society. The two men had been treating a snowy owl under anesthesia, and the owl had not recovered from the anesthesia by the time they had to leave for their appointment with the director. They did not dare to leave it unattended while recovering from anesthesia, so they took the owl with them to the meeting. The director of the humane society was so impressed with their work on the owl that she gave them the names of foundations that became important sources of revenue for the Raptor Center.

This was a critical time for the Raptor Center as Patrick Redig was graduating from the College of Veterinary Medicine and would have to leave without funds sufficient to give him a staff appointment. Dr. Duke increased his efforts to obtain more funds and, in 1974, the Mardag Foundation offered to provide matching funds to enable the Raptor Center to keep Dr. Redig on staff. The U.S. Department of Interior, through its Division of Fisheries and Wildlife, also helped by making a continuous annual grant of $5,000. Finally, Dean Ewing allotted $5,000 one year from the college's budget to the center.

The Raptor Center received about 200 birds in 1975. This number has increased until it has now reached between 300 and 400 birds per year. By 1986, the center had treated 3,600 raptors, including 500 bald eagles. The recovery rate at the Raptor Center is about 65 percent, with approximately 40 percent of the birds being returned to the wild. The center's fame has spread and is recognized world-wide for its excellent work. Persons interested in caring for injured or ill wild birds have come from foreign countries to study the methods used at the center.

Space, facilities, equipment, and staff have been a problem since the center was created. In 1988, a generous donation from Mr. and Mrs. Don Gabbert funded the construction of the Raptor Building, which is designed exclusively for raptors and consists of nearly 14,000 square feet of space. The Raptor Building was constructed at a cost of $2,400,000.

The staff has increased from just two to nine members. The annual budget has increased to $350,000. Dr. Redig is program director, and Dr. Duke has continued on as a member of the Board of Directors. Barb Walker is the center's coordinator. The U.S. Division of Fisheries and Wildlife has continued to allot $5,000 each year since 1985, and the state of Minnesota provides $40,000 each year to support the center. The remainder of the funds needed to meet the $350,000 budget are raised from private contributions from foundations, businesses, and individuals.

In reviewing the growth and development of the College of Veterinary Medicine at the University of Minnesota, one cannot help but marvel at the steady and effective growth that the college has experienced since 1947. While the appropriations have not always matched the requests, the college has relied on and received important state findings to make its growth and success possible. See Exhibit IV-4.

EXHIBIT IV-4

SUMMARY OF REQUESTS AND APPROPRIATIONS FOR PHYSICAL FACILITIES OF THE COLLEGE OF VETERINARY MEDICINE

1947 $600,000 appropriated for the establishment of a school of veterinary medicine: $400,000 to be used for buildings and equipment and $200,000 for supplies, expenses, and salaries.

1949 $600,000 appropriated for first unit of Veterinary Science Building.

1955 $600,000 appropriated for second addition to Veterinary Science Building.

1957 $600,000 appropriated for Diagnostic Laboratory; $100,000 appropriated for Veterinary Science Building ($300,000 matching funds received from NIH).

1959 $550,000 requested for addition to Veterinary Science Building; no appropriation.

1961 $616,000 requested and appropriated for additional two floors on Veterinary Science Building ($294,000 matching funds were obtained from NIH).

1965 $1,500,000 requested for addition to Veterinary Clinic Building; $1,000,000 appropriated, $500,000 obtained from Title I funds.

1967 $720,000 requested and appropriated for addition to Diagnostic and Research Laboratory; $97,000 requested for Veterinary Medicine Building planning; $171,000 appropriated for Animal Science and Veterinary Medicine Phase I planning; $522,000 appropriated to make up remaining deficiency of addition to Veterinary Clinic Building.

1971 $120,000 requested and appropriated for preliminary planning for Phase II; $10,000,000 requested and appropriated for Phase I Animal Science — Veterinary Medicine facility.

1973 $480,000 requested, and $300,000 appropriated for construction plans for Phase II.

1975 No legislative request — delayed due to status of Wisconsin decision on regional education.

1977 $17,706,000 requested for construction; no appropriation.

1978 Legislation developed to appropriate $17,000,000 for Phase II construction given that Wisconsin passed legislation committing that state to a regional program. Following the decision in Wisconsin not to develop a regional program, the University was instructed to present plans in 1979 for facilities to accommodate 80 students per class.

1979 $12,500,000 requested for Phase II construction; $13,600,000 was appropriated to complete the project.

Source: Courtesy of Dr. Dale K. Sorenson.

EARLY WOMEN GRADUATES OF THE COLLEGE OF VETERINARY MEDICINE

No women applied for enrollment in the first class at the College of Veterinary Medicine. However, JoAnne Schmidt and Griselda (Bee) Wolf applied for admission to and were accepted as members of the class of 1952. Both women were initially rejected when they applied for admission to the class that entered in the fall of 1948. At the time, the Admissions Committee believed that women would not be able to complete the required course work for the veterinary degree. Veterinary medicine was thought to be too physically demanding for women, and the veterinary practitioners and clientele were generally reluctant to accept women veterinarians.

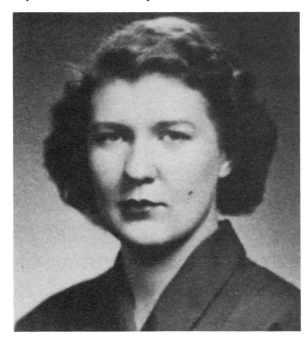

JoAnne Schmidt O'Brien.

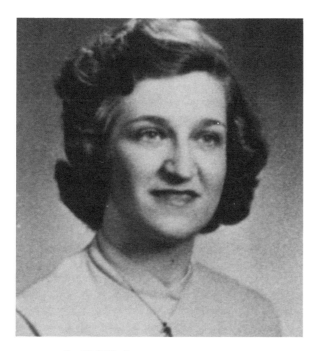

Bee Wolf Hanlon.

Furthermore, the Admissions Committee believed the attrition rate of women students would be high due to marriage and family responsibilities. If a woman student was accepted and later dropped out due for these reasons, she would have taken the place of a male student who would have remained in school and become a member of the profession.

These two women were highly qualified candidates for admission. JoAnne Schmidt had wished to pursue veterinary medicine since she was a junior in high school and had learned there were women veterinarians. She went on to complete one year of pre-veterinary medicine at the University of Illinois. Since Illinois had not yet opened their school of veterinary medicine, Schmidt returned to Minnesota to complete her pre-veterinary courses at the university. She had hopes of enrolling in the new college. Schmidt was a dog breeder and an experienced handler of dogs. Because of her background, she was offered employment at a large collie kennel in St. Paul. The employment at the collie kennel was important as it would provide her with living and tuition expenses while attending veterinary school.

Bee Wolf had graduated from Montana State University with a bachelor's in entomology. Following graduation in 1943, she worked as an entomologist in Southern California studying the transmission of equine encephalitis. She was stationed at the Hooper Foundation in the University of California Medical School in San Francisco where she worked under the famed research veterinarian Dr. Karl F. Meyer. In 1944, Bee enlisted in the U.S. Navy and was attached to an epidemiology unit at the Naval Hospital in San Diego, California. During World War II, Wolf met a woman in San Diego who was a medical doctor in charge of an animal hospital at the Balboa Park Zoo. That doctor introduced Wolf to animal medicine and inspired her to go into that field. Following her discharge, Wolf took up residence in Minnesota with her husband. Upon hearing of the new veterinary school and completing the required husbandry courses, she applied for admission at the college.

In 1948, both women applied for enrollment in the college for the fall quarter. At the time, neither woman knew that the other had applied for admission to the college. Wolf returned to Montana for summer employment with the forest service. Schmidt remained in St. Paul where she continued to manage the kennel. At the end of August, neither of these women had been notified of any action on their application for admission. Schmidt went to see Dr. Martin Roepke, chair of the Admissions Committee, to inquire about her application. He informed her they were not accepting women to veterinary medicine that year. At approximately the same time, Wolf received a letter in Montana notifying her that women were not being accepted in the veterinary curriculum.

Schmidt informed her employer, Mrs. Viola Bantle, of the Admission Committee's decision not to accept women. Mrs. Bantle, a prominent resident of St. Paul and an alumnus of the University of Minnesota, was outraged. She immediately spoke to her influential friends about the decision. Mrs. Bantle's friends included members of the Board of Regents, trustees and alumni of the university, bank presidents and directors, and other distinguished persons. Letters and telephone calls poured in to the university administration.

Schmidt was subsequently advised to meet with Henry Schmitz, dean of the College of Agriculture, Forestry, and Home Economics, who told her that he had received a great volume of mail in support of her admission. He also indicated his daughter, Mary, who worked in the

Division of Veterinary Medicine, had kept him informed of the latest news in the school. When Dean Schmitz inquired of the Admissions Committee about Schmidt's rejection, he was informed that she was not a resident of Minnesota and therefore did not qualify for admission. Dean Schmitz advised Schmidt to petition for the status of an emancipated minor so she could become a resident. He promised in the meantime to work with the administration of the veterinary school on this issue.

Shortly after this meeting and four days before classes began, Schmidt was notified of her acceptance to the college. Wolf also received a telegram inviting her to attend class that fall. Schmidt and Wolf met for the first time at their 8 o'clock class on the first day of classes. They developed a close friendship that has continued ever since.

The classrooms at the college had originally been equipped for the 48 men who had already been accepted. With the admission of Wolf and Schmidt, the 1948 entering class had 50 students. To accommodate the two women students, two chairs were added to the classrooms.

Because of the short notice, as well as the overall shortage of space, funds for teaching, and laboratory facilities, no provisions were made for women students. Throughout their student days in veterinary medicine, Schmidt and Wolf had to cope with many indignities. Beginning with their freshman year in Old Anatomy, and continuing through their sophomore year in Temporary East of Haecker and their last two years in the Veterinary Clinic, they had lockers and changed clothes in the ladies restroom. They also had to spend time studying, exchanging notes, and eating their lunch in these public facilities. It was not for many years and until many more women students were enrolled that the facilities were finally modified to accommodate women.

After the initial shock, the men students more or less accepted having women in their classes. The women asked no favors and none were given. Schmidt and Wolf each performed exceptionally well throughout the four years and graduated in the upper third of their class.

Following graduation, Dr. Schmidt practiced in the Anti-Cruelty Society Clinic in Chicago, Illinois. There she gained valuable experience and, after her marriage in 1959, she practiced in Washington, D.C., and in Jacksonville, North Carolina. In 1972, she became the owner of a small animal hospital in Washington, D.C. Her clients included such prominent individuals as Senator Howard Baker, J. Edgar Hoover, John Foster Dulles, several ambassadors, and cabinet members. She served as a member of the Board of Veterinary Examiners in Washington, D.C., for many years.

Since her retirement in 1987 after 35 years in practice, Dr. Schmidt O'Brien has continued to pursue her hobby of breeding and raising Chow dogs. She has also served on the committee that wrote the judging standards for this breed and has been invited to judge Chow shows throughout the United States and abroad.

Dr. Bee Wolf Hanlon remained at the university where she completed the master's program in veterinary medicine. She specialized in radiology and completed the requirements for board examinations in veterinary radiology. In 1969, she passed the examinations and became the first woman Diplomate of the American College of Radiology.

Dr. Bee Hanlon advanced in rank from instructor to professor at the College of Veterinary Medicine where she taught undergraduate and graduate students. In 1970, she was the U.S. representative to the International Veterinary Radiology Association. A year later, she was elected president of the American Radiology Society. She has taken a quarter leave to Bristol, England, to study radiology, and she has also spent a sabbatical year in the radiology department at the Royal Veterinary College in Stockholm, Sweden. Dr. Hanlon retired after 33 years at the university. However, she continues to perform consulting work and is active in the Minnesota Veterinary Historical Museum.

The acceptance of Drs. Schmidt O'Brien and Bee Wolf Hanlon in the veterinary curriculum was not followed by an immediate increase in the number of women veterinary students at Minnesota. Prior to 1970, in some years no women were accepted and, in other years, anywhere from one to three women received their D.V.M. In 1970, the number of women who graduated increased to six. The names of women who graduated from the College through 1970 are listed in Exhibit V-5.

EXHIBIT V-5

WOMEN GRADUATES OF THE COLLEGE OF
VETERINARY MEDICINE

JoAnne Schmidt O'Brien	1952
Griselda (Bee) Wolf Hanlon	1952
Ruth Krueger	1956
Ann Holt	1958
Barbara J. Follstad	1960
Francine Gough	1960
Donna DenBoer	1961
Susan Daniels	1964
Geraldine Osterberg	1964
Evelyn Groth	1965
Edith M. Lucas	1965
Judy Soderstrom	1965
Ellen L. Ferdon	1966
Alice L. Larson	1966
Margo Myers	1967
Alvina Cook	1968
Bonnie Gustafson	1968
Sharon Wachs	1969
Linda Gandrud	1970
Arleen Larson	1970
Diane Lauritsen	1970
Judy Ann McBain	1970
Patricia Schultz	1970
Priscilla Stockner	1970

The number of women students continued to gradually increase. By 1975, 24 percent of the students in the College of Veterinary Medicine were women. Since the 1980s, about half of the students at the College have been women.

MINNESOTA STUDENT CHAPTER OF THE AMERICAN
VETERINARY MEDICAL ASSOCIATION

The American Veterinary Medical Association sponsors student chapters in veterinary colleges. The first veterinary class at the College of Veterinary Medicine formed the Minnesota Student Chapter (SCAVMA) in the fall of 1947. Ithel Schipper served several terms as president. The organization held its first Christmas Party in 1947 at a total cost of less than $10.00.

The goals of the SCAVMA are to make the veterinary student's life more pleasant, to further educational experience, and to help improve the veterinary college overall. The Chapter has acted as a voice for the student body and has established a student bookstore.

The National Organization of Student Chapters of the AVMA holds expositions for its members. In 1973, the Minnesota Student Chapter hosted the Third National Exposition and, in 1986, hosted the sixteenth such exposition, where there were 100 hours of lectures and 100 hours of "wet labs." Approximately 1,300 persons attended. Although the exposition was a tremendous undertaking for the students, the guests had an enjoyable as well as educational visit.

PHI ZETA — KAPPA CHAPTER

Signatures of Charter Members of Kappa Chapter, Phi Zeta (honorary veterinary fraternity) signed June 13, 1952.

Phi Zeta is the National Honor Society of Veterinary Medicine. It was founded in 1925 at Cornell University and has local chapters at numerous veterinary colleges.

In 1951, Dr. Willard L. Boyd appointed an ad hoc committee to investigate the establishment of an honorary professional veterinary fraternity at the University of Minnesota. The members of the committee included Drs. A. F. Sellers, as chair; Harvey H. Hoyt; and Alvin Weber. The committee recommended establishing a chapter of Phi Zeta. Following an informal meeting of faculty members who were members of Phi Zeta at other veterinary colleges, the college contacted the headquarters of National Phi Zeta and successfully petitioned for the creation of the Kappa Chapter at the University of Minnesota.

A committee was formed to select the members to be initiated at a banquet on June 13, 1952. The committee consisted of Drs. Harvey Hoyt, as chair, H. C. H. Kernkamp; Ralph Kitchell; Clarence Stowe; and George Mather. The initiation banquet was held in the Faculty Club Rooms in the Coffman Memorial Union. Dr. Earl A. Hewitt of Iowa State University, secretary-treasurer of the National Society, represented Phi Zeta at the banquet. Dr. Hewitt presented the charter to the Kappa Chapter and installed the charter members. He also installed the new initiates as members of the chapter. In October of 1952, the newly formed Kappa Chapter of Phi Zeta held its first meeting. Dr. A. F. Sellers was elected president, Dr. Donald W. Johnson, vice president, and Dr. Ralph L. Kitchell, secretary-treasurer.

The chapter agreed to sponsor an annual lecture in veterinary medicine. Drs. H. C. H. Kernkamp and John P. Arnold were appointed to arrange the first lecture. Since that time, the Kappa Chapter has also held spring initiation and banquets, sponsored lectureships, and awarded prizes for excellence in research.

VETERINARY TECHNICIANS

Veterinarians in the United States have used assistants in their practice since the time of the first graduate veterinarians. Assistants were first used on a part-time basis during busy periods such as in the spring to help with the castration of horses and treatment of obstetrical cases. The assistants would hold the twitch on a horse for restraint or would pull the rope in obstetrical cases. Assistants would carry the instrument and medicine bags for the veterinarian, clean instruments, and help in the office. Assistants were men and, in Minnesota, many were retired farmers.

As veterinary medicine advanced, assistants were called upon to perform more technical tasks. Development of small animal practices, advances in surgery and radiology, and greater reliance on laboratory work increased the need for assistants in large and busy practices. Veterinarians also began to hire women as well as men to work as assistants.

With the increased demand for trained veterinary assistants, institutions developed to offer training programs for assistants. These programs were created to train technicians to assist veterinarians in the examination of patients, medical treatment, vaccinations, radiology, and surgery. The programs also trained students in office procedures such as scheduling, receiving patients, and record keeping. At first, the students were called "animal technicians," but the title was subsequently changed to "veterinary technicians."

UNIVERSITY OF MINNESOTA, WASECA

The first veterinary technician program in Minnesota was offered at the technical agricultural college campus of the University of Minnesota in Waseca in 1971. Dr. W. Clough Cullen was director of the veterinary technician program. The two-year program consisted of seven quarters: five quarters were spent taking courses on campus; one quarter was spent on a selected veterinary practice, laboratory, or zoo; and one quarter was spent at the College of Veterinary Medicine on the St. Paul Campus of the University of Minnesota, where students would go through a clinical rotation in the Veterinary Teaching Hospital. During the quarter at the college, the students took field trips to research laboratories, commercial pharmaceutical and biological laboratories, licensed dog shows, zoos, and animal research centers such as the Mayo Clinic at Rochester. The program covered subjects in both large and small animals, zoo animals, laboratory animals, birds, and laboratory work.

Since the first class of 14 graduated in 1973, the veterinary technician classes have increased in size until classes of about 60 were graduated each year. The faculty originally consisted of one veterinarian plus support staff. The faculty subsequently grew to four veterinarians plus support staff. Veterinarians on the faculty included Drs. Wilbur Leibrand, as director, Karen Brandt; Janet Donlin; and Larry Sinn.

The Veterinary Technician Program was accredited by the Committee on Animal Technician Activities of the American Veterinary Medical Association. Upon graduation, the students received the Associate in Applied Degree with a major in Veterinary Technology. They were qualified to take the Minnesota Veterinary Technician Certification Examination or similar examinations in other states.

When the University of Minnesota began to have budget problems and required departments to cut expenses, the Veterinary Technician Program at Waseca reduced to the point where Dr. Betsy Torgeson was the only veterinarian on the faculty. Notwithstanding these efforts, the program was altogether eliminated when the Waseca Campus was closed on June 30, 1992.

WILLMAR TECHNICAL COLLEGE

The Willmar Technical College, which is part of the Minnesota Technical College System, began to offer a Veterinary Technician Program in the fall of 1992. The courses are similar to those offered in the Waseca Veterinary Technicians Program. Dr. Betsy Torgeson is the lead instructor in the program. Mr. Steve Hormann, an experienced veterinary technician, is another instructor in the program. The Willmar Technical College was able to obtain most of the equipment used in the Veterinary Technician Program from the Waseca Campus of the University of Minnesota.

MEDICAL INSTITUTE OF MINNESOTA

The Medical Institute of Minnesota was founded in 1961 to train medical technicians. The facilities include the main campus on Nicollet Avenue in Minneapolis and additional space in St. Paul and Brooklyn Center.

In 1975, the Veterinary Technician Program at the Medical Institute of Minnesota began with Dr. Henry Philmon as program director. Twenty-four students were accepted in the institute's first class. The institute offers both day and night programs. The day program consists of seven quarters while the night program is made up of fourteen quarters.

The program covers both large and small animals, birds, zoo animals, radiology, and laboratory work. Approximately 65 percent of the students' time is spent in classroom work and 35 percent is spent in laboratories. Once the course work at the institute is completed, the students take one quarter of clinical training in an approved veterinary facility.

The Veterinary Technician Program at the Medical Institute has grown from 24 students in 1975 to approximately 40 students in each class in the 1990s. Dr. Jeffrey Hall is the present program director, and Dr. Mark Gluck is assistant director.

The institute's program is accredited by the Committee on Veterinary Technician Activities of the American Veterinary Medical Association. The graduates receive Associate of Science Degree in Veterinary Technology, and are qualified to take the Minnesota Veterinary Technician Certification Examination or similar examinations in other states.

GRADUATING CLASS PHOTOGRAPHS

COLLEGE OF VETERINARY MEDICINE

UNIVERSITY OF MINNESOTA

1951 to and Including the class of 1993

In Chronological Order

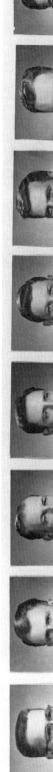
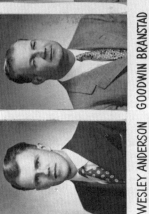
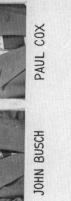
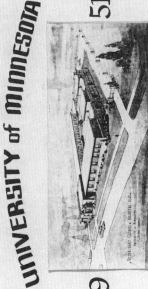
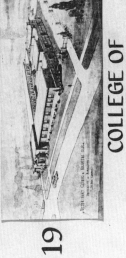
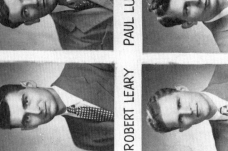
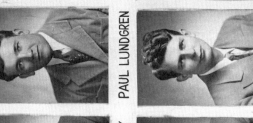
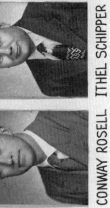
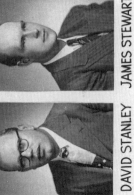

UNIVERSITY of MINNESOTA

19 51

COLLEGE OF
VETERINARY MEDICINE

WILLIAM GLADITSCH

STANLEY JEPSON

GLEN NELSON

JAMES STEWART

JOHN FOGARTY

BRUCE HOHN

WALTER MACKEY

DAVID STANLEY

VERNIE DAHL

ITHEL SCHIPPER

PAUL COX

CONWAY ROSELL

JOHN BUSCH

LESTER REDDER

GOODWIN BRANSTAD

ROBERT PYLE

WESLEY ANDERSON

PAUL LUNDGREN

DEAN WILLARD BOYD

KENNETH PALMER

ARCH ALEXANDER

DONALD HICKS

ROBERT LEARY

VERN OLSON

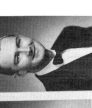

UNIVERSITY of MINNESOTA 1952
College of Veterinary Medicine

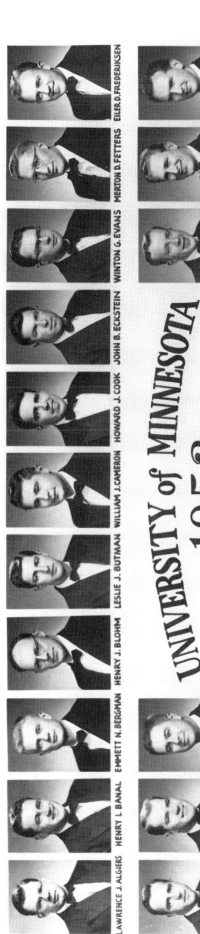
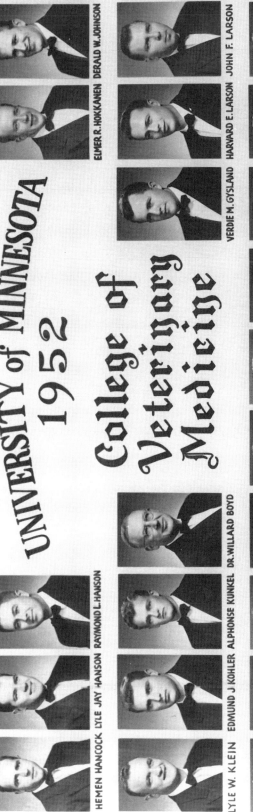
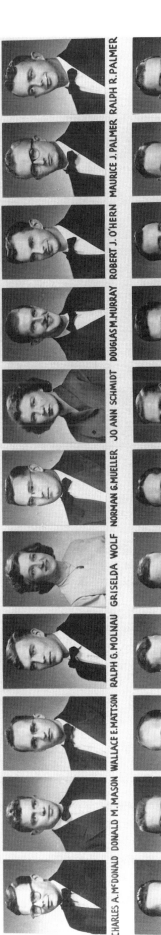
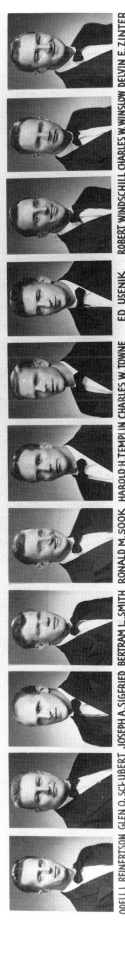
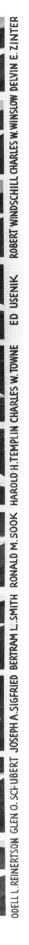

EILER D.FREDERIKSEN MERTON D.FETTERS WINTON G.EVANS JOHN B.ECKSTEIN HOWARD J.COOK WILLIAM J.CAMERON LESLIE J.BUTMAN HENRY J.BLOHM EMMETT N.BERGHAN RAYMOND L.HANSON LYLE JAY HANSON HEMEN HANCOCK HENRY L.BANAL LAWRENCE J.ALGIERS

DEAN R.KINGREY DERALD W.JOHNSON ELMER R.HOKKANEN VERDIE M.GYSLAND

LESTER L.LARSON JOHN F.LARSON HARVARD E.LARSON

RALPH R.PALMER MAURICE J.PALMER ROBERT J.O'HERN DOUGLAS M.MURRAY JO ANN SCHMIDT NORMAN G.MUELLER GRISELDA WOLF RALPH G.MOLNAU WALLACE E.MATTSON DONALD M.MASON CHARLES A.McDONALD

DELVIN E.ZINTER CHARLES W.WINSLOW ROBERT WINDSCHILL ED USENIK CHARLES W.TOWNE HAROLD H.TEMPLIN RONALD M.SOOK BERTRAM L.SMITH JOSEPH A.SIGFRIED GLEN O.SCHUBERT ODELL L.REINERTSON

DR.WILLARD BOYD ALPHONSE KUNKEL EDMUND J KOHLER LYLE W.KLEIN

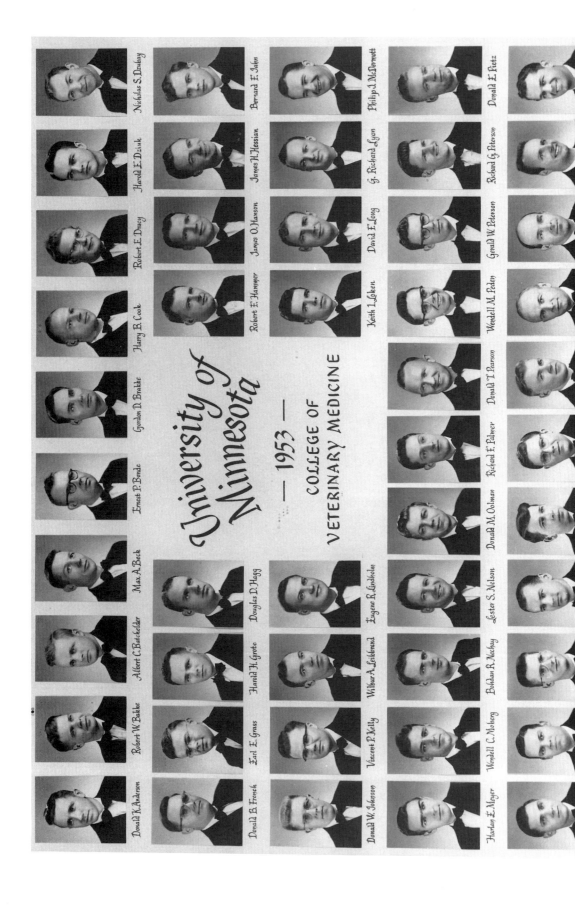

University of Minnesota

— 1953 —

COLLEGE OF VETERINARY MEDICINE

Donald K. Anderson Robert W. Bakke Max A. Beck Albert C. Batchelder Ernest P. Bonde Gordon D. Brakke Harry B. Cook Robert E. Dracy Harold E. Dink Nicholas S. Drubay

Donald B. French Earl E. Grass Harold H. Grote Douglas D. Hagg Robert E. Hanuyer James O. Hanson Keith L. Loken David F. Long G. Richard Lyon Bernard F. Jahn James H. Hessian Philip J. McDermott

Donald W. Johnson Vincent P. Kelly Wilbur A. Leibbrand Eugene R. Lindholm Donald M. Oolman Donald T. Pearson Wendell M. Peden Gerald W. Peterson Richard G. Peterson Donald E. Pietz

Harlan E. Meyer Wendell C. Moberg Bohdan R. Neohuy Lester S. Nelson Leroy W. Thom Richard F. Palmer Wallace M. Wass Philip J. Whalen Rufus F. Weidner Stanford J. Wilson

Milton L. Pietz Francis F. Siegfried Robert H. Steinkraus Harold L. Strandberg Elroy M. Thom Leo A. Zehrer

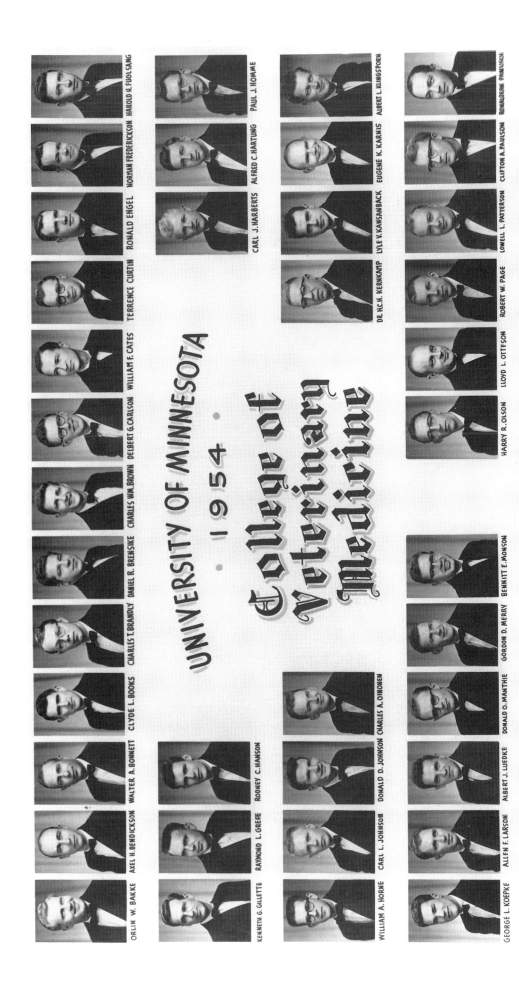

UNIVERSITY OF MINNESOTA
· 1 9 5 4 ·

College of Veterinary Medicine

ORLIN W. BAKKE • AXEL H. BENDICKSON • WALTER A. BONNETT • CLYDE L. BOOKS • CHARLES T. BRANDLY • DANIEL R. BRENSIKE • CHARLES WM. BROWN • DELBERT G. CARLSON • WILLIAM F. CATES • TERRENCE CURTIN • RONALD ENGEL • NORMAN FREDERICKSON • HAROLD H. FUGLSANG

KENNETH G. GILLETTE • RAYMOND L. GREEF • RODNEY C. HANSON • PAUL J. HOMME

WILLIAM A. HORNE • CARL L. JOHNSON • DONALD D. JOHNSON • CHARLES A. OIHONEN

CARL J. HARBERTS • ALFRED C. HARTUNG

DR. H.C.H. KERNKAMP • LYLE V. KANSANBACK • EUGENE K. KARNIS • ALBERT L. KLINGSPORN

GEORGE L. KOEPKE • ALLEN F. LARSON • ALBERT J. LUEDKE • DONALD O. MANTHIE • GORDON D. MERRY • BENNITT E. MONSON

HARRY R. OLSON • LLOYD L. OTTESON • ROBERT W. PAGE • LOWELL L. PATTERSON • CLIFTON A. PAULSON • RONALD GENE PAWLUSCH

JOHN C. SCHLOTTHAUER • CHARLES R. SHREFFLER • CHARLES E. STEVENS • LOREN L. STOCK • MELVIN W. STROMBERG • DAN E. SUTHER • I. LELAND THAL • ROBERT F. WALSER • DONALD R. WENGER • DANIEL A. WEST • EUGENE L. WHITFORD • ROGER L. WINANS • JAMES R. ZOSEL

UNIVERSITY OF MINNESOTA
1955
School of Veterinary Medicine

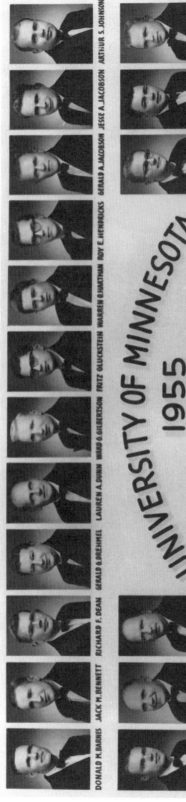
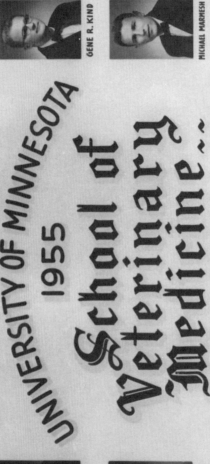
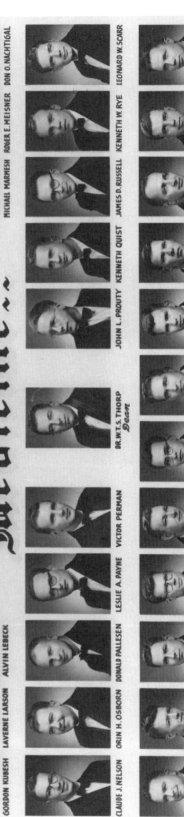
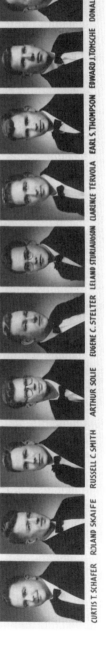

DONALD M. BARNES
JACK M. BENNETT
RICHARD F. DEAN
GERALD G. DREHMEL
LAUREN A. DUNN
WARD G. GILBERTSON
FRITZ GLUCKSTEIN
WARREN O. HARTNAM
ROY E. HENDRICKS
GERALD A. JACOBSON
JESSE A. JACOBSON
ARTHUR S. JOHNSON

DEAN F. JOHNSON
MARK JUREK
JOHN L. KETOLA
GENE R. KIND
JAMES F. KRIER
HOWARD H. KRUEGER

GORDON KUBESH
LAVERNE LARSON
ALVIN LEBECK
MICHAEL MARMESH
ROGER E. MEISNER
DON O. NACHTIGAL

JOHN L. PROUTY
KENNETH QUIST
LEONARD W. SCARR

DR. W. T. S. THORP
Dean

LESLIE A. PAYNE
VICTOR PERMAN
KENNETH W. RYE

CLAUDE J. NELSON
ORIN H. OSBORN
DONALD PALLESEN
ARTHUR SOLIE
EUGENE C. STELTER
LELAND STURLAUGSON
CLARENCE TERVOLA
EARL S. THOMPSON
EDWARD J. TOMSCHE
DONALD L. WELCH
HUGH C. WILLIAMS
WILLIAM A. ZWIENER

CURTIS T. SCHAFER
ROLAND SKAIFE
RUSSELL C. SMITH
JAMES D. RUSSELL

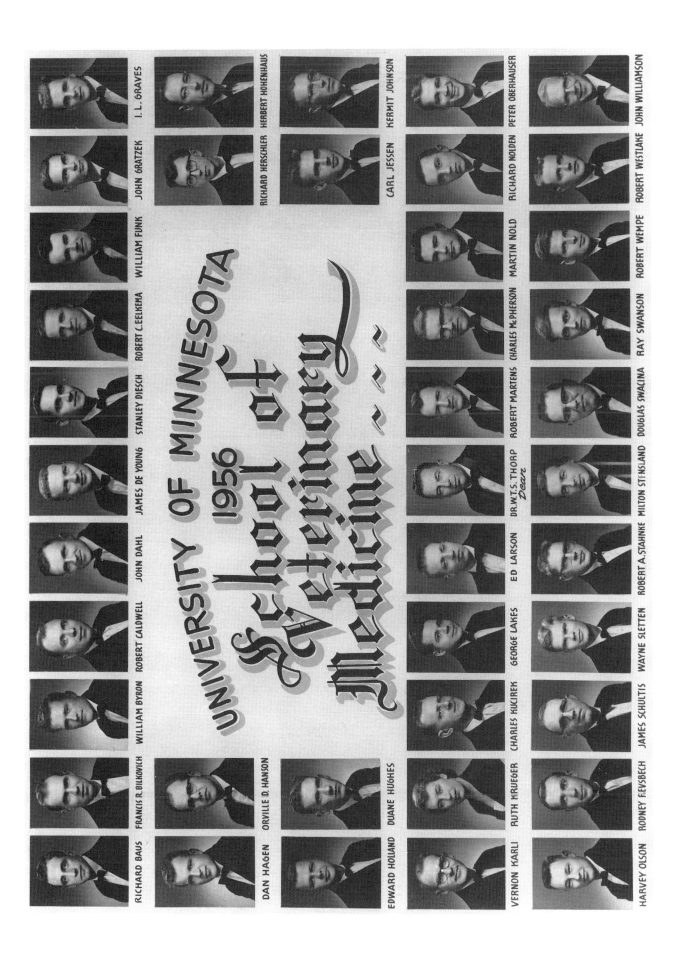

UNIVERSITY OF MINNESOTA
1956
*School of
Veterinary
Medicine*

DR. W.T.S. THORP
Dean

RICHARD BAUS · FRANCIS R. BILKOVICH · WILLIAM BYRON · ROBERT CALDWELL · JOHN DAHL · JAMES DE YOUNG · STANLEY DIESCH · ROBERT C. EELKEMA · WILLIAM FUNK · JOHN GRATZEK · I. L. GRAVES

DAN HAGEN · ORVILLE D. HANSON · RICHARD HERSCHLER · HERBERT HOHENHAUS

EDWARD HOLLAND · DUANE HUGHES · CARL JESSEN · KERMIT JOHNSON

VERNON KARLI · RUTH KRUEGER · CHARLES KUCIREK · GEORGE LAKES · ED LARSON · ROBERT MARTENS · CHARLES McPHERSON · MARTIN NOLD · RICHARD NOLDEN · PETER OBERHAUSER

HARVEY OLSON · RODNEY FEVSBECH · JAMES SCHULTIS · WAYNE SLETTEN · ROBERT A. STAHNKE · MILTON STENSLAND · DOUGLAS SWACINA · RAY SWANSON · ROBERT WEMPE · ROBERT WESTLAKE · JOHN WILLIAMSON

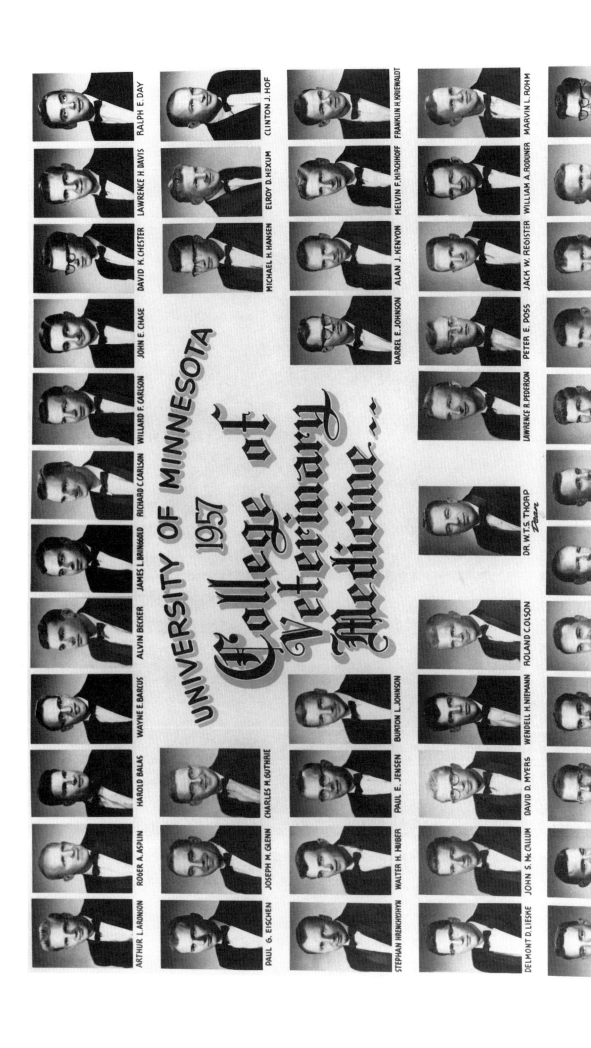

UNIVERSITY OF MINNESOTA
College of Veterinary Medicine
1957

RALPH E. DAY

LAWRENCE H DAVIS

DAVID K. CHESTER

JOHN E. CHASE

WILLARD F. CARLSON

RICHARD C.CARLSON

JAMES L BRINGGOLD

ALVIN BECKER

WAYNE E. BARCUS

HAROLD BALAS

ROGER A. ASPLIN

ARTHUR L. ARONSON

CLINTON J. HOF

ELROY D. HEXUM

MICHAEL H. HANSEN

CHARLES M. GUTHRIE

JOSEPH M. GLENN

PAUL G. EISCHEN

FRANKLIN H. KRIEWALDT

MELVIN F. KIRCHHOFF

ALAN J. KENYON

DARREL E. JOHNSON

BURTON L. JOHNSON

PAUL E. JENSEN

WALTER H. HUBER

STEPHAN HRENCHDHYN

MARVIN L. ROHM

WILLIAM A. RODUNER

JACK W. REGISTER

PETER E. POSS

LAWRENCE R. PEDERSON

DR. W.T.S. THORP
Dean

ROLAND C.OLSON

WENDELL H. NIEMANN

DAVID D. MYERS

JOHN S. McCALLUM

DELMONT D. LIESKE

STUART WYAND

DONALD A. WITZEL

GENE WHEELER

WILLIS J. WESLEY

ROBERT A. WESCOTT

RONALD E. WERDIN

DONALD L. STRANDBERG

STANLEY C. SKADRON

LA VERNE SCHUGEL

CHARLES G.SCHLOTTHAUER

ROBERT C. SARTORI

GERALD M. ROSEN

UNIVERSITY OF MINNESOTA
1958
College of Veterinary Medicine

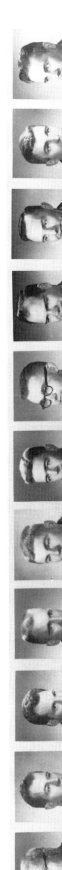
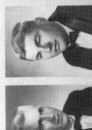
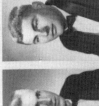
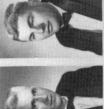
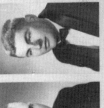
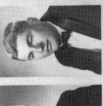
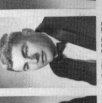
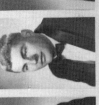
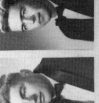
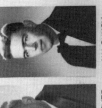
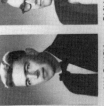
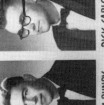
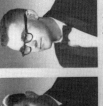
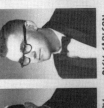
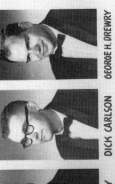
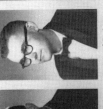
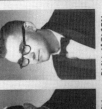
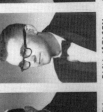
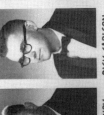
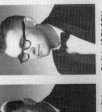
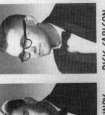
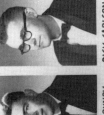
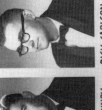
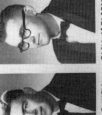
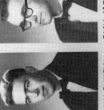
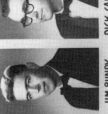
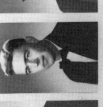
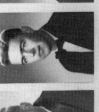
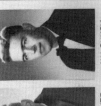
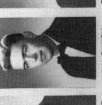
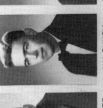
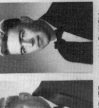
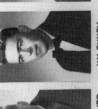
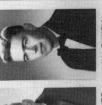
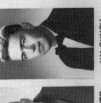
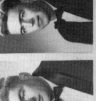
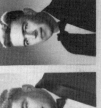
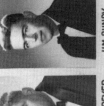
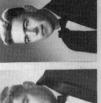
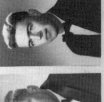
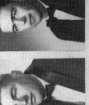
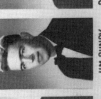
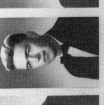
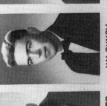
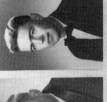
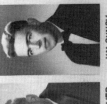
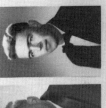
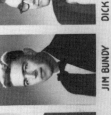
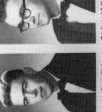
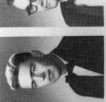
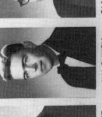
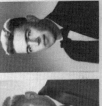

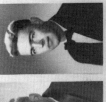
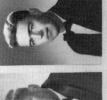

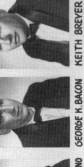

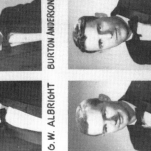

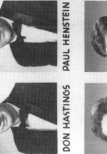
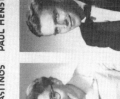
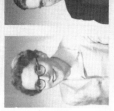
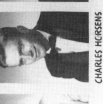
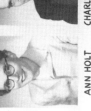
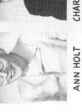
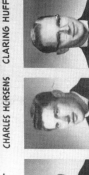
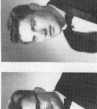
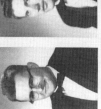
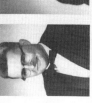
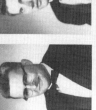
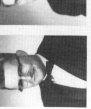
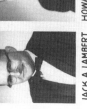
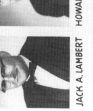
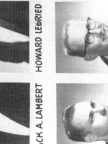
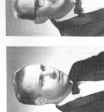
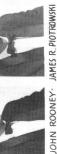

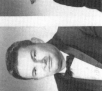
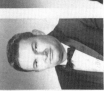
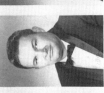
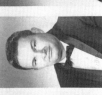
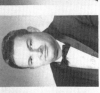

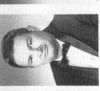

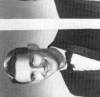

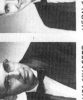
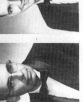
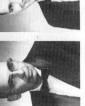
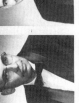
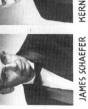
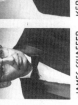
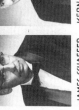
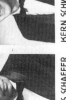

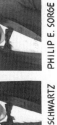
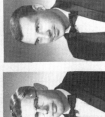
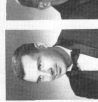
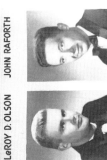

- MAURICE HANIFY
- LAWRENCE W. FERRIGAN
- DONALD A. ELLIS
- GEORGE H. DREWRY
- DICK CARLSON
- JIM BUNDY
- KEITH BREYER
- GEORGE K. BACON
- WENZEL ARMSTRONG
- BURTON ANDERSON
- G. W. ALBRIGHT

- OSCAR HILDEBRANDT
- GARY HIGGINS
- DARREL JOEL
- CLARING HUFF
- CHARLES HERSENS
- PAUL HENSTEIN
- DON HASTINGS
- ANN HOLT

- HAROLD J. KURTZ
- JOHN KOMAREK
- WARREN NYSTROM
- ROBERT NORTHROP
- DR. W. T. S. THORP, Dean
- GEORGE MORGAN
- THOMAS E. LUCAS
- HOWARD LeGRIED
- JACK A. LAMBERT

- JOHN RAFORTH
- LeROY D. OLSON
- CLAYTON TORBERT
- LESTER SWANSON
- RODERICK STENZEL
- JOHN STRACHE
- PHILIP E. SORGE
- KERN SCHWARTZ
- JAMES SCHAEFER
- JAMES R. PIOTROWSKI
- JOHN ROONEY

- ROGER WILSNACK
- RICHARD WESCOTT

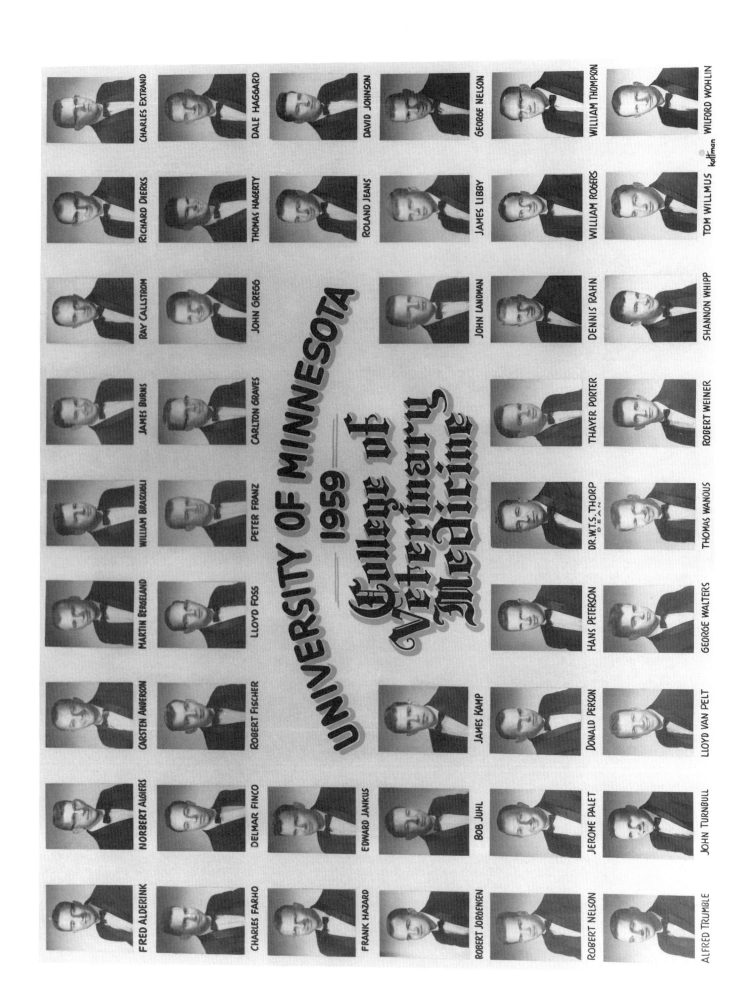

UNIVERSITY OF MINNESOTA
1959
College of Veterinary Medicine

FRED ALDERINK   NORBERT ALGHERS   CARSTEN ANDERSON   MARTIN BERGELAND   WILLIAM BRASCUGLI   JAMES BURNS   RAY CALLSTROM   RICHARD DIERKS   CHARLES EXTRAND

CHARLES FARHO   DELMAR FINCO   ROBERT FISCHER   LLOYD FOSS   PETER FRANZ   CARLTON GRAVES   JOHN GREGG   THOMAS HAGERTY   DALE HAGGARD

FRANK HAZARD   EDWARD JANKUS   JAMES KAMP   DAVID JOHNSON   ROLAND JEANS

ROBERT JORGENSEN   BOB JUHL   DONALD PERSON   HANS PETERSON   DR.W.T.S.THORP DEAN   THAYER PORTER   JOHN LANDMAN   JAMES LIBBY   GEORGE NELSON

ROBERT NELSON   JEROME PALET   LLOYD VAN PELT   GEORGE WALTERS   THOMAS WANOUS   ROBERT WEINER   DENNIS RAHN   WILLIAM ROGERS   WILLIAM THOMPSON

ALFRED TRUMBLE   JOHN TURNBULL   SHANNON WHIPP   TOM WILLMUS   WILFORD WOHLIN

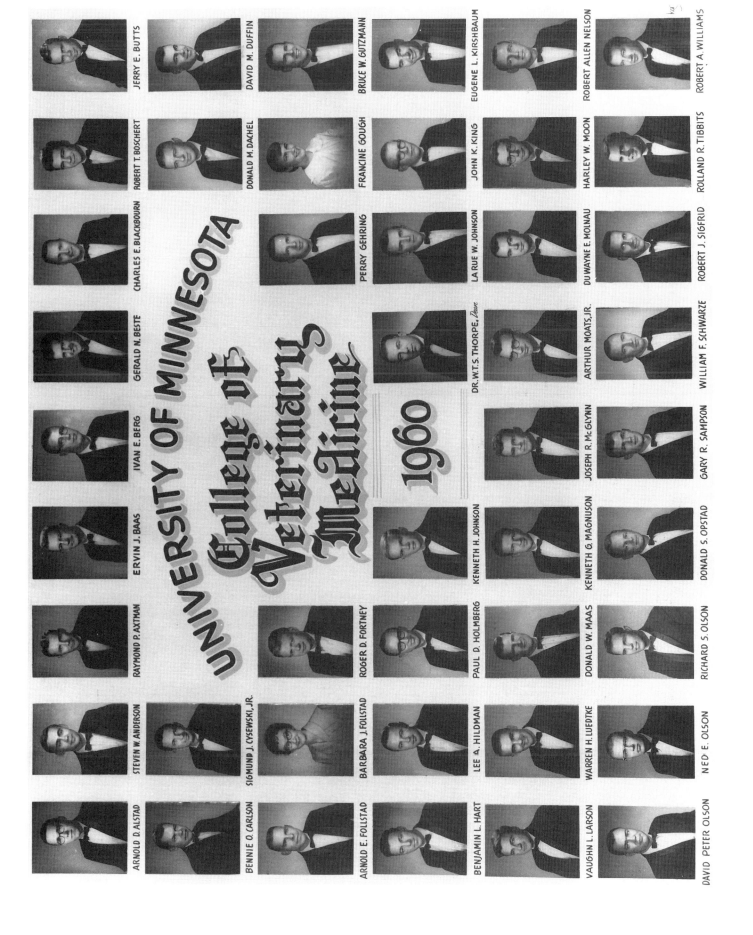

UNIVERSITY OF MINNESOTA
College of Veterinary Medicine
1960

JERRY E. BUTTS

DAVID M. DUFFIN

BRUCE W. GUTZMANN

EUGENE L. KIRSHBAUM

ROBERT ALLEN NELSON

ROBERT A. WILLIAMS

ROBERT T. BOSCHERT

DONALD M. DACHEL

FRANCINE GOUGH

JOHN K. KING

HARLEY W. MOON

ROLLAND R. TIBBITS

CHARLES E. BLACKBOURN

PERRY GEHRING

LA RUE W. JOHNSON

DU WAYNE E. MOLNAU

ROBERT J. SIGFRID

GERALD N. BESTE

DR. W.T.S. THORPE, Dean

ARTHUR MOATS, JR.

WILLIAM F. SCHWARZE

IVAN E. BERG

JOSEPH R. McGLYNN

GARY R. SAMPSON

ERVIN J. BAAS

KENNETH H. JOHNSON

KENNETH G. MAGNUSON

DONALD S. OPSTAD

RAYMOND P. AXTMAN

ROGER D. FORTNEY

PAUL D. HOLMBERG

DONALD W. MAAS

RICHARD S. OLSON

STEVEN W. ANDERSON

SIGMUND J. CYSEWSKI, JR.

BARBARA J. FOLLSTAD

LEE A. HILDMAN

WARREN H. LUEDTKE

NED E. OLSON

ARNOLD D. ALSTAD

BENNIE O. CARLSON

ARNOLD E. FOLLSTAD

BENJAMIN L. HART

VAUGHN L. LARSON

DAVID PETER OLSON

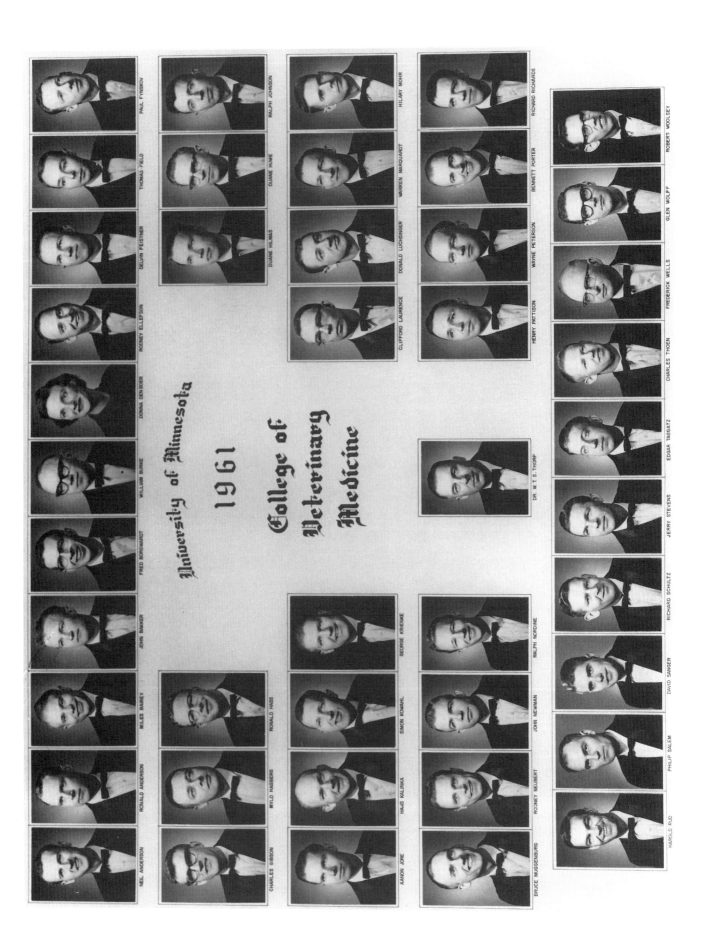

University of Minnesota

1961

College of Veterinary Medicine

NEIL ANDERSON · RONALD ANDERSON · MILES BABBEY · JOHN BAKKER · FRED BORGWARDT · WILLIAM BURKE · DONNA DEN BOER · RODNEY ELLEFSON · DELVIN FEISTNER · THOMAS FIELD · PAUL FYKSON

CHARLES GIBSON · MYLO HAGBERG · RONALD HASS · CLIFFORD LAURENCE · DONALD LUCHSINGER · WAYNE PETERSON · HILARY MOHR · WARREN MARQUARDT · RALPH JOHNSON · DUANE HILMAS · BENNETT PORTER · RICHARD RICHARDS

AARON JORE · HANS KALINKA · SIMON KOWAHL · GEORGE KRIEWME · DR. W.T.S. THORP · HENRY PATTISON

BRUCE MUGGENBURG · RODNEY NEUBERT · JOHN NEWMAN · RALPH NORDINE · PHILIP SALEM · DAVID SANGER · RICHARD SCHULTZ · JERRY STEVENS · EDGAR TAGGATZ · CHARLES THOEN · FREDERICK WELLS · GLEN WOLFF · ROBERT WOOLSEY

HAROLD RUD

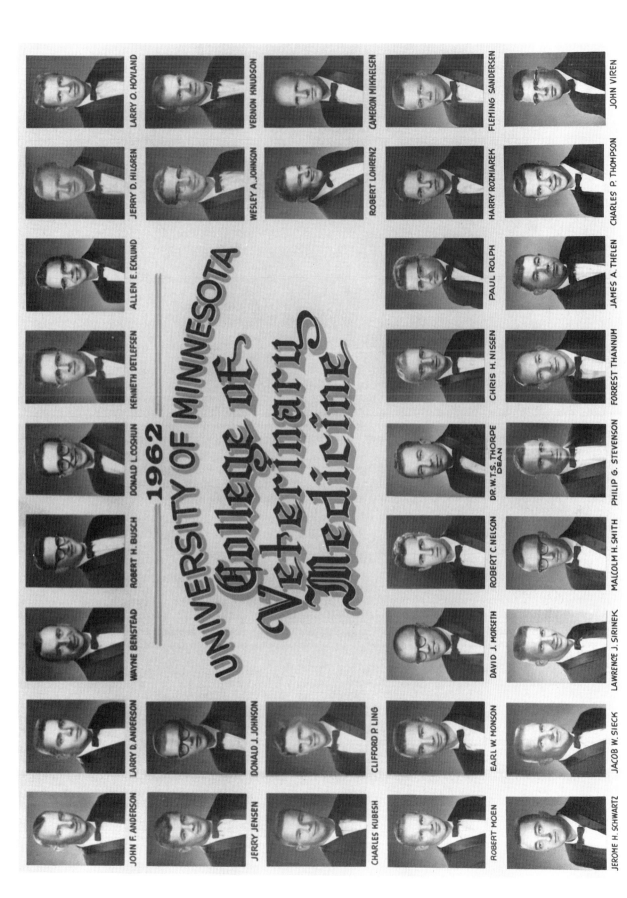

1962
UNIVERSITY OF MINNESOTA
College of Veterinary Medicine

LARRY O. HOVLAND

VERNON KNUDSON

CAMERON MIKKELSEN

FLEMING SANDERSEN

JOHN VIREN

JERRY D. HILGREN

WESLEY A. JOHNSON

ROBERT LOHRENZ

HARRY ROZMIAREK

CHARLES P. THOMPSON

ALLEN E. ECKLUND

PAUL ROLPH

JAMES A. THELEN

KENNETH DETLEFSEN

CHRIS H. NISSEN

FORREST THANNUM

DONALD L. COSHUN

DR. W.T.S. THORPE
DEAN

PHILIP G. STEVENSON

ROBERT H. BUSCH

ROBERT C. NELSON

MALCOLM H. SMITH

WAYNE BENSTEAD

DAVID J. MORSETH

LAWRENCE J. SIRINEK

LARRY D. ANDERSON

DONALD J. JOHNSON

EARL W. MONSON

JACOB W. SIECK

CLIFFORD P. LING

JOHN F. ANDERSON

JERRY JENSEN

CHARLES KUBESH

ROBERT MOEN

JEROME H. SCHWARTZ

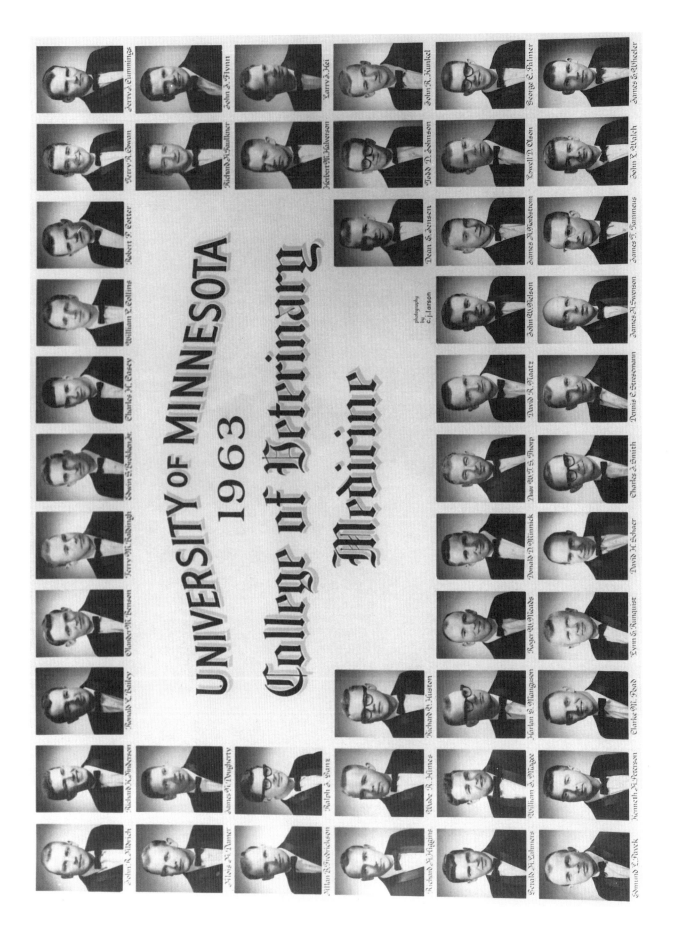

UNIVERSITY OF MINNESOTA
1963
College of Veterinary Medicine

photography by
C. J. Larson

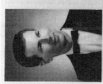 Ronald Ferguson

 James N. Gleason

 Robert E. Kickman

 Kenneth S. Krueger

 Geraldine Osterberg

 Howard A. Stryker

 Melvin E. Fahning

 David A. Espeseth

 Susan Daniels

 Robert Cleary

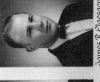 James R. Claesgens

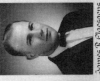 John Breiland

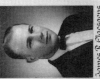 James Andrews

 Wilhelm Hanstad

 Dale Foss

 Dennis Goltz

 John T. Hervet

 Florian Edermann

 Gregory S. Peterson

UNIVERSITY OF MINNESOTA
1964
College of Veterinary
Medicine

photography
by
c.j. larson

 Ronald D. Kuecker

 James D. Mortimer

 Jerome Westweber

 James Moe

 Robert S. Stukel Jr.

 Harold O. Miller

 Wesley E. Schroeder

 Dan W. S. Thorp

 James McLeod

 Ronald D. Ree

 Kermit Lyngaas

 Michael S. Rasmussen

 Donald Janceck

 Glen S. Loosbrock

 Duane A. Purtilo

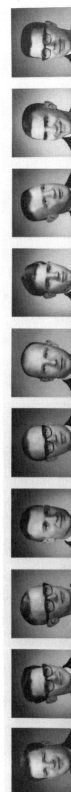
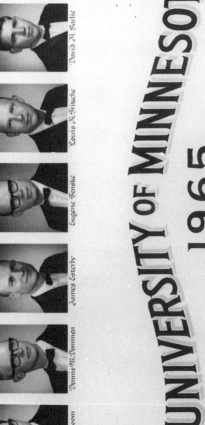
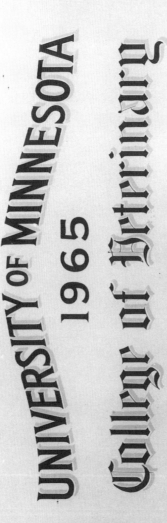

UNIVERSITY OF MINNESOTA
1965
College of Veterinary Medicine

photography
by
c.j.larson

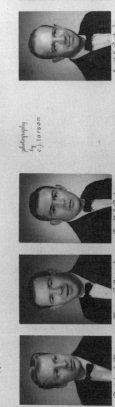
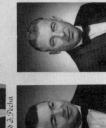

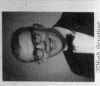

Ronald G. Goos
Larry D. Ecmar
Charles F. Echman
David H. Garlie
Louis N. Fritsche
Eugene Fenske
James Esterly
Dennis McDennnan
Gilbert Beerboom
Milton C. Bauer, Jr.
Larry Baudin
Eldon Buazin

Douglas Edvenson
George D. Ihrke, Jr.

Leonard Knoll
Stan Kleven

Patrick J. Manning
Charles P. Maier, Jr.

Jerome Schmidt
Conrad B. Schm*t
Alan Segen

Russell Urbanksan

Clair D. Souc*
James Starley
George R. Roth
Richard R. Ruhlig
Emil C. Roth, Jr.
Vernon Vallery
Dean W. C. Thorp
Gerald A. Reha
Larry R. Traynor
Norman E. Osgood
Stan E. Thompson
Dwight S. Olson
Alfred Senting
Gerald A. Nidelson
David J. Spong

Evelyr Troth
James B. Johnson
Philip A. Lucas
Douglas R. Jensen
Edith N. Lucas
Charles R. Meiners
Gale E. Nastrom

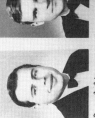

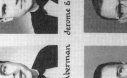

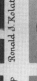

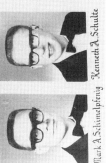
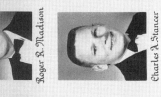

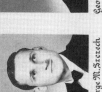

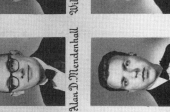

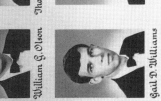
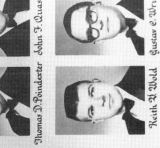

UNIVERSITY OF MINNESOTA

1966

College of Veterinary Medicine

Robert A. Pietl
Gerard A. Pahl
Byron L. Buehli
Gerald F. Francich
Paul L. Berge
Roger W. Boser
Bertram R. Berg
Raymond O. Benson
Alfred W. Anderson
Jerome E. Ahrendt
Dean A. Aberman

Richard E. Faivre
Duane A. Erickson
Edward D. Halls
John G. Fritsche
Thomas A. Lang
David H. Lamphere
John F. Quast
Thomas D. Poindexter
Gustav E. Wruck
Keith D. Wold

William G. Olson
Gail D. Williams
Alan D. Mendenhall
James E. Warling

Dean W.T.S. Thorpe

George A. Twitero
George M. Szczech
Earl H. McCauley
James A. Swenberg
Roger R. Madison
Charles A. Stancer
John B. Luther
Kenneth A. Schulte
Alice L. Larsen
Mark A. Schimelpfenig

Ronald F. Dubbe
Larry E. Eitts
Louie A. Fries
Ellen L. Jerdon
Ronald J. Kolata
David G. Klomp

UNIVERSITY of MINNESOTA

1967

College of Veterinary

Medicine

Dean W.T.S. Thorpe

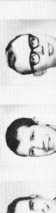 Cameron Gilts

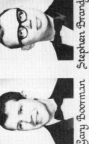 Offiong Eden

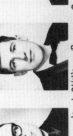 Raymond Diemer

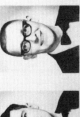 Gary Diehl

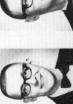 Gordon de Vries

 Paul Dettloff

 Russell Currier II

 William Burnap

 Stephen Brandjord

 Gary Boorman

 Galen Adkins

 Robert Fischar

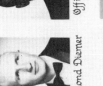 Todd Fetsch

Richard Gebhart, Kenneth Greiner

Douglas Hammer Eugene Holmgren David Jacobs Richard Klimmek Margo Myers

John Loda Donald Mac Martin Tom Mehlhoff William Miller

Leonard Fogelson Lloyd Garrett

David Halvorson, Gordon Hamann

Charles Kratt George Krzaczynski Gary Kuehn

Glenn Kolb

Donn Oelschlager Patrick O'Neil Norman Purrington James Rundquist Bernard Schwetz

Frank Voelker Lyle Vogel

Donald Vezina

Brian Sotvola

Robert Stone

Richard Stalmach

Gary Steen

Kenneth Speltz

Ian Shaw

George Sedgwick

Earl Wahlstrom, Robert Waterman

Studio of The Dayton Company

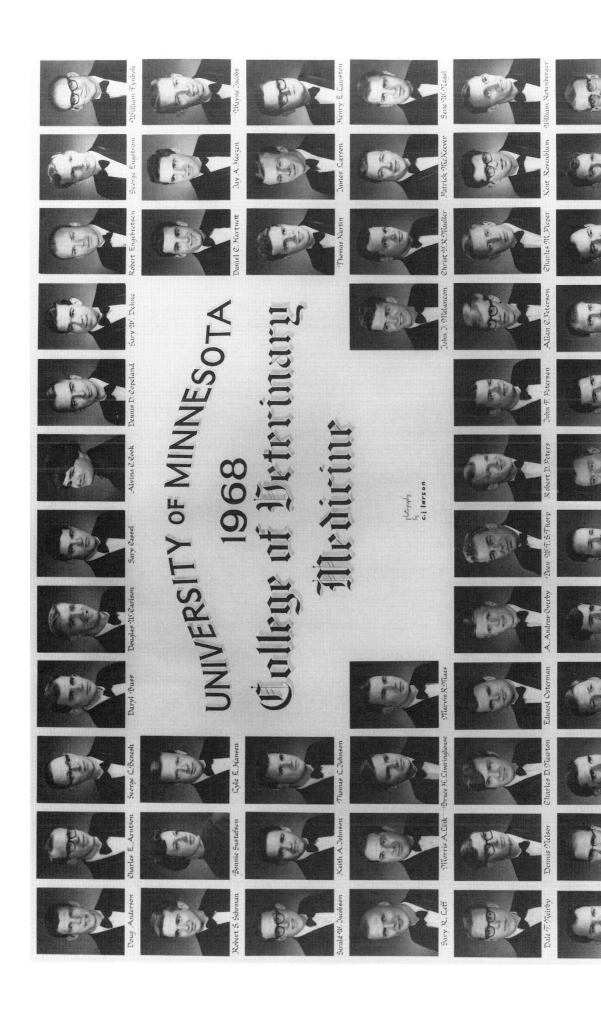

UNIVERSITY OF MINNESOTA
1968
College of Veterinary Medicine

photography by
c.j larson

William Tynboh
Dwayne Jacobs
Henry E. Lawston
Gene McNagel
Glen Zebarth

George Engstrom
Jay A. Hagen
James Larson
Patrick McKeever
Kent Rosenblum
Bradford C. Yoke

Robert Engebretsen
Daniel C. Hartnett
Thomas Kurtin
Christ M. R. Mueller
Charles M. Pieper
James C. Philkus

Gary W. Delue
John J. Melancon
Allan C. Peterson
Richard H. Watkins

Dennis D. Copeland
John F. Peterson
DeWayne H. Walker

Alvina C. Cook
Robert D. Peters
Robert J. Schure

Gary Cassel
Dean W. T. S. Thorp
Adrian F. VanDellen

Douglas W. Carlson
A. Andrew Overby
James Tripp

Daryl Buss
Marvin R. Haas
Edward Osterman
Jerald D. Sprau

Charles E. Arntson
Lyle E. Hansen
Thomas C. Johnson
Bruce H. Liveringhouse
Charles D. Newton
Ronald J. Scheuring
George Schumber

Doug Anderson
Robert S. Sohrman
Gerald W. Jacobson
Gary R. Leff
Morris A. Eisk
Dennis Nelson
Dale T. Kirby
Thomas A. Rutz

Bennie Gustafson
Keith A. Johnson

UNIVERSITY OF MINNESOTA
1969
College of Veterinary Medicine

Photo by Schmiding Patrick Studio

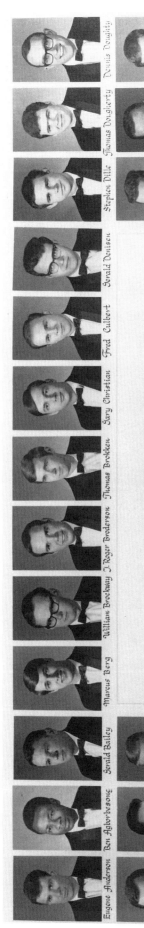
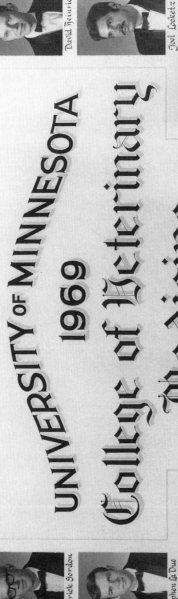
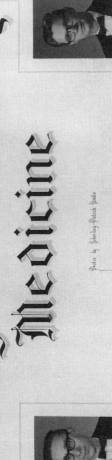
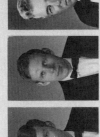

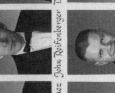

Dennis Doughty — Thomas Dougherty — Stephen Dille — Donald Denison — Fred Culbert — Gary Christian — Thomas Brokken — J. Roger Broderson — William Brockway — Marcus Berg — Gerald Bailey — Frederick Gordon — Stephen La Due

Duane Rissner — William Isaacson — David Heinrich — Joel Loeketz

Mike McMenomy — Lee McDonald — Francis Mills — Douglas Mason

Robert Nesvold — Loyal Monson — Kenneth Rosenberg — Patrick Rooney — John Rolfson — Charles Rhodes — Dean W.T.S. Thorp — John Reifenberger — Terrence Rapacz — Andrew Peterson — Peter Olson — Alan Olson — Joseph Norquist

Ronald Schreiber — Anthony Scheiber — Warren Wilson — Thomas Winter — Loren Will — James Wege — Sharon Wadis — Robert Thompson — Dennis Sweet — Jamie Swanson — David Stewart — Henry Stelling — Philip Soustegard — Donald Skaife

Eugene Anderson — Ben Agborbesong — Mark Engelbreth — James Farnham — John Rohpanen — Laverne Krista — Roger Magnusson — William Maher — James Majka — Donald Maki

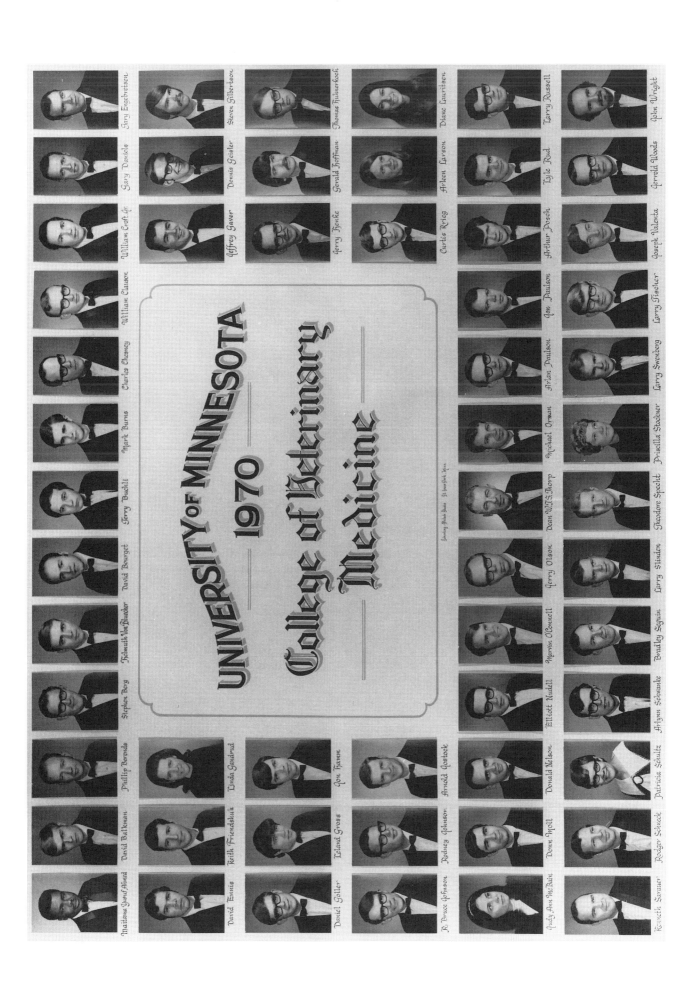

UNIVERSITY OF MINNESOTA
1970
College of Veterinary Medicine

Gary Engebretson

Steven Gilbertson

Thomas Rudrowkoch

Diane Lauritsen

Larry Russell

John Wright

Gary Daniels

Dennis Geisler

Gerald Hoffman

Arlene Larson

Lyle Rud

Gerrold Woods

William Croft Jr.

Jeffrey Gever

Jerry Henke

Curtis Krieg

Arthur Posch

Joseph Valenta

William Clausen

Jon Paulson

Larry Fischer

Charles Chesney

Brian Paulson

Larry Swenberg

Mark Burns

Michael Orman

Priscilla Stockner

Jerry Buchli

Dean W.F.S. Thorp

Theodore Specht

David Bourget

Jerry Olson

Larry Studen

Richmik Van Bluecher

Marvin O'Connell

Bradley Segura

Stephen Berg

Elliott Nadell

Arlynn Schwanke

Phillip Berends

Linda Gaudrud

Jon Hamm

Arnold Gostock

Donald Nelson

Patricia Schultz

David Bakkenen

Keith Friendshuh

Leland Gross

Rodney Johnson

Denn Wyatt

Rodger Scheck

Mattana Jusuf Abwad

David Ennis

Daniel Goller

R. Bruce Johnson

Judy Ann McBain

Kenneth Savauer

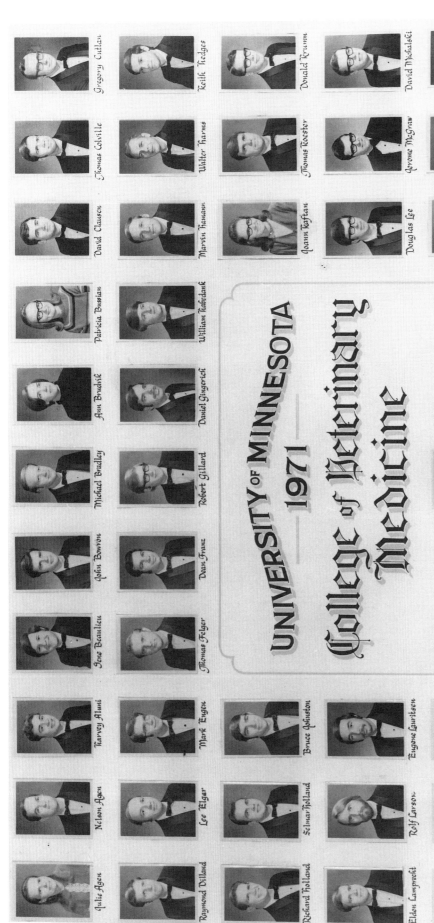
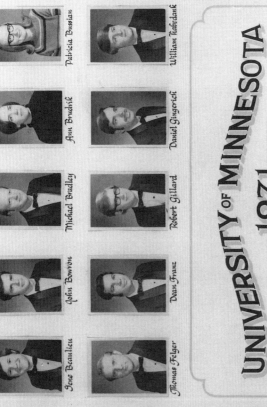
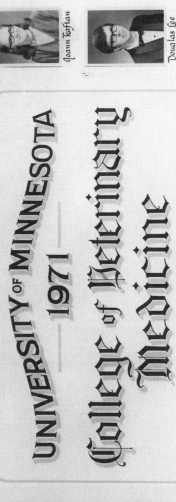
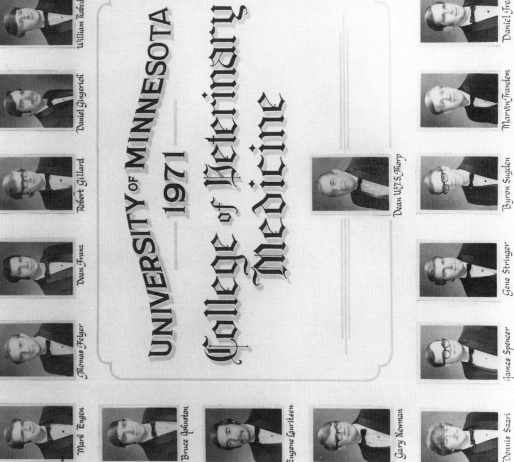
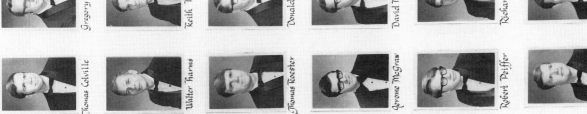
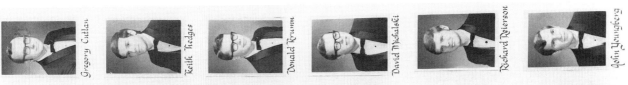

UNIVERSITY OF MINNESOTA
1971
College of Veterinary Medicine

Gregory Cutlan · Keith Tedges · Donald Krumm · David Michalski · Richard Rierson · John Youngberg

Thomas Colville · Walter Tharms · Thomas Koester · Jerome McGraw · Robert Peiffer · Roland Wohlin

David Clausen · Marvin Thimann · Joann Raftain · Douglas Lee · Wayne Ode · Paul Venne

Patricia Bussian · William Rabedank · Daniel Gingerich · Daniel Treat

Ann Brudvik · Daniel Gingerich · Marvin Frandsen

Michael Bradley · Robert Gillard · Dean W.T.S. Thorp · Byron Sugden

John Bowron · Dean Franz · Gene Stringer

Gene Beaulieu · Thomas Felger · James Spencer

Harvey Alumi · Mark Engen · Bruce Johnston · Eugene Lauritsen · Gary Newman · Dennis Saari

Nelson Agen · Lee Elgar · Selmar Holland · Rolf Larson · Roger Nelson · Marc Rothstein

Julie Agen · Raymond Dilland · Richard Holland · Eldon Lamprecht · John Neitzke · Ronald Riis

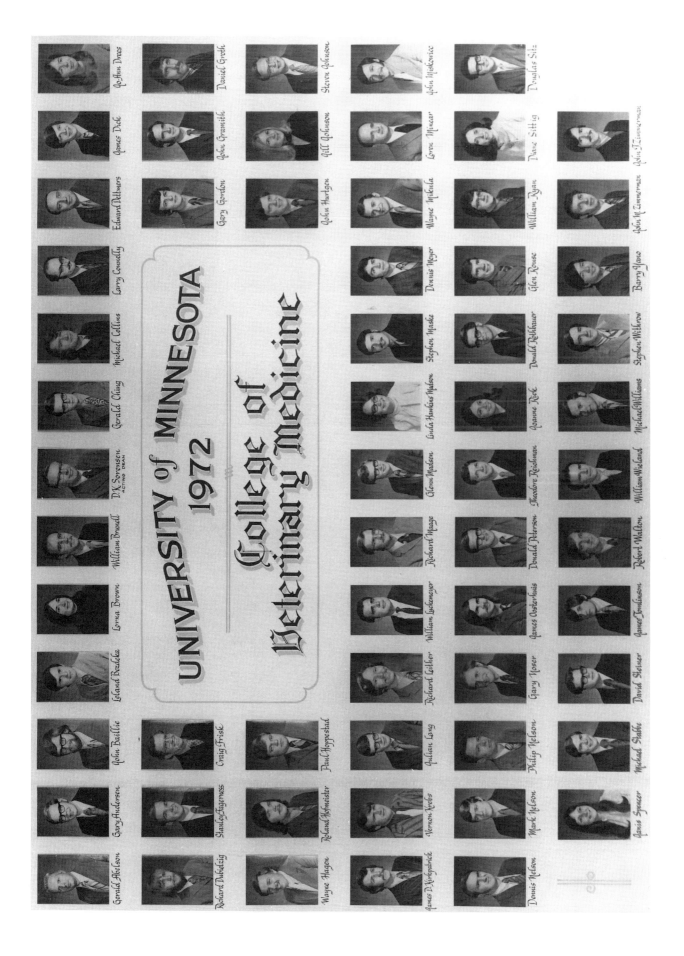

UNIVERSITY of MINNESOTA
1972

College of
Veterinary Medicine

D.K. Sorensen, ACTING DEAN

Jo-Ann Drees
James Dick
Edward Dettmers
Larry Connelly
Michael Collins
Gerald Ching
William Brunell
Lorna Brown
Leland Bradeka
John Baillie
Craig Frisk
Gary Anderson
Stanley Fagerness
Robert Dubielzig
Wayne Hagen
Roland Hofmeister
Paul Hoppestad
Julius Lang
Vernon Krois
Philip Nelson
Mark Nelson
James Kirkpatrick
Dennis Nelson
Denise Spencer
Michael Stahl
David Steiner
James Tomlinson
Robert Walton
William Wieland
Michael Williams
Stephen Withrow
Gary Noser
Richard Leither
William Luckemeyer
James Oosterhuis
Donald Peterson
Theodore Reichman
Donald Reitkauer
Joanne Rott
Linda Hawkins Madsen
Glenn Madsen
Richard Maage
Stephen Maske
Glen Rouse
Donald Meyer
Wayne Mikula
William Ryan
Barry Jano
John W. Zimmerman
Steven Johnson
Will Johnson
John Hartgen
Gary Gordon
John Gramith
Daniel Groth
Lorne Mincar
Diane Sittig
John Mjolkowice
Douglas Sitz
John T. Zimmerman

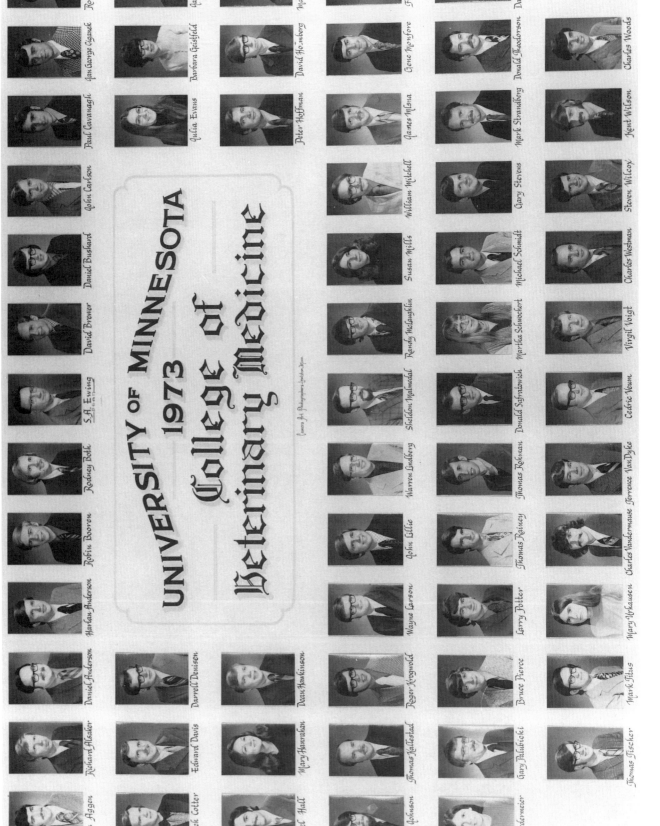

UNIVERSITY OF MINNESOTA
1973
College of
Veterinary Medicine

Camera Art Photographers—Lewiston, Minn.

Ronald Clappier

Jan George Ciganek
James Geistfeld

Paul Cavanagh
Barbara Geistfeld
David Homberg
Mary Isaacson

John Carlson
Julia Evans
Peter Hoffman
Gene Monfore
Francis Muggli

David Brewer
James Nelsen
Mark Strandberg
Donald Theodorson
Danny Thornborrow

Rodney Both
William Mitchell
Gary Stevens
Kent Wilson

S.A. Ewing
Susan Mills
Michael Schmidt
Steven Wilcox

Robin Booren
Randy McLaughlin
Charles Westman
Charles Woods

Harlan Anderson
Sheldon Nyalmedal
Martha Schwoerbt
Virgil Voigt

Warren Lindberg
Donald Safratowich
Cedric Venn

Thomas Robinson
Terrence VanDyke

Daniel Anderson
Darrell Denison
Dean Hawkinson

John Lillie
Thomas Rainey

Wayne Carson
Larry Potter
Charles Vandermause
Mary Urhausen

Richard Alsaker
Edward Davis
Mary Hanrahan

Roger Krogwold
Bruce Pierce
Gary Palubicki
Mark Titus

Lynn Aggen
Patrick Cotter
Daniel Hall

Thomas Hallestad
Gary Johnson
Thomas Tischer

Janice Niedermeier

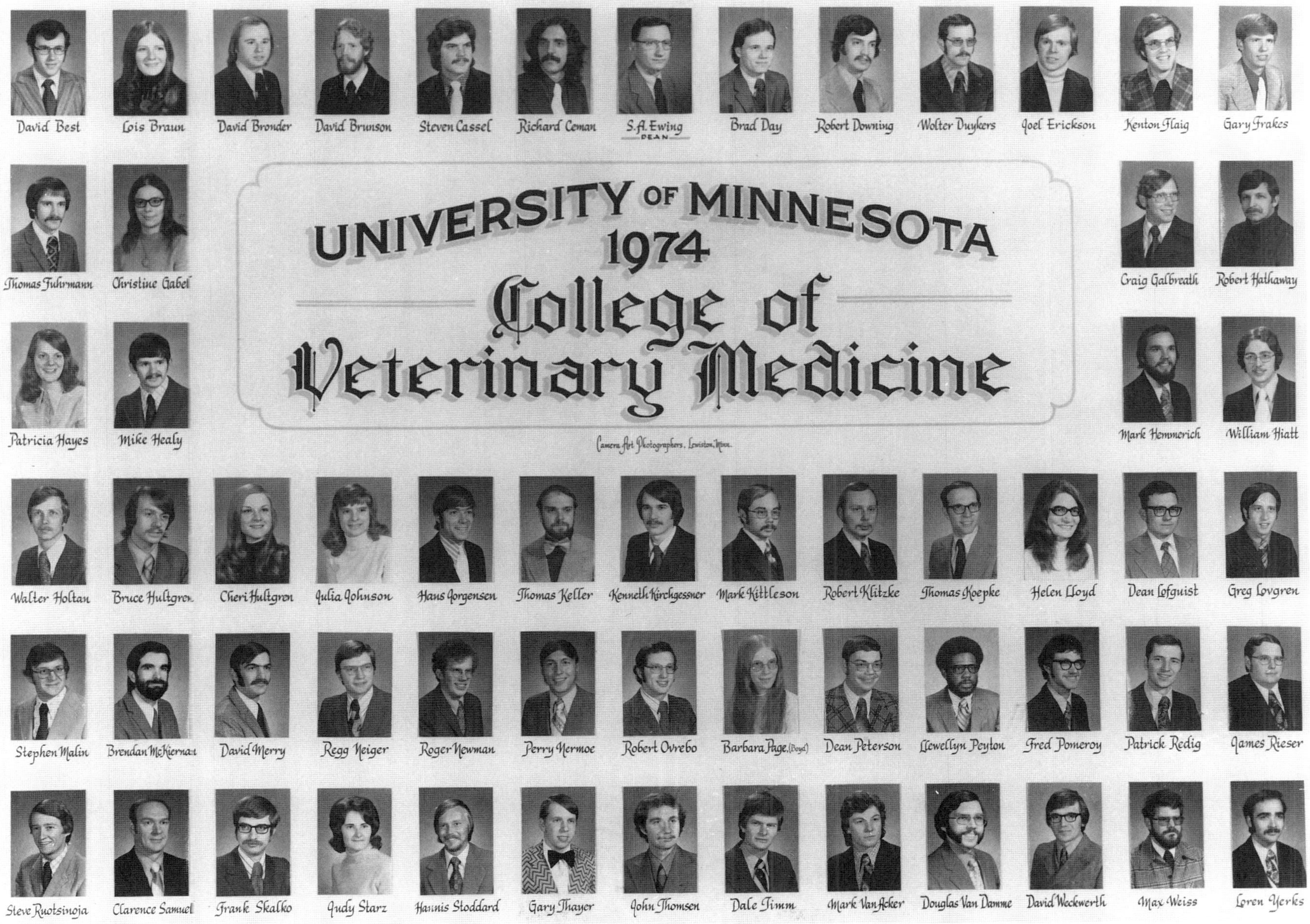

UNIVERSITY OF MINNESOTA
1974
College of Veterinary Medicine

S.A. Ewing, DEAN

Camera Art Photographers, Lewiston, Minn.

David Best
Lois Braun
David Bronder
David Brunson
Steven Cassel
Richard Coman
Brad Day
Robert Downing
Walter Duykers
Joel Erickson
Gary Frakes

Thomas Fuhrmann
Christine Gabel
Craig Galbraith
Robert Hathaway
Kenton Haig

Patricia Hayes
Mike Healy
Mark Homonorich
William Hiatt

Walter Holian
Bruce Hultgren
Cheri Hultgren
Julia Robinson
Hans Jorgensen
Thomas Keller
Kenneth Kordgessner
Mark Kittleson
Robert Klitzke
Thomas Koepke
Helen Lloyd
Greg Lovgren
Dean Lofgquist

Stephen Malin
Brendan McKiernan
David Merry
Rega Weiger
Roger Newman
Perry Mermae
Robert Orrebo
Barbara Page (Prof.)
Dean Peterson
Llewellyn Peyton
Fred Pomeroy
Patrick Redig
James Rieser

Steve Rudisinaja
Clarence Samuel
Frank Skalko
Judy Starz
Harris Stoddard
Gary Thayer
John Thomson
Dale Trimm
Mark VanAcker
Douglas Van Damme
David Wadsworth
Max Weiss
Loren Werks

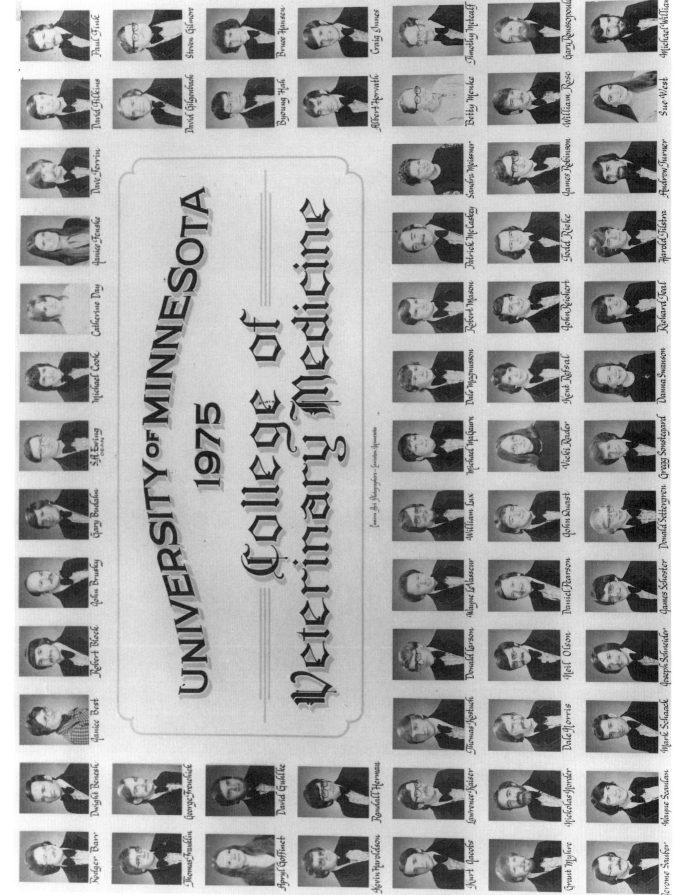

UNIVERSITY OF MINNESOTA
1975
College of Veterinary Medicine

Camera Art Photographies — Lewiston, Minnesota

Paul Fink
David Filkins
Dave Ferrin
Janice Fenske
Catherine Day
Michael Cook
S.H. Ewing DEAN
Gary Budahn
John Brusky
Robert Bleck
Janice Best

Steven Gilmore
David Grigorbach
Byoung Hah
Albert Horvath
Rodger Barr
Dwight Benesh
George Frenchick
David Gullikke
Randall Herman

Bruce Hansen
Craig Innes
Timothy Metcalf
Betty Wenke
William Rose
Gary Roussopoulos
Michael Williams

Sue West
Andrew Turner
Harold Tilstra
Richard Teal
Danna Swanson
Gregg Soustegard
James Schuster
Mark Schaack
Wayne Scanlan
Jerome Sauber

Sandra Weissner
Patrick McCaskey
Robert Mason
Michael Mabaum
Wayne Schlasner
Donald Larson
Thomas Kostuch
Lawrence Kaiser
Kevin Haroldson

James Robinson
Todd Ricke
John Reichert
Kent Refsal
Vicki Rador
John Quast
Daniel Pearson
Neil Olson
Dale Norris
Nicholas Norder
Kurt Jacobs
Grant Myhre

Donald Settergren
Joseph Schneider
Dale Magnusson
William Lex
Thomas Kostuch

Thomas Franklin
Apryl Goffinet
Kevin Haroldson

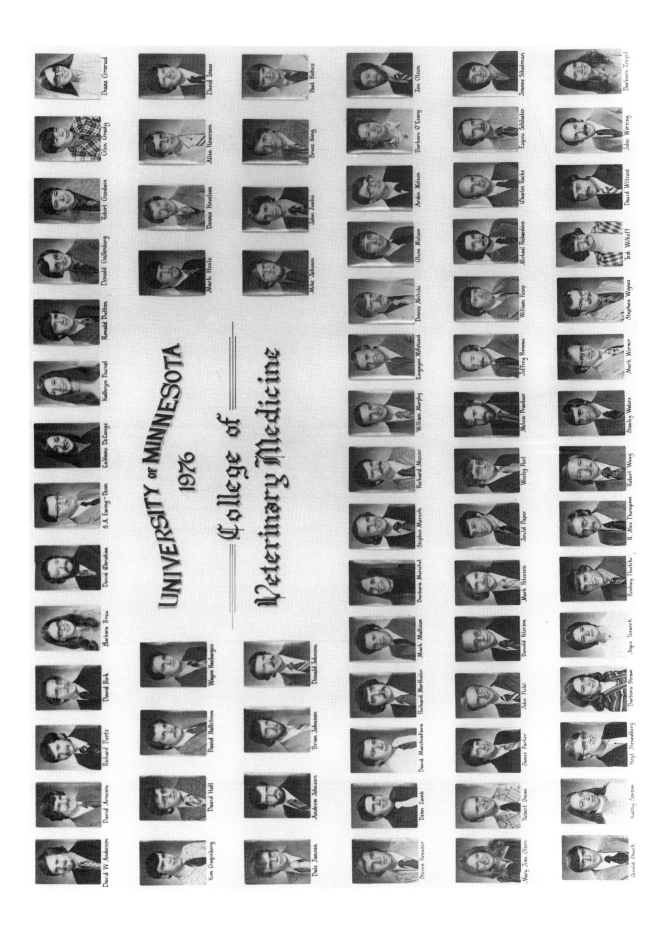

UNIVERSITY OF MINNESOTA
1976
College of
Veterinary Medicine

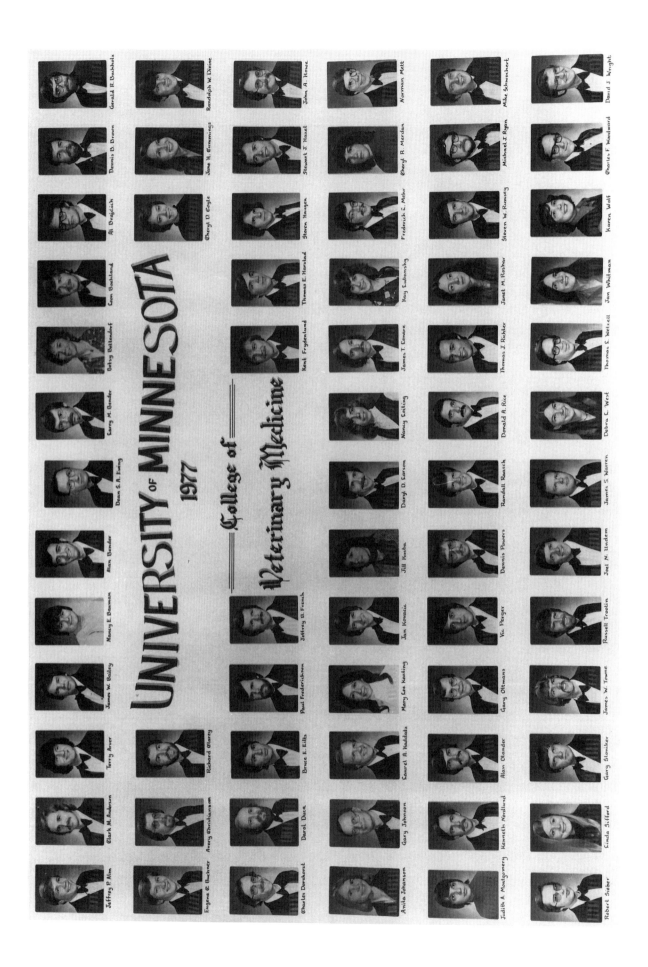

UNIVERSITY OF MINNESOTA
1977
College of
Veterinary Medicine

Jeffrey P. Alm
Charles Dorshorst
Judith A. Montgomery
Robert Sieber

Clark M. Anderson
Eugene E. Buckner
Avery Christianson
Linda Sifford

Terry Arver
Richard Olasey

Anita Johanson
Kenneth Nordlund

Darel Duca
Bruce E. Eilts
Paul Frederickson
Gary Johnson
Alan Olander

James W. Bailey
Nancy E. Bauman
Jeffrey B. French

Laurel A. Kaddatz
Mary Lee Keating
Gary Oltmans

Alan Bender
Dean S. A. Ewing

Jan Kovacic
Vic Panzer
James W. Towne

Larry M. Gender
Betsy Battendorf

Jill Kuehn
Dennis Powers
Gary Slemiker
Russell Trooien

Leon Gachland
Al Drajeich

Nancy Leiting
Daryl D. Larson
Randall Roesch
Joel N. Undem

Cheryl D. Engle

Thomas J. Richter
Donald A. Rice
James S. Warren

Thomas E. Morstad
Kay Lubensky
Janet M. Roshar

Gerald R. Buchholz
Randolph W. Divine

Kent Frydenlund
Frederick L. Mohr
Steven W. Ramsey

Dennis B. Brown
Jane N. Cummings

Steven Haugen
Cheryl R. Merdan
Michael J. Ryan

Al Drajeich

Stewart J. Hazel
John A. Howe

Thomas E. Wetzell
Debra L. West
Jan Whitman
Karen Wolf

Norman Mett

James T. Lewenz

Charles F. Woodward
David J. Wright
Mike Schwochert

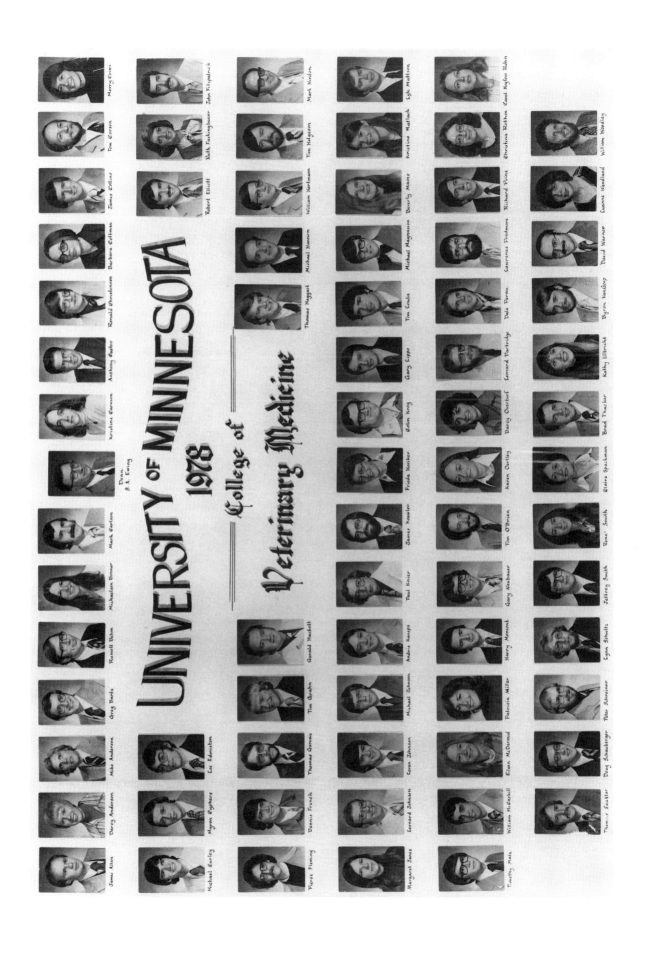

UNIVERSITY OF MINNESOTA
1978

Dean
B. A. Ewing

College of
Veterinary Medicine

James Allen

Darcy Anderson

Mike Anderson

Greg Barta

Russell Behm

Michaelene Benner

Mark Carlson

Kristina Carlson

Anthony Castro

Ronald Christianson

Barbara Coffman

James Collins

Tom Carlson

Merry Crini

Michael Curley

Myron Cryhers

Lee Edmisten

Robert Elliott

Ruth Fashingbauer

John Fitzpatrick

Flora Fleming

Dennis French

Thomas Gereau

Tim Grahn

Gerald Hackett

Thomas Haggart

Tim Helgeson

Mark Hinzon

Michael Hannon

William Hartman

Gary Epps

Gary Krula

Tim Krula

Michael Magnuson

Beverly Mains

Kristine Matlack

Lyle Mattson

Margaret Jones

Leonard Johnson

Karen Johnson

Michael Johnson

Andrea Kamps

John Krog

Frieda Kessler

Karen Oorley

Darcy Overlurf

Lawrence Predmore

Dale Persa

Leonard Partridge

Richard Prine

Christina Rothen

Carol Bayless Rehm

Timothy Matz

Doug Schaubergar

Thomas Seutter

William McfacksII

Eileen McDermid

Patricia Miller

Harry Mement

Gary Neubauer

James Kessler

Paul Krica

Tim O'Brien

Claire Spackman

Brad Thacker

Kathy Ulbricht

Byron VanDorp

David Warner

Luanne Wandland

Peter Schreiner

Lynn Schultz

Jeffrey Smith

Rene' Smith

William Woedley

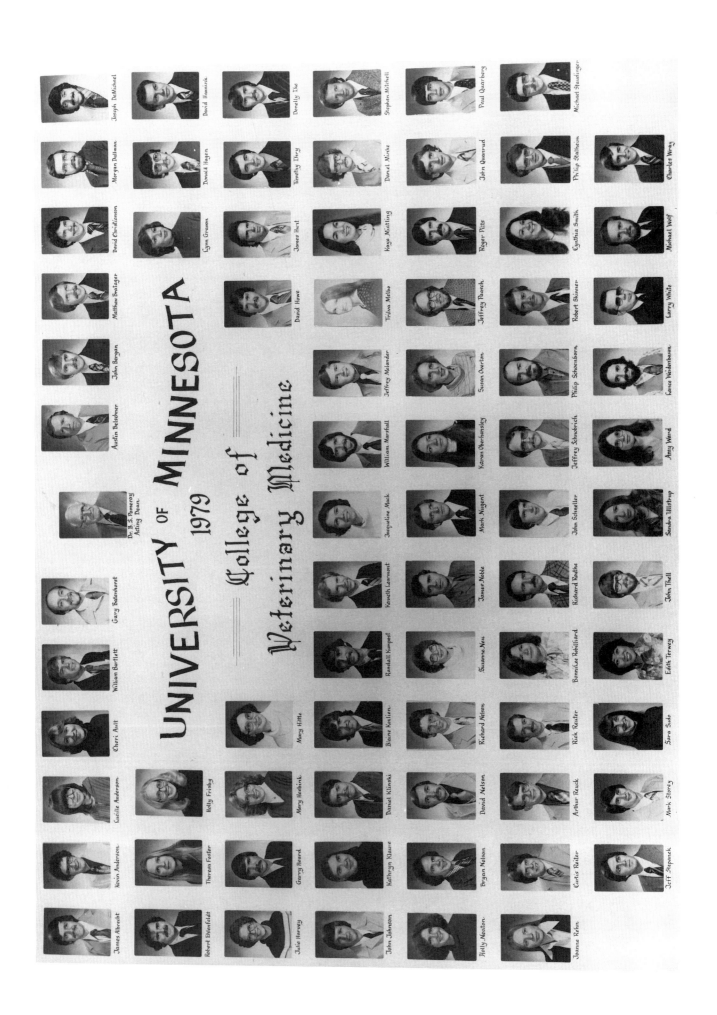

UNIVERSITY OF MINNESOTA
1979
College of
Veterinary Medicine

Dr. B. S. Pomeroy
Acting Dean.

Joseph DeMichael
David Hamink
Dorothy Ike
Stephen Mitchell
Paul Quarberg
Michael Staudinger

Morgan Dallman
Donald Hagen
Timothy Ihrig
Daniel Minke
John Quamrud
Philip Stalheim
Charles Wray

David Christianson
Lynn Gruson
James Hurt
Kaye Mietling
Roger Pitts
Cynthia Smith
Michael Wolf

Matthew Brolsager
David Howe
Triloa Melbo
Jeffrey Raasch
Robert Skinner
Larry White

Austin Belschner
John Bergan
Jeffrey Melander
Susan Overton
Philip Schoenborn
Lance Weidenbaum

Gary Batenhorst
William Marshall
Karen Oberhansley
Jeffrey Schnobrich
Amy Ward

William Bartlett
Jacqueline Mack
Mark Nugent
John Schneiter
Sandra Ullstrup

Cheri Ault
Kenneth Learmont
James Noble
Richard Radtke
John Thell

Mary Hittle
Randall Kumpost
Susanne Neu
Bonnie Lee Rohlilzard
Edith Terwey

Blaine Kosloen
Richard Nelson
Rick Reuter
Sara Sudo

Lucille Anderson
Holly Frisby
Mary Heebink
Daniel Klinski
David Nelson
Arthur Rauck
Mark Storey

Kevin Anderson
Theresa Foster
Garry Heard
Kathryn Klause
Bryan Nelson
Curtis Reiter
Jeff Stepanek

James Albrecht
Robert Ehlenfeldt
Julie Harvey
John Johnson
Holly Newton
Joanne Rehm

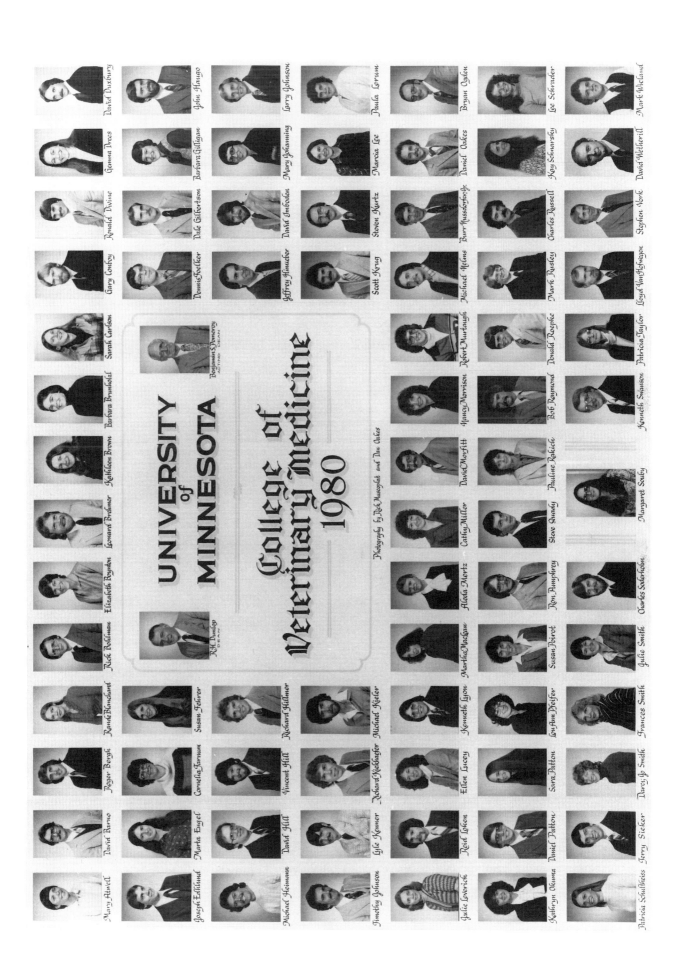

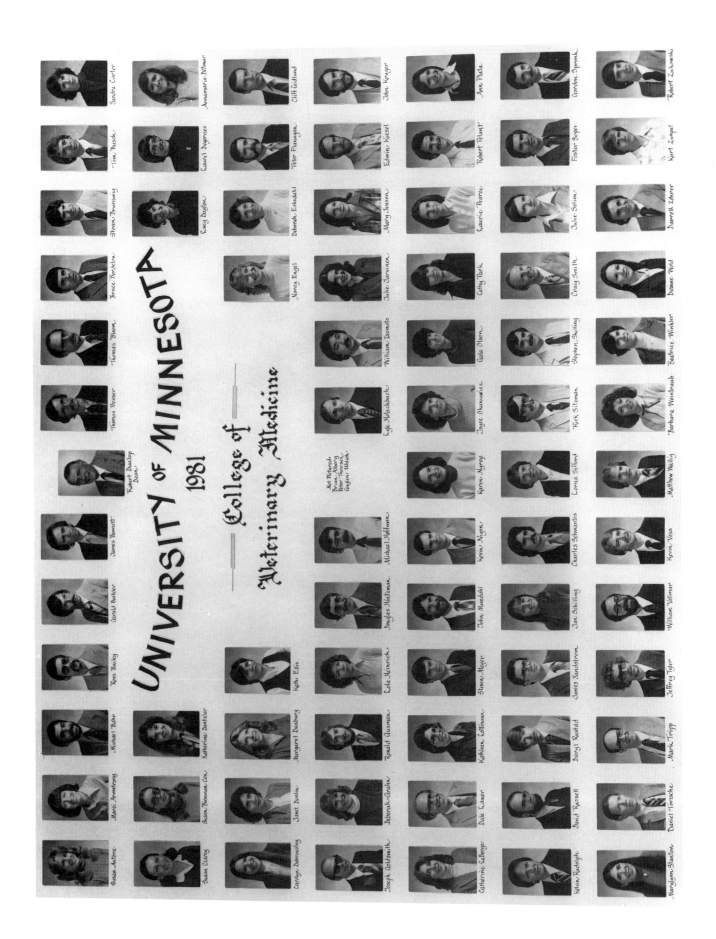

UNIVERSITY OF MINNESOTA
1981
College of
Veterinary Medicine

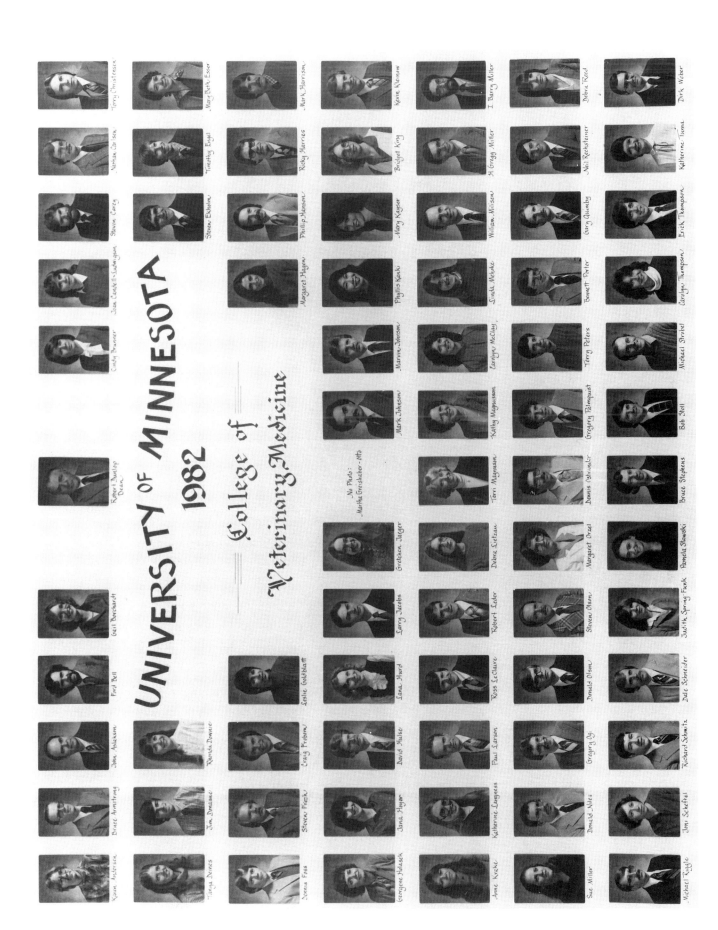

UNIVERSITY OF MINNESOTA
1982
College of
Veterinary Medicine

Robert Dunlop, Dean

Karen Andersen
Bruce Armstrong
John Aaldsson
Ford Bell
Earl Borchardt
Cindy Brawner
Jean Cockrell-Suchovsky
Steven Carey
Nathan Carlson
Terry Christensen

Tanya Denns
Jim Dresser
Rhonda Downie
Jim Drasann
Mary Beth Esser
Timothy Engel
Steven Ekstein
Mark Harrison

Nonus Foss
Steven Frein
Craig Probow
Leslie Goldblatt
Ricky Harries
Philip Hanson
Bridget King
Mary Kayser
Kevin Klonow
Margaret Hagen

Georgene Holasek
Jana Hyer
David Hulse
Lana Hurd
Larry Jacobs
Gretchen Jager
No Photo:
Marika Grrishaber-Otto
Mark Johnson
Marvin Johnson
Phyllis Kaski
William Milison
H. Gregg Miller
I. Barry Miller

Ann Krahe
Katherine Langness
Paul Larson
Ross LeClaire
Robert Leder
Debra Lietzau
Terri Magnuson
Kathy Magnusson
Carolyn McCllay
Linda Metcke
Gary Quamby
Neil Rechsteiner
Debra Reed

Sue Miller
Donald Niles
Gregory Oj
Donald Olson
Steven Olson
Margaret Orzel
Dennis Ostrander
Gregory Palmquist
Terry Peters
Bennett Porter
Carolyn Thompson
Katherine Tuona
Dirk Weber

Michael Riggle
Joni Scheffel
Richard Schmitz
Dale Schneider
Judith Spring Funk
Pamela Slawski
Bruce Stephens
Bob Stoll
Michael Strobel
Erick Thompson

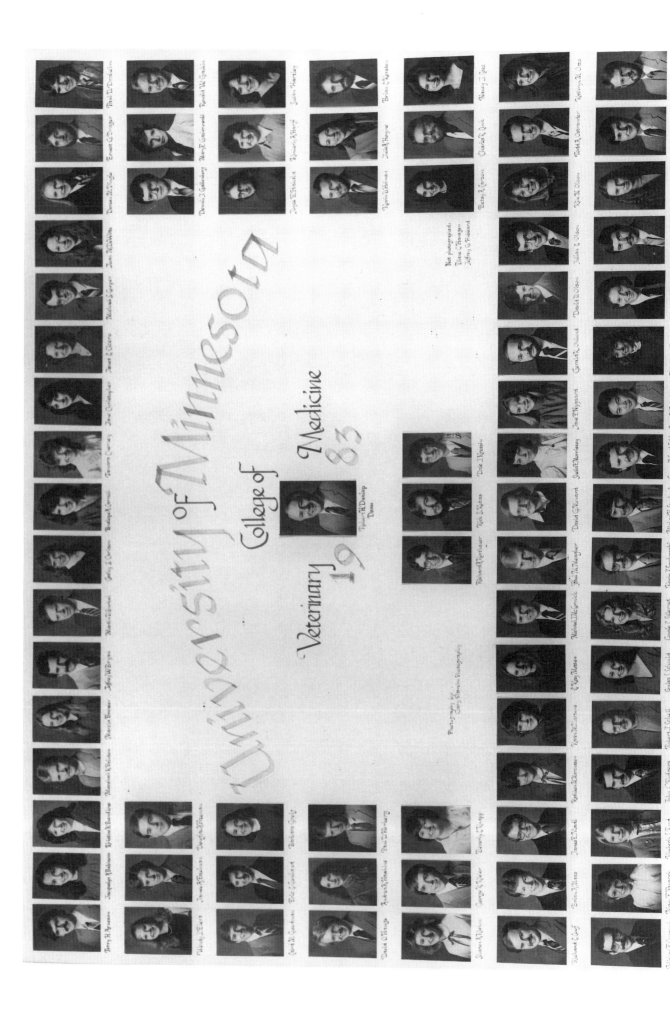

University of Minnesota

College of

Veterinary Medicine

19 83

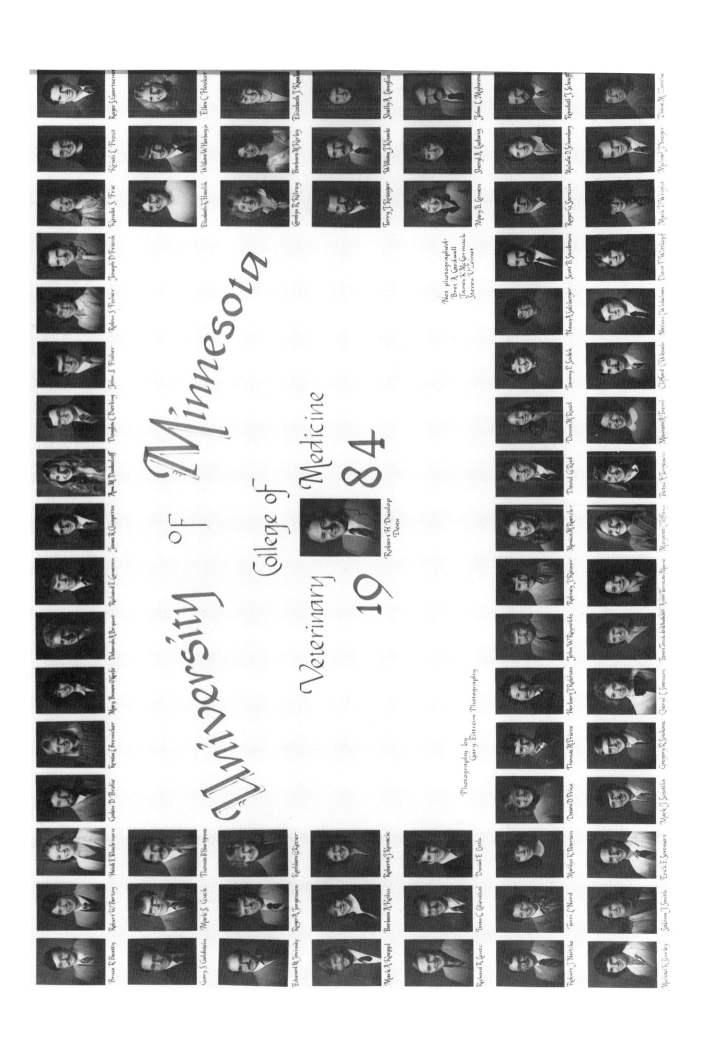

University of Minnesota

College of Veterinary Medicine

19 84

Robert H. Dunlop
Dean

Photography by
Gary Ettinger Photography

Not photographed:
Bret A. Cardwell
Travis K. McCormack
Steven V. Zenner

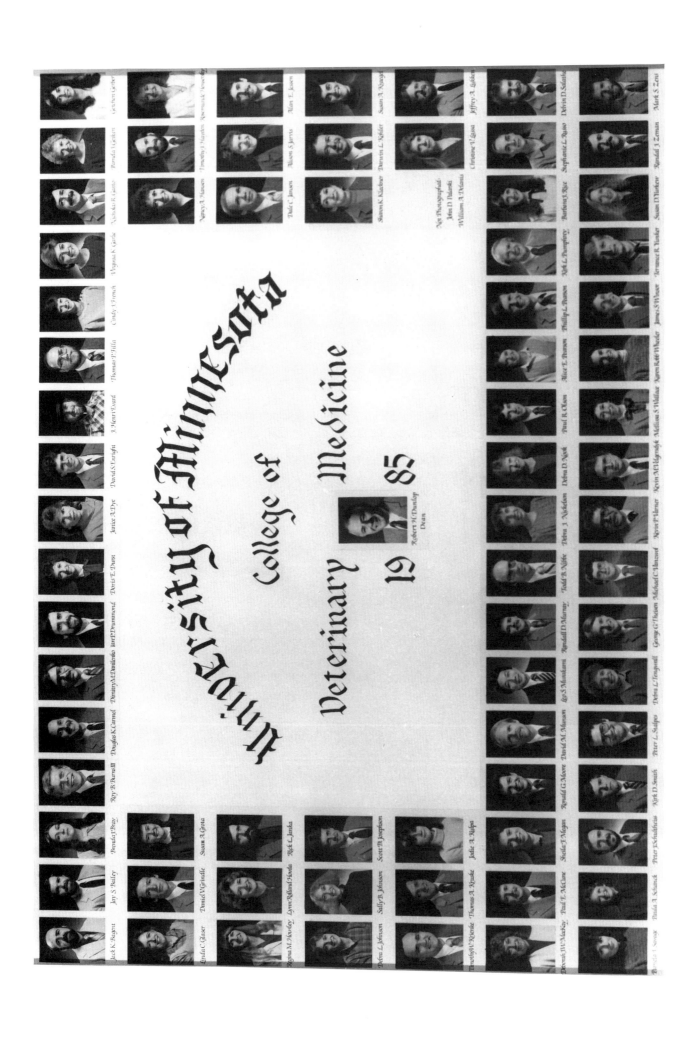

University of Minnesota

1986

College of Veterinary Medicine

R.H. Dunlop
Dean

Jeffrey C. Abott
Susan Abott
Denise L. Albert
Evelyn Arthur
Kevin Wayne Barcus
Michael Bernard

Valerie Caskey
Sheila E. Connelly

Geoffrey Buhr
Melinda R Burgwardt
Cindi Casagranda

Laura Lynn Bougie
Jane L. Brackken

Thomas S. Bowersox

Jacqueline R Davidson
Dana Dane

Mark S. DeKoning
Mary Sue Dierckins
Therese M. Dieringer

Ann Enright
Deborah D. Ekstrom

Russell Eurl

Nancy Fairman
Lois Finsmith
Mary L. Fitzgerald
Lisa K. Fruechte
William E. Graham
Lucy A. Grina
Betsy Goucette
Virginia M. Goett
Mary S. Girtz

Patricia Anne Kuehn
Gary Kotecki
Joelle Marie Hymel
Billy M. Hargis
Barbara L. Guy

Richard Larson
Jean L. Lifgren
David D. LoGiudice
Kathryn E. Marr
John S. Myers, Jr.
Randy A. Musack
Daniel P. Murray
Eric A. Mattson
Anne Mattson

Barbara. O'Brien
Jane Norrgard
Norbert Nigon
Debra Nielsen
Linnea J. Newman

Nina M. Rados
William Rice
Bruce Schnabel
Michael A. Scott
Keith H. Soring
Sherrie Jo Solberg
Jill Stachdpole
Richard Sielicki

Debra Teachout
JoAnn W. Taurog
Constance D Tarasek
Janine L. Suailes
Patricia Sperling
Jane Anne Sprangers

Steven F. Timm
Jerry Torrison
Kellay Tousley
David H. Vandegritt
Lynn Weaver
Mark J. Werner
Keith A. Wilson
Gregory Windschill
Jeffrey Winkelman

Paul J. Vatso
Robert L. Wright
Linda A. Wolf

University of Minnesota
College of Veterinary Medicine
1987

R.H. Dunlop, Dean

Frank Buckingham
Curtis Brown
Gary Bramel
Jeff Bohn
Kathie Bjork
Cindy Bergquist
Caroline Bakily
Carol Bachman
Bruce Akey
Catherine Adams

Scott Dee
Deborah Cox
Bruce Coston
Suzanne Cook
Dawn Carlson
Patricia Burns

Alan Flory
Mark FitzSimmons
Stephanie Ferguson
Leah Fauskar
Barbara Farrell
Lorelei Ecklund
Shawn Dutton
Mark Drew

Douglas R. Kern
Vicki Keltner-Domeier
Susan Jones
Kent Nelson
Michael Herman
Ted Johnson
Miriam Hay
Donna Haugen
Gregory Harms
Allan Harmening
Michael Griep
Donelda Coy
Donald Glassman
Gregg Laurence
Jennifer Larsen
Paul Koskinen

Glen Otto
Douglas A. Kern
Jean Nemzek
Deborah Mood
Rod Moberg
Amanda Miller
Jamie Meagher
Daina Rosen
Jeffrey Lindstrom
Douglas LeMay
Christopher Lee
Brian Reed
Bradley Peterson
Allen Pederson
Mary Pariso

Larry Shofner
Gloria Schnell
Janet Schnell
Therese Schneider
David Sauter
Mary Sahagian
Arthur Rutscher
Margaret Root
Nancy Rohland
Eric Thorsgard
Virginia Thorne
Robert Tanaka
Susan Stanius
Paul Sjoberg

Daniel Lilverberg
Elizabeth Wysocki
William Warvin
Margaret Watkins
Lucy Ward
Philip Walch
Nancy Vincent
Paul Tippery

Kathryn Ott

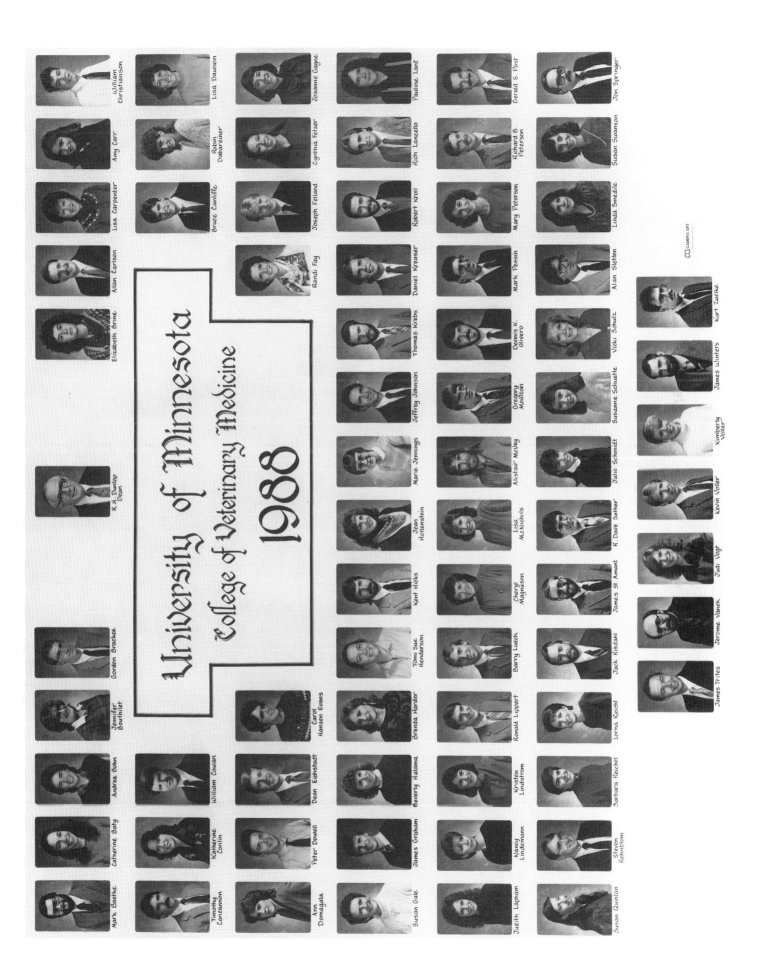

University of Minnesota
College of Veterinary Medicine
1988

R.A. Dunlop, Dean

William Christianson
Lisa Dawson
Josanne Gagne
Pauline Lant
Gerald S. Post
Jon Springer

Amy Carr
Robin Dabareiner
Cynthia Fetzer
Rich Lancello
Richard B. Peterson
Susan Swanson

Lisa Carpenter
Bruce Cunliffe
Joseph Fetland
Robert Kroll
Mary Petersen
Linda Smedile

Allan Carlson
Randi Fay
Daniel Kreuser
Mark Pessin
Alan Sletten
Kurt Zuelke

Elizabeth Brine
Thomas Krebs
Dennis K. Olivero
Vicki Schulz
James Winters

Jeffrey Johnson
Gregory Moulton
Susanne Schuette
Kimberly Voller

Marie Jennings
Alistair McVay
Julie Schmidt
Kevin Voller

Jean Hollenstein
Lisa McNichols
R. Dave Sather
Judi Vogt

Kent Hicks
Cheryl Magnuson
James St. Amant
Jerome Vanek

Tomi Sue Henderson
Barry Lueck
Jack Risdahl
James Trites

Brenda Harder
Ronald Lippert
Lorna Reichl

Beverly Haloma
Kristen Lindstrom
Barbara Reichel

Carol Hansen Evans
Nancy Lindemann
Steven Rehnblom

Dean Eichstadt
William Cowan
Katherine Conlin

Peter Dowell

Gordon Bracke
Jennifer Bouthilet

James Graham

Andrea Bohn
Catherine Baty
Mark Baetke

Timothy Concannon
Ann Domagala
Susan Gale
Judith Lapham
Susan Quinlan

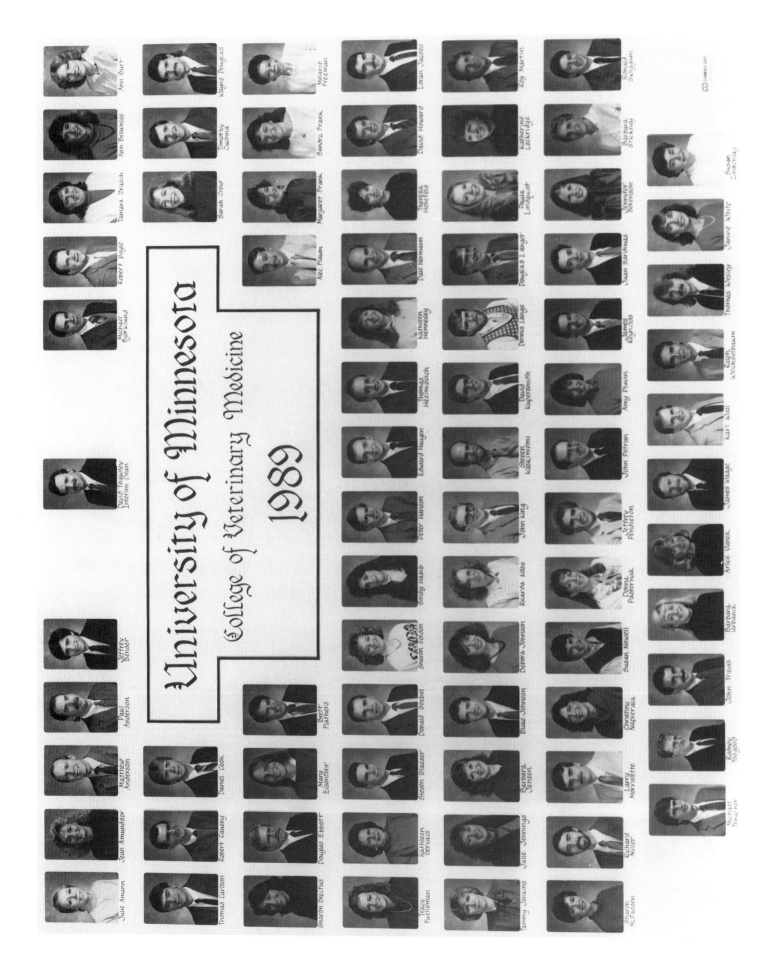

University of Minnesota
College of Veterinary Medicine
1989

David Thawley
Interim Dean

Ann Burt

Ann Brownlee

Tamara Brasch

Robert Boyle

Michael Bjorklund

Wayne Douglas

Timothy Cwiklia

Sarah Crour

Melanie Freeman

Sandra Frank

Margaret Frank

Alec Flaum

Loran Jacobs

David Howard

Theresa Howells

Duc Hermann

Katherine Lockridge

Paula Lindquist

Douglas L Langer

Jennifer Stevenson

Juan Sardinas

Barbara Strickland

Kathleen Hennessy

Dennis Lange

James Reynolds

Thomas Hecmovich

David Kuptersmith

Amy Plaunt

Edward Haugen

Steven Kaskinemi

John Petran

Peter Hanson

John King

Jeffrey Pendleton

Sindy Habib

Ricarda Kifea

Donna Pasternak

Sharon Belden

Debora Johnson

Susan Newell

Donald Goebel

Blake Johnson

Christine Napierala

Steven Glaeser

Barbara Jensen

Larry Morrissette

Kathleen Gervais

Julie Jennings

Richard Miller

Douglas Ebbott

Mary Eisenlohr

Robert Causey

Brett Fluthers

Daniel Cook

Paul Anderson

Jeffrey Bender

Matthew Anderson

Jean Amundson

Thomas Carlson

Sharon Declus

Tracy Fuelleman

Tammy Jenkins

Sharon McFadden

Susan Zielinski

Janine White

Thomas Wesley

Ralph Weindelbaum

Kurt Wall

James Wedge

Arlice Varek

Barbara Urbanik

John Traxus

Rodney Tobgood

Michael Thacker

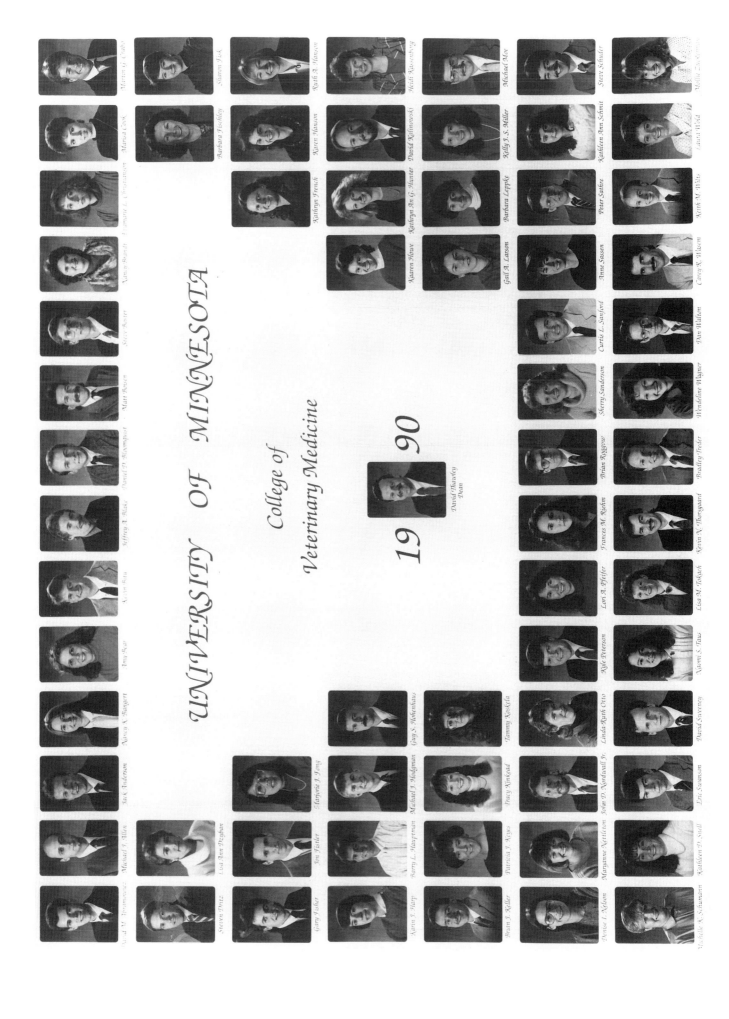

UNIVERSITY OF MINNESOTA

College of
Veterinary Medicine

19 90

David Thawley
Dean

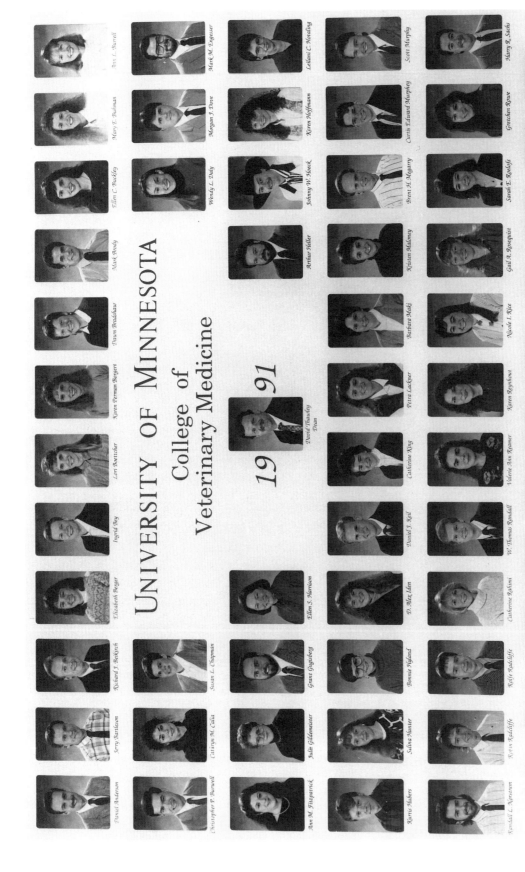

UNIVERSITY OF MINNESOTA
College of
Veterinary Medicine

19 91

David Thawley
Dean

Ann L. Burrell

Mary E. Bushman

Ellen C. Buckley

Mark Brody

Dawn Bradshaw

Karen Perman Bogert

Lori Boettcher

Ingrid Beg

Elizabeth Berger

Richard J. Bekierk

Jerry Bartleson

Daniel Anderson

Christopher P. Burwell

Susan L. Chapman

Catarzyn M. Cislia

Julie Gildemeister

Grant Gogisberg

Ellen S. Harrison

Mark M. Engesser

Morgan S. Dove

Wendy L. Daly

Arthur Heller

D. Alex Iden

Daniel J. Keil

Bonnie Hyland

Selina Hunter

Ann M. Fitzpatrick

Kurtis Hubers

Johnny W. Hoeck

Karen Hoffmann

Leilani C. Hotaling

Kristen Maloney

Barbara Maki

Petra Lackner

Catherine King

Valerie Ann Kramer

Catherine Rahimi

Rolfe Radcliffe

Robin Radcliffe

Randall L. Korstrom

Curtis Edward Murphey

Brent H. Megarry

Nicole I. Rice

Gail A. Rosequist

Karen Reynhout

W. Thomas Rendall

Scott Murphy

Gretchen Rowe

Sarah L. Rodolfs

Laura Toddie

Tracey L. Terrio

Fred Terrell

Brett Terhaar

Jody Skartvedt

Lisa Sell

Teri R. Schweiss

Donald P. Schrep

Harry R. Sachs

Anne L. Voytovich

Jonathan Van Berkom

Karen Tuma

University of Minnesota

College of Veterinary Medicine

19 92

 LeAnn L. Hilbrecht
 Debra A. Allerkamp
 Ann F. Barksdale
 Jody P. Bearman
 Ann Bower
 Layne B. Daniels
 David Patt
 David Patt
 Mark L. Debner
 Kevin Dill
 Dennis L. Donohue
 Theresa A. Donohue
 Melissa Dudley

 Sandra Edgar-Sargent
 David T. Edinger
 Angela M. Erickson
 Mark Gowdy-Jaafing
 Walt Grambow
 Victoria C. Hamer

 Lesley A. Frogh
 Elizabeth Hennessy
 Kim Hiller
 Francine Hofmeister

 Melissa C. Henry
 Ben Leavens
 Randall L. Lindemann
 Pete Litynski

 Elizabeth LaFond

 Natalie J. Pursel
 Julie Roguski Leckey
 Paul Ruen
 Tina Ruiz

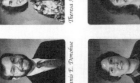 Elisabeth M. Faulkner
 Ann Marie Fischer
 Liz Friedman

 Diane Hansen
 Donna Heaney
 Janet Helms

 Katie C. Hom
 Leslie A. Jackson
 Jean Jarvis
 Patrick J. Jannrich
 Sandra L. Fox
 Alison A. Kinnunen
 Karen M. Heineman
 Kim F. Krivit

 David Thawley, Dean

 Richard Lornig
 Mei-yao C. Lewis
 David McClenahan
 Thomas G. Metzdorff
 David J. Mitzelfeldt
 Steve Olson
 Joan R. Onffroy
 Scott Kuecker

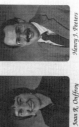 Marvin D. Slabaugh
 David R. Stagg
 Brian C. Sullivan
 Aimee Sutherland

 Helen L. Suthill
 Ron Titterington
 Pan J. Un
 Henry J. Peeters
 Henry J. Peeters

University of Minnesota
College of Veterinary Medicine

19 93

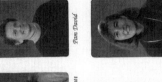

David Thawley
Dean

 Kari L. Anderson

 Christine Mary Baysinger

 Karyn E. Beringo

 Lorin R. Bilhorn

 Catherine M. Brown

 Ann S. Busalacchi

 Houstoun Clinch

 Christopher E. Corn

 Mary P. Craig

 Vicki Johnson Datt

 Tricia M. Delhamer

 Pam David

 Jane E. Flathers

 Diane M. Forner

 Barbara M. Grebart

 Paul R. Gauer

 Sharyl L. Fulop

 Cheryl A. Freske

 Juliette Hanson

 Jim H. Hanson

 Linda Heaton

 Catherine E. Hibbitt

 Christopher M. Holenstein

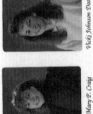 Esther Hope

 Patricia Holz

 Susan M. Keil

 Kelly L. Krambs

 Sarah Lathrop

 Linda Lauper

 Laura C Lefkowitz

 Linnea Rae Lentz

 Roxanne L. Mahan

 Michael C. McCaw

 Lindsay Kaye Merkel

 Martin F. Mohr

 Diane M. Murray

 Jane M. Olin

 Kimberly M. Olson

 Robert Orr

 Kim K. Peterson

 Nancy L. Peterson

 Nancy Rinkardt

 Joseph A. Sousa

 Eric Sienz

 Meg Sulzen

 Kelly Tart

 Daniel L. Terhaar

 Sharon Witensky

 Vickie M. Wang

 David Ween

 Mary Virginia Weuer

 Martha A. Weber

 Barbara Weiss

Not Pictured:
Tracey Cronin

Maureen Schlueter

Kenneth T. Lian Jr.

APPENDIX I

Graduate Veterinarians in Minnesota by 1900

Name	Location Of Graduation	School & Year		Year of License
Adamson, J.H.	St. Paul	CVC	1893	
Allen, Frank	St. Paul	AVC	1889	
Amos, W.	Owatonna	OVC	1889	1893
Anderson, J.P.	Rochester	OVC	1888	1893
Annand, J.G.	Duluth	OVC	1891	1893
Barrett, A.V.	Waterville	WES		1895
Bartrum, G.S.	Lanesboro	OVC	1881	
Brimhall, S.D.	Rochester	UP	1889	1893
Burnham, C.O.	Stillwater	NWV	1887	1893
Butler, J.S.	Minneapolis	OVC	1880	1893
Butters, J.S.	Renville	OVC	1894	1896
Casserly, W.H.	St. Paul	CVC	1893	
Chute, R.N.	Faribault	CVC	1892	1893
Coffeen, R.H.	Stillwater	CVC	1896	1906
Connelly, V.M.	Minneapolis	OVC	1891	1899
Cook, J.L.	Duluth	OVC	1887	1902
Cotton, C.E.	Minneapolis	UP	1893	1897
Craige, E.	Fairmont	OVC	1894	
Dallimore, G.A.	St. Paul	OVC	1879	1893
Dietz, J.H.	Owatonna	OVC	1891	1893
Douglas, J.M.	Hendrum	OVC	1894	1894
Eaton, R.D.	Minneapolis	CVC	1893	1893
Eckles, C.F.	St. Charles	CVC	1890	1902
Erb, N.E.	Faribault	OVC	1888	
Falconer, T.	Alexandria	OVC	1894	1894
Findlay, J.J.	Duluth	OVC	1888	1893
Frank, E.T.	Warren	CVC	1897	1897
Girard, D.G.	Zumbrota	CVC	1889	
Golden, J.W.	Redwood Falls	CVC	1895	1895
Gould, J.N.	Worthington	CVC	1893	1893
Gould, J.W.	Fairmont	CVC	1893	1893
Graham, Chris.	St. Paul	UP	1882	
Harris, J.G.	Duluth	MON	1889	1903
Hay, L.	Faribault	OVC	1896	1899
Hela, H.A.	Wadena	OVC	1900	1906
Illstrup, F.A.	Willmar	CVC	1893	1895

Name	Location Of Graduation	School & Year		Year of License
Kalb, E.S.	Rochester	OVC	1893	1893
Kennedy, J.T.	St. Paul	OVC	1888	1903
Keyes, A.A.	Minneapolis	MON	1885	1893
Kirby, R.W.	St. Paul	CVC	1887	1893
Kjerner, R.	Chatfield	OVC	1896	1902
Kuhns, W.A.	Chaska	OVC	1899	1904
Lambrechts, B.	Granite Falls	RVC	1883	1893
Lambert, J.M.	St. Peter	CVC	1895	1895
Langevin, H.	Crookston	MON	1879	1894
La Pointe, R.	St. Peter	MON	1885	1900
Leech, G.Ed.	Winona	CVC	1900	1902
Lees, A.F.	Red Wing	OVC	1889	1902
Leffingwell, M.F.	Austin	CVC	1892	1905
Lyford, C.C.	Minneapolis	MON	1877	1893
Lyon, R.C.	Hutchinson	MCK	1891	1893
Mack, C.A.	Stillwater	OCV	1891	
		MCK	1892	
Mason, R.C.	Winona	NWV	1885	1893
Metzgar, A.E.	Minneapolis	CVC	1893	
McDonald, D.M.	Minneapolis	MON	1891	1901
McKay, John	Duluth	OVC	1895	1902
McKenzie, K.J.	Northfield	OVC	1892	1893
McGillivary, G.	Roseau	OVC	1885	1893
McLaughlin, J.J.	Blue Earth	ISU	1890	1893
McLellan, F.W.	St. Paul			
Milligan, G.W.	Faribault	OVC	1892	1893
Mueller, Emil	New Ulm	CVC	1892	1893
Murray, S.J.	LeSueur	OVC	1894	1895
O'Neil, D.O.	St. Cloud	CVC	1890	1893
Peters, R.C.	Litchfield	CVC	1896	1898
Pomeroy, B.A.	St. Paul	MON	1883	1893
Price, R.	St. Paul	MON	1881	1893
Rennicks, G.T.	Sauk Centre	CVC	1885	1904
Rennil, J.A.		OVC	1900	1903
Reynolds, M.H.	St. Paul	ISU	1889	1897
Rydell, Oscar	Wheaton	CVC	1898	1898
Schwartzkoff, O.	St. Paul	IVC	1880	
Schmitz, J.J.	Lambert	CVC	1892	1894

Name	Location Of Graduation	School & Year		Year of License
Scott, J.A.	Waverly	CVC	1893	1894
Sexton, M.J.	Minneapolis	OVC	1895	1899
Sheppard, J.N.	Barnesville	OVC	1892	1903
Sigmond, C.J.	Pipestone	OVC	1893	
Soneral, Wm.	Cambridge	CVC	1897	1899
Spence, A.	Hallock	OVC	1893	1893
Sproule, W.A.	Mankato	OVC	1889	1902
Standish, W.M.	Mankato	OVC	1885	1903
Sutzin, J.	Minneapolis	CVC	1893	1893
Treacy, M.J.	St. Paul	RVC	1874	
Ward, S.H.	St. Cloud	OVC	1894	1894
Whitbeck, S.A.	Caledonia	ISU	1891	1906
Whitcomb, M.H.	Austin	CVC	1892	
White, Robt.	St. Paul	OVC	1879	1893
Wrigglesworth, T.	Duluth	OVC	1882	
Youngberg, Anton	Lake Park	OVC	1892	

APPENDIX II

Non-Graduate Veterinarians in Minnesota by 1900
Under "Grandfather Clause"

Name	**Location**	**Year Granted License**
Anderson, T.E.	Maple Plain	1893
Ash, F.	Faribault	1893
Ashmidt, J.	St. Paul	1893
Ayers, J.H.	Minneapolis	1893
Bacon, W.S.	Minneapolis	1893
Baker, B.F.	Elgin	1893
Beaulinx, D.	Luverne	1893
Bernard, D.	Warren	1893
Bill, J.J.	Madelia	1893
Bird, J.L.	Worthington	1893
Bissell, H.H.	Cannon Falls	1893
Blankenburg, A.	Lakefield	1894
Bleyl, A.	New Richland	1893
Bolton, A.H.	St. Paul	1893
Bossant, W.D.	St. Peter	1893
Britton, E.L.		1893
Burrows, C.F.	Lake Crystal	1893
Butler, Clayton	Madelia	1893
Canfield, M.F.	Long Prairie	1893
Chambers, S.J.	Detroit?	1893
Clark, D.	Clear Lake	1893
Close, J.W.	Little Falls	1893
Cole, A.W.	Spring Valley	1893
Colgan, E.P.	Wells	1893
Confer, S.C.	Barnum	1893
Cooley, L.A.	Austin	1893
Coons, W.H.	Ivanhoe	1893
Cottrell, W.H.	Houston	1893
Crossland	Little Falls	1893
Cummins, A.L.	Eagle Lake	1893
Crows, W.H.		1893
Dahlstrom, G.	Winnebago	1893
Davis, C.S.	Buffalo	1893
Davis, M.F.	Taopi	1895
Dean, G.S.	Worthington	1893
Dean, J.A.	Shakopee	1893
DeGill, ?	Stewart	1893

Name	Location	Year Granted License
Dick, Sr., J.S.	Minneapolis	1893
Dodds, R.M.	Mankato	1893
Durburger, O.	Shakopee	1893
Eastman, W.S.	Marshall	1893
Endersbe, A.R.	Pine River	1893
Erickson, O.S.	Milan	1893
Filmore, H.G.	St. Cloud	1894
Finney, J.W.	Rochester	1893
Fitzimmons, W.	Sebeka	1893
Frye, J.H.	Forest Lake	1893
Gilkey, E.B.	Prior Lake	1894
Graham, H.	Hallock	1893
Grass, J.J.	Owatonna	1893
Grey, L.C.	Kerkhoven	1893
Hake, W.W.		1893
Halverson, E.A.		1893
Hanson, A.W.	Hartland	1893
Havorka, W.J.	St. Paul	1893
Hellen, John	Minneapolis	1893
Horton, D.C.	Benson	1895
Horton, John	Minneapolis	1893
Ingalls, H.	Coleraine	1893
Kochne, A.G.	New Ulm	1893
Knapp, J.K.	Madison Lake	1893
Kraemer, C.A.	Dawson	1893
Kraemer, P.H.	Sauk Centre	1893
Leut, A.	Springfield	1893
Lipp, M.	New Ulm	1893
Lydick, C.H.	Anoka	1893
Lyke, J.E.	Kasson	1893
McCagen, W.H.	Clear Lake	1893
McCullough, H.	Minneapolis	1893
McKee, D.W.	Monticello	1893
Metzger, W.J.	Minneapolis	1893
Nell or Nelle, H.	Lewiston	1893
Nelson, P.	Willmar	1893
Neukon, Wm.	Ada	1894
Newman, Wm.	Princeton	1893
Northrup, G.L.	Slayton	1893
O'Brien, ?	Minneapolis	1893
Ohlin, C.O.	North Branch	1893

Name	Location	Year Granted License
Orr, G.O.	Jordan	1893
Parker, C.H.	Minneapolis	1893
Paulson, D.M.	Sacred Heart	1893
Pew, F.	Stewartville	1893
Place, J.H.	Waseca	1893
Porter, Bennet	Albert Lea	1893
Ray, F.J.	Minneapolis	1893
Reider, M.	St. Cloud	1893
Roberts, W.M.	Winnebago	1893
Rockwell, J.F.	Austin	1893
Rogers, O.H.	Minneapolis	1893
Ross, J.	St. Paul Park	1893
Roth, John	Lamberton	1893
Satre, R.J.	Clarkfield	1893
Sauby, J.O.	Elbow Lake	1893
Schjoll, K.B.	Rushford	1893
Scott, M.S.	Faribault	1893
Scruby, H.	Melrose	1893
Senescall, J.A.	Ortonville	1893
Sheldahl, R.L.	Pipestone	1893
Sherman, H.	St. Paul	1893
Smith, D.D.	New Richland	1893
Soeffkir(?), H.	Arlington	1893
Solem, O.H.	Windom	1893
Soneral, Same	Sauk Centre	1894
Standish, A.M.	Arthyde	1893
Stowell, L.B.	Minneapolis	1893
Stratton, J.P.	Belle Plain	1893
Stromme, G.A.	Lanesboro	1893
Taylor, J.N.	Preston	1895
Teal, C.W.	Thief River Falls	1893
Thompson, D.L.	Minneapolis	1893
Thompson, H.F.	Minneapolis	1893
Thompson, W.M.	Adrian	1893
Van Dework, ?	Fair Haven	1893
Walz, J.D.	Sauk Rapids	1894
Warninger, J.	Bemidji	1894
Weillger, W.E.	Maple Grove	1894
Whiting, A.F.	Ortonville	1893
Zindell, Albin	Lamberton	1896

APPENDIX III

Biographies of Pioneer Veterinarians
Practicing in Minnesota in 1900

ADAMSON, J.H., (OVC, 1893), St. Paul, Minnesota. Born in 1858 in Chicago, Illinois; died on October 25, 1887 in St. Paul, Minnesota. Dr. Adamson taught anatomy at the U.S. College of Veterinary Surgeons, Washington, D.C., before entering practice in St. Paul in 1893. While treating a horse, Dr. Adamson was kicked in the abdomen. The blow resulted in perforation of his intestine from which he died a short time later.

ALLEN, Frank, (AmVC, 1889), St. Paul, Minnesota. Date and place of birth unknown; died in 1944 in St. Paul, Minnesota. Dr. Allen began practicing in St.Paul in 1889. For a time, he was veterinarian for the St. Paul Fire Department.

AMOS, Walter, (OVC, 1888), Owatonna, Minnesota. Born in 1864 in Guelph, Ontario, Canada; died on October 5, 1912, in Owatonna, Minnesota. Dr. Amos taught school in Canada before entering veterinary college. After receiving his veterinary degree, he located in Owatonna in 1888, and practiced there until his death at the age of 48. He was very active in his profession and often appeared on programs of MVMA. He was MVMA president from 1908 to 1909. He also served on the Board of Veterinary Medicine from 1908 until his death in 1912. Dr. Amos also was very active in community affairs. He was a prominent member of the Ancient Order of Workman. Dr. Amos suffered from tuberculosis and, while helping at a corn show in Owatonna, he sat in a draft that caused him to catch cold which progressed to pneumonia and caused his death.

ANDERSON, John P., (OVC, 1888), Rochester, Minnesota. Born on October 7, 1863, in Guelph, Ontario, Canada; died on October 20, 1928, in Rochester, Minnesota. Dr. Anderson began his practice in Rochester, Minnesota, in March of 1890, and remained in practice there until 1924 when he was forced to retire due to poor health. He was a charter member of the MVMA and served as president from 1910 to 1911. Dr. Anderson was a brother-in-law of Drs. Charles and William Mayo and Christofer Graham of the Mayo Clinic.

ANNAND, James G., (CVC, 1891), Wabasha, Minnesota. Born in 1867 in Lake City, Minnesota; died in Wabasha, Minnesota, date unknown. He began practice in Duluth, Minnesota in 1891, and later moved his practice to Wabasha, Minnesota. Dr. Annand worked on a temporary assignment for the Board of Animal Health from 1900 to 19043. He was a charter member of the MVMA and served as secretary in 1904.

BRIMHALL, Simon D., (UP, 1889), Rochester, Minnesota. Born in Dakota County, Minnesota in 1863; died in 1941 in Battle Creek, Michigan. Dr. Brimhall began practice in Minneapolis, Minnesota in 1889 and worked for the State Board of Health on animal health problems from 1897 to 1903. He was praised for his use of the laboratory to make diagnoses. When the Board of Animal Health was formed in 1903, he worked a field veterinarian for the Board from 1903 to 1904. He was a veterinarian with the Mayo Foundation in Rochester, Minnesota, from 1906 to 1913. Dr. Brimhall later practiced in Rochester until his retirement in 1938 when he moved to Battle Creek, Michigan. Dr. Brimhall was a charter member of the MVMA and served as the first president from 1897 to 1898.

BUTLER, J.S., (OVC, 1881), Minneapolis, Minnesota. Dates and places of birth and death unknown. Dr. Butler began a practice in Renville, Minnesota, in 1881. During the mid-1890's, he turned the practice over to Dr. J.R. Butters and relocated to Minneapolis, Minnesota, where he remained until at least 1906. He is reported to have subsequently relocated to Willmar, Minnesota, for a time and later to Raleigh, North Carolina. He was a member of the MVMA and served on the Board of Veterinary Medicine in 1889.

BUTTERS, J.R., (OVC. 1894), Renville, Minnesota. Born on January 17, 1871, in Metherwill, Ontario, Canada; died on December 13, 1948, in Willmar, Minnesota. Dr. Rutters was a student in the veterinary curriculum at the University of Minnesota in 1891. When this program was discontinued, he transferred to the Ontario College of Veterinary Medicine. He may have began practice in Waverly, Minnesota, in 1894, and later taken over Dr. Butler's practice in Renville. Dr. Butters and his wife celebrated their Golden Wedding Anniversary in 1947. He was a member of the MVMA and the Masonic Lodge.

CHUTE, Ernest N., (CVC, 1892), Fairmont, Minnesota. Born in 1872 in Fairmont, Minnesota; died on December 11, 1949, in Fairmont, Minnesota. Dr. Chute began a practice in Madison, Minnesota in 1892, before moving to Fairmont, Minnesota. He retired from practice in 1943. He was a charter member of the MVMA. Dr. Chute was also a member of the Minnesota National Guard from which he retired with the rank of captain and was very active in the Masonic Lodge.

COFFEEN, Robert J., (CVC, 1896), Stillwater, Minnesota. Born on December 30, 1864, in Columbus, Ohio; died on February 10, 1971, at the age of 106 in Stillwater, Minnesota. As a young boy, Dr. Coffeen worked in Buffalo Bill's Wild West Show. As he grew older, he gained quite a reputation as a wrestler in the midwest. In 1896, he began to practice in Albert Lea, Minnesota. In 1916, he became a field veterinarian for the Board of Animal Health. He resigned from this position after a few years and began a practice in Stillwater, Minnesota. Dr. Coffeen was the veterinarian for the St. Croix Lumber Co. He traveled to various logging camps to treat its horses. During World War I, at the age of 52, he talked his way into obtaining a first lieutenant's commission in the Army Veterinary Corps. At this age, he was a marvelous physical specimen and had the appearance of a much younger person. He was mustered out of the service in 1919 with the rank of captain. He was a member of the MVMA and served as president from 1923 to 1924. Dr. Coffeen was a member of the Board of Veterinary Medicine from 1916 to 1949 and served as secretary during many of those years. He was mayor of Stillwater from 1923 to 1927. On his 100th birthday, his friends honored him with a festive party.

COTTON, Charles E., (UP, 1893), Minneapolis, Minnesota. Born in Prescott, Wisconsin on September 18, 1871; died on April 21, 1954 in Minneapolis, Minnesota. Dr. Cotton was enrolled in the ill fated curriculum at the University of

Minnesota in 1891. When the curriculum was discontinued he transferred to the University of Pennsylvania to complete his veterinary degree work. As a student, he participated in the tuberculosis testing of the first herd of cattle in the United States. After graduation, Dr. Cotton practiced in Minneapolis from 1893 to 1918. While in practice, he tested cattle for tuberculosis in the Minneapolis and St. Paul areas. He was largely responsible for Minneapolis' requirement that milk sold within the city limits must be from cattle free of tuberculosis. He left private practice in 1918 to become secretary and executive officer of the Board of Animal Health. He was appointed a member of the first Board of Animal Health and remained on the Board until he was appointed secretary and executive officer. Dr. Cotton served in the Army Veterinary Corps from 1915 to 1918 and was mustered out with the rank of colonel. He was a charter member of the MVMA and president from 1909 to 1910. He was president of the AVMA in 1916 and a member of its Executive Board from 1920 to 1925. He was president of the U.S. Animal Health Association in 1936 and received the International Veterinary Congress Prize in 1952.

DALLIMORE, George Ambrose, (OCV, 1879), St. Paul, Minnesota. Born on April 11, 1848, in Toronto, Ontario, Canada; died on December 18, 1923, in St. Paul, Minnesota. After his death from apoplexy, he was buried in Faribault, Minnesota. Dr. Dallimore came from Canada in 1880 to start a practice in Faribault, Minnesota. He brought with him a pure bred Clydesdale stallion. He claimed this animal was the first of its breed in Southern Minnesota. Dr. Dallimore was elected to the Minnesota House of Representatives from the 24th District. In 1884, Dr. Dallimore moved to St. Paul, Minnesota, where he continued to practice. He was a charter member of the MVMA and a member of the Board of Veterinary Medicine from 1911 to 1915. He was also a member of the Masonic, Knights of Pythias and Odd Fellows Lodges.

DOUGLAS, Joseph Moffet, (OVC, 1894), Hendrum, Minnesota. Born on December 29, 1866, in Minnesota; died of diabetes on October 29, 1918, place unknown. He practiced all of his professional life at Hendrum and left a widow with nine children.

ECKLES, Charles F., (CVC; 1890), St. Charles, Minnesota. Born on May 9, 1864, in Eyota, Minnesota; died on November 11, 1933, in St. Charles, Minnesota. Dr. Eckles practiced all of his professional life in St. Charles and was very active in community affairs. He served several terms on the village council and was a member of the Odd Fellows and Moose Lodges. He had been ill with a cardiac problem for several months before he died of a heart attack.

ERB, Nelson S., (OVC, 1888), Faribault, Minnesota. Born on March 9, 1861, in Canada; died on August 19, 1944, in Faribault, Minnesota. Dr. Erb started a practice in Faribault after graduation in 1888. He practiced until about 1896 when Dr. Leopold Hay took over his practice. Dr. Erb then began working for a railroad company and remained with the company until 1909 when he purchased an interest in the Faribault Engine Mfg. Co. He eventually became secretary and manager of the company. He was elected to two-year terms as mayor of Faribault in 1910, 1915 and 1933. He was postmaster of Faribault from 1923 to 1924. He was also a charter member of the MVMA and served as president from 1898 to 1899. He was active in the Faribault Commercial Club and was a member of the Masonic and Elk Lodges.

FALCONER, Thomas, (OVC, 1894), Alexandria, Minnesota. Born on July 16, 1858, in Luchnow, Ontario, Canada; died on September 2, 1930, in Alexandria as the result of a skull fracture received in an automobile accident. Dr. Falconer came to North Dakota in 1877 and was a student in the veterinary curriculum at the University of Minnesota in 1891. When the curriculum was abolished, he transferred to the Ontario Veterinary College to obtain his veterinary degree. Dr. Falconer practiced for a very short time in North Dakota before moving to Glenwood, Minnesota in 1894. In 1902, he relocated a in Alexandria, Minnesota. He was a member of the MVMA and the AVMA.

FINLAY, James J., (OVC, 1888), Duluth, Minnesota. Born on August 18, 1860 in Aberdeen or Edinburgh, Scotland; died on September 23, 1938, in Duluth, Minnesota. Dr. Finlay practiced all of his professional life in Duluth. He was a member of the MVMA and of the Twelfth International Veterinary Congress. He was also a member of the Scottish Clan Stewart.

FRANK, Edward T., (CVC, 1897), Warren, Minnesota. Born on March 21, 1867, in Omro, Wisconsin; died on March 21, 1934, in Warren, Minnesota. Dr. Frank came to Warren in 1897 and practiced there all of his professional life (with the exception of 1904 when he took graduate studies at the Kansas City College of Veterinary Medicine). He was a member of the MVMA and served as president from 1917 to 1918. Dr. Frank was very active in community affairs. He helped organize the Marshall County Agricultural Society and served as its secretary for many years. Dr. Frank also was active in horse racing and had a fine horse by the name of Radium. He raced the horse himself and, according to family history, Radium finished second to Dan Patch in a race in which Dan Patch set a new world record. Radium was given credit for forcing Dan Patch run fast enough to set the record.

GOULD, John N., (CVC, 1893), Worthington, Minnesota. Born on December 13, 1869 in Fairmont, Minnesota; died on February 27, 1932, in Worthington, Minnesota. Dr. Gould was a student at the Northwestern Veterinary College in Minneapolis when it burned in 1889. He then entered the Chicago Veterinary College with his father. After receiving his veterinary degree in 1893, Dr. John N. Gould practiced in Jackson, Minnesota, for less than a year before moving to Worthington, Minnesota. He served as a private in the U.S. Army from 1898 to 1903. On May 7, 1917, he was commissioned first lieutenant in the U.S. Army to serve in World War I. He retired as a major on May 12, 1922. Dr. Gould was a charter member of the MVMA and was president from 1901 to 1902. In Worthington, he served as alderman, president of the village council, member of the Board of Education and member of the Worthington Civic and Commerce Association. He was a member of the Masonic Lodge and Kiwanis.

GOULD, John Whipple, (CVC. 1893), Fairmont, Minnesota. Born in 1844 in Vermont; died on March 16, 1910, in Worthington, Minnesota. Dr. Gould served in the Civil War and later settled on a land claim in Martin County. He was the father of Dr. John N. Gould with whom he attended the Chicago Veterinary College. In 1893, after receiving his veterinary degree, Dr. John Whipple Gould returned to practice in Fairmont. During John Whipple's terminal illness, he was taken to Worthington where he was cared for by his son.

GRAHAM, Christofer, (UP, 1892), Rochester, Minnesota. Born on April 3, 1856, in Cortland, New York; died on June 20, 1952, in Rochester, Minnesota. Dr. Graham early life exemplifies the hardships endured in obtaining higher education during those times. As a boy, Dr. Graham walked 7 miles from his parents home to the nearest school. His attendance was sporadic—sometimes as little as 3 months during a school year. When he was 20 years old, he entered a private school. After attending for only 6 months, he taught in a country school from 1879 to 1881. Dr. Graham then returned to a private school to complete his pre-college education. In 1882, he enrolled at the University of Minnesota where he was classified as a sub-freshman. His academic progress was interrupted for 6 to 9 months while he taught school to earn money to continue his education. He received his B.S. in 1887 and taught for 2 years at Shattuck School in Faribault, Minnesota. He eventually enrolled in the University of Pennsylvania Veterinary College when he received his veterinary degree in 1892. Dr. Graham returned to the University of Minnesota on an interim appointment as an instructor on the Agricultural Experiment Station staff. This position filled the void left by the resignation of Dr. Schwartzkoff. Dr. Graham remained on the staff for one year and then entered the University of Pennsylvania Medical School. He graduated in 1894 and joined the staff at the Mayo Clinic at Rochester, Minnesota, where he earned a worldwide reputation in internal medicine. He became Head of the Department of Internal Medicine in 1909 and remained in that position until he retired in 1919. Dr. Graham never lost his interest in veterinary medicine. He often attended veterinary meetings and the summer clinics. He had a farm near Rochester and developed one of the best Holstein-Friesian herds in the midwest. He also bred high quality Percheron and Shire horses.

HANISH, Joseph A., (OVC, 1891), Lake City, Minnesota. Born on June 10, 1867, in La Crosse, Wisconsin; died on April 12, 1901, in Lake City, Minnesota. Dr. Hanish moved with his parents to Lake City when he was two years old. His father sent him to the Ontario Veterinary College to fulfill his boyhood desire to be a veterinarian. After receiving his veterinary degree, Dr. Hanish began practice in Lake City. In 1899, he subsequently started a practice in Zumbrota. He only stayed in Zumbrota for one year and then returned to Lake

City where he remained for the rest of his life. He was a charter member of the MVMA and a member of the AVMA. He also belonged to the Ancient Order of United Workmen and the Sons of Herman Lodge. Dr. Hanish never married. He died as the result of "acute muscular rheumatism" which caused him great suffering. He was only 38 years of age when he died.

HAY, Leopold, (OVC, 1896), Faribault, Minnesota. Born on June 16, 1873, in Russia; died on March 12, 1928, in Faribault, Minnesota. When Dr. Hay was 7 years of age, his Scottish parents moved from Russia to Scotland. He attended the University of Edinburgh and, to satisfy his requirement for military duty, he served in the Queen's Cavalry. After completing his military duty, he went to Canada and enrolled in the Ontario Veterinary College. After graduation in 1896, he went to Faribault, Minnesota, and took over the practice of Dr. Nelson Erb. Dr. Hay was a member of the MVMA and served as its president from 1904 to 1905. He also was a member of the Board of Veterinary Medicine and served as secretary for many years. At the time of his death, he was the Dairy Inspector for the City of Faribault. He was also a member of the Masonic, Osman Temple, United Workman and Elk Lodges.

ILLSTRUP, Frederick A., (CVC, 1893), Willmar, Minnesota. Born in 1868 in Buffalo, Minnesota; died on June 5, 1911, in Willmar, Minnesota. Dr. Illstrup began his practice out of state before returning to Minnesota. He moved to Willmar in 1895 where he remained until his death. Dr. Illstrup was treating an animal on a farm when he suffered a fatal heart attack.

KALB, Edward L., (OVC, 1893), Rochester, Minnesota. Born on November 13, 1872, in Rochester, Minnesota; died on August 2, 1914, in Rochester, Minnesota. As a young man, Dr. Kalb worked in his older brother's drug store. After the death of his brother, he decided to become a veterinarian because of his love for horses. Dr. Kalb practiced all of his professional life in Rochester and was elected alderman in 1905. He was a member of the MVMA, AVMA, Knights of Pythias, Independent Order of Workmen and Elk Lodge.

KIRBY, Burrows K., (OVC, 1886), St. Paul, Minnesota. Born in 1848 in Warickshire, England; died in 1928 in St. Paul, Minnesota. Before attending veterinary college, Dr. Kirby owned and operated a pharmacy in Elk River, Minnesota. At one time, he also was Register of Deeds for Sherburne County, Minnesota. After receiving his veterinary degree, Dr. Kirby opened a veterinary practice in St. Paul and was veterinarian for the City's Department of Health. He was a member of the MVMA and served on the Board of Veterinary Medicine from 1893 to 1900.

KJERNER, Rudy, (OVC, 1896), Chatfield, Minnesota. Born on November 1, 1870, in Rochester, Minnesota; died on February 10, 1933, in Rochester, Minnesota. Dr. Kjerner came to Chatfield in 1896 and practiced until his death (with the exception of one year spent at Dogden, North Dakota). During the last 10 years of his professional life, he mainly tested cattle for the Board of Animal Health.

KUHNS, Walter A., (OVC, 1899), Chaska, Minnesota. Born on March 12, 1872, in Boston, Massachusetts; died on September 19, 1935, in Chaska, Minnesota. Dr. Kuhns was a noted musician before becoming a veterinarian. At the age of 6, he began taking violin lessons and, by age 9, he was performing in Boston theaters. He went to Germany and France to study under European masters. Dr. Kuhns returned to America when he was 19 or 20 years old and became a member of the New York Sympathy Orchestra. After a short time with the orchestra, he decided to become a veterinarian. He went to Canada to obtain his degree. He subsequently took graduate work at Harvard University and operated a small animal clinic in Boston for a short period of time. In 1899, he located in Paynesville, Minnesota, for a very short time and then accepted a contract commission with the British Army during the Boer War in Africa. He made three trips with horses from the port of New Orleans, Louisiana, to South Africa. When Dr. Kuhns finished his contract with the British Army, he moved from Paynesville to Chaska where he practiced until his death.

LAMBRECHTS, Bernard, (RVC, 1853), Granite Falls, Minnesota. Born on April 15, 1828, in Christiana, Norway; died on March 20, 1907, in Granite Falls, Minnesota. Dr. Lambrechts was the first college trained veterinarian to practice in

Minnesota. Dr. Lambrechts received his veterinary degree from the Royal Veterinary and Agricultural University, in Copenhagen, Denmark. After graduation he served as veterinary surgeon for the Norweigian Army for 12 years. He subsequently worked for two years on the eradication of contagious diseases for the Norweigian Government. He emigrated to the United States in 1867, and practiced in Wisconsin, Iowa and Texas before coming to Minnesota in 1872. He first located at Willmar, and, in 1890, moved to Montevideo. In 1900, he received his M.D. from St. Louis University and relocated in Granite Falls later that year. During his career, he also studied for two years in Vienna, Austria. Dr. Lambrechts was a charter member of the MVMA and served on the Board of Veterinary Medicine from 1901 to 1905. He was the father of Dr. T. Lambrechts of Montevideo who graduated from the McKillip Veterinary College in 1901.

LANGEVIN, Hector, (McG, 1879), Crookston, Minnesota. Born on January 10, 1860 in Quebec Province, Canada; died on December 23, 1940 at Crookston, Minnesota. Dr. Langevin began his practice at Crookston in 1880, and continued to practice there until a few years before his death. He was active in his profession and was a charter member of the MVMA. Dr. Langevin was well educated in history and literature. He was regarded as one of the most broadly educated veterinarians of his era. He was the father of Dr. Elmer Langevin who graduated from the McKillip Veterinary College in 1912 and who also practiced in Crookston

LaPOINTE, J.T., (McG, 1886), St Peter, Minnesota. He was born on August 31, 1860, in St. Scholastique, Quebec, Canada; died on January 19, 1923, in St. Peter, Minnesota. Dr. LaPointe practiced for a short time in North Carolina and West Virginia before coming to St. Peter in 1888.

LEECH, G. Ed., (CVC, 1891), Winona, Minnesota. He was born on September 17, 1857, in Delavan, Wisconsin; died of pneumonia on June 4, 1947, in St. Paul, Minnesota. After receiving his veterinary degree, Dr. Leech practiced for a short time in Milwaukee and then relocated to Winona in 1891. When Winona required that all milk sold in the city must be from tuberculosis free cattle, Dr. Leech was authorized by the Board of Animal Health to test the cattle supplying milk to the city.

Dr. Leech moved to St. Paul, Minnesota, in 1940 where he remained until he retired to Delavan, Wisconsin. He was visiting in St. Paul when he contracted pneumonia and died in 1947. He was a member of the AVMA, and served as secretary of the MVMA from 1909 to 1915. He was also a member of the Masonic Lodge.

LEES, Arnold F., (OVC, 1889), Red Wing, Minnesota. Born on December 21, 1866, in London, England; died on March 17, 1957, in Red Wing, Minnesota. Dr. Lees came to Canada as a young man and, after receiving his veterinary degree, started a practice in Red Wing, Minnesota, in 1889. He was an avid horse racing fan who owned his own horses. Dr. Lees often raced his own horses. He was the author of several articles on racing and on veterinary surgery. He was a member of the MVMA and served as its president from 1905 to 1906. He also served on the Board of Veterinary Medicine. In his later years, he often worked for the Board of Animal Health as a per diem veterinarian testing cattle for tuberculosis and brucellosis.

LYFORD, Charles Chambers, (C.C.), (McG, 1877), Minneapolis, Minnesota. Born on August 21, 1853, in Roscoe, Illinois; died on June 15, 1925, in Roscoe, Illinois. Dr. Lyford was a very well educated veterinarian. He received his B.S. in agriculture from the University of Illinois in 1875, his veterinary degree in 1877 from McGill University, and his M.D. from McGill University in 1879. At McGill University, he studied for a time under the famous physician, Sir William Osler. He also did graduate work at the Royal Veterinary College in London. Dr. Lyford came to Minneapolis in 1880. He was the founder and president of the Northwestern Veterinary College which was later destroyed by fire in 1889. He was City Veterinarian of Minneapolis from 1881 to 1890. Dr. Lyford was a charter member of the MVMA and served as president from 1902 to 1903. He also served as vice president of the AVMA in 1901. Dr. Lyford was a prolific writer and often appeared on local and national veterinary programs where he delivered papers and surgical demonstrations. Dr. Lyford was a lover of fast horses and maintained a stable of trotting horses. Dr. Lyford drove his horses in several races. Many of his fine horses were destroyed in the fire at the Northwestern Veterinary College. In later years, Dr. Lyford moved to Graceville,

Minnesota, and to Osseo, Minnesota, before retiring to Roscoe, Illinois.

McGILLIVARY, George, (OVC, 1885), Roseau, Minnesota. Born on April 21, 1856, in Whitby, Ontario, Canada; died on February 10, 1938, in Roseau, Minnesota. After receiving his veterinary degree, Dr. McGillivary practiced in Pipestone, Minnesota, and in Browns Valley, Minnesota, before relocating to Roseau, Minnesota. He was a member of the MVMA and served as president from 1907 to 1908. He was active in community affairs and served several terms on the Roseau School Board.

McKAY, John M., (OVC, 1895), Duluth, Minnesota. Born in 1872 in Scotland; died on November 3, 1948, in Duluth, Minnesota. Dr. McKay operated a livery stable on the west side of Duluth for many years. He was a lover of horses and had a stable of race horses. He was widely known for his ability to drive horses in races on the ice of Lake Superior. He was the father of Dr. John M. McKay, Jr., who took over his practice.

McKENZIE, K.J., (OCV, 1892), Northfield, Minnesota. Born on August 6, 1868 in Picton, Nova Scotia, Canada; died on January 30, 1946, in Northfield, Minnesota. Dr. McKenzie was a student in the short-lived veterinary curriculum at the University of Minnesota in 1891. He transferred to the Ontario Veterinary College to receive his veterinary degree. In 1892, he began a practice in Redwood Falls, Minnesota, and, in about 1896, moved to Northfield, Minnesota. He was a charter member of the MVMA and served as secretary for a time. He served as president of MVMA from 1903 to 1904. He was also a member of the Board of Veterinary Medicine, serving as its president and secretary. Dr. McKenzie was a horse racing fan and served as superintendent of the horse department at the Rice County Fair for many years. He, along with Dr. Alexander, Dr. Lee and Dr. Higbee, often attended county fair horse races. Dr. McKenzie served on the village council of Northfield for 12 years and was the city's mayor from 1926 to 1932. He was a member of the Masonic Lodge and the Osmon Temple.

McLOUGHLIN, J.J., (ISU, 1890), Blue Earth, Minnesota. Born on April 13, 1866, in Hamilton County, Iowa; died on January 16, 1934, in Blue Earth, Minnesota. Dr. McLoughlin began practice in Rush City, Minnesota, after receiving his veterinary degree in 1890. In 1891, he moved to Blue Earth, Minnesota, where he practiced all of his remaining professional life. Dr. McLaughlin served as a member of the Board of Education and Board of Public Works, as well as the mayor, of Blue Earth.

MUELLER, Emil, (OVC, 1892), New Ulm, Minnesota. Born on September 8, 1869, in Brown County, Minnesota; died on December 5, 1938, in New Ulm, Minnesota. Dr. Mueller started a practice in New Ulm Minnesota after receiving his veterinary degree in 1892. He served on the New Ulm Council for eight years and was president of the Council for three of those years. He was also mayor of New Ulm for eight years and a director on the Brown County Fair Board. Dr. Mueller was president of the Farmers and Merchants State Bank of New Ulm at the time of his death. He was active in politics and a member of the Republican Party. He was a member of the Masonic and Knights of Templar Lodges.

PETERS, H.C., (OVC, 1896), Litchfield, Minnesota. Born on February 6, 1866, in Greenleaf Township, Meeker County, Minnesota; died on August 24, 1930, in Litchfield, Minnesota. He had the reputation in the Litchfield area of answering farm calls regardless of the weather (sub-zero temparatures, snow, blizzard), the condition of the roads, or the time of the day or night. Dr. Peters was a member of the MVMA.

POMEROY, Benjamin A., (McG, 1883), St. Paul, Minnesota. Born in July 5, 1861, in Compton, Quebec, Canada; died on January 12, 1956, in St. Paul, Minnesota. Dr. Pomeroy came to St. Paul and started a practice in 1894. When the City of St. Paul began requiring milk sold within the city limits be from tuberculosis free cattle, Dr. Pomeroy tested many of the cattle. In nearly 70 years of practice, Dr. Pomeroy saw his practice change from treating almost exclusively large animals (mostly horses) to primarily small animals. Dr. Pomeroy was veterinarian for the Prevention of Cruelty to Animals Society from 1893 to 1898, and a member of the Board of Examiners for Horseshoers for 1903 to 1905. He was a member of the AVMA, and served as president of the MVMA from 1938 to 1939. Dr. Pomeroy was the father of three sons who became veterinarians: Benjamin S., Iowa State University, 1933; Harold,

Colorado State University, 1848; and James, Kansas State University, 1949. Dr. Pomeroy's grandson, Dr. Fred W. Pomeroy, University of Minnesota, 1974, has continued the practice started by his grandfather.

PRICE, Richard, (McG, 1881), St. Paul, Minnesota. Born on May 18, 1856 in Dublin, Ireland; died on April 3, 1909, in St. Paul. Dr. Price was sent to England as a boy in 1864 to attend school. He attended Hampton and Chester before entering Leamington College. In 1871, at the end of his third year at the college, he went to the Wimbledon School with the intend to eventually enter the army. Due to changed circumstances, he subsequently went to Germany in 1872 and spent two years in the principal cities of that country. After returning to Ireland for a short time, Dr. Price went to Montreal, Canada in 1878, and entered McGill University. He received his veterinary degree and came to St. Paul, Minnesota, in April of 1881. Dr. Price started a practice in St. Paul, and remained there during his professional life. He did investigative work on animal disease for the State Health Department from 1884 through the 1890's. Dr. Price taught medicine and surgery in the Northwestern Veterinary College. He was a charter member of the MVMA and served as president from 1905 to 1906. He was the father of Dr. Richard H. Price who continued his father's practice.

REYNOLDS, Myron H., (ISU, 1889), St. Paul, Minnesota. Born on November 1, 1865, in Wheaton, Illinois; died on January 5, 1929 in St. Paul, Minnesota. Dr. Reynolds was broadly educated in medicine. After receiving his veterinary degree in 1889, he received an M.D. from the Iowa College of Physicians and Surgeons in 1891 and a degree from the Iowa College of Pharmacy the same year. In 1892, Dr. Reynolds was hired to join the speakers staff of the Farmer's Institute which was part of the School of Agriculture at the University of Minnesota. He remained an Iowa resident during this period of employment and traveled to Minnesota for his speaking engagements. In 1893, Dr. Reynolds was appointed veterinarian on the staff of the School of Agriculture. When more veterinarians were added to the staff, Dr. Reynolds became professor and head of the Division of Veterinary Medicine at the University. He held that position until he was replaced in 1917. Dr. Reynolds continued as a professor in the division until his death in 1929. He was a member of the Minnesota Board of Health in 1897 and, when the Board of Animal Health was created in 1903, he was appointed a member and remained on the Board until 1921. Dr. Reynolds helped obtain passage of the Practice Acts. He was a charter member of the MVMA and president from 1899 to 1900. He also was a member of the AVMA, served on many of its committees, and was elected vice president in 1902. He appeared on many professional programs presenting papers and giving demonstrations. He was a member of the American Animal Health Association and the International Tuberculosis Committee. He wrote a textbook entitled "Veterinary Studies" for agricultural students.

RYDELL, Oscar, (CVC, 1894), Wheaton, Minnesota. He was born on April 23, 1869, in Rud, Vasa, Stocken Parish, Varmland, Sweden; died on March 28, 1936, in Wheaton, Minnesota. Dr. Rydell immigrated to the United States when he was 19 years of age. After receiving his veterinary degree, he practiced in River Falls, Wisconssin, until 1898 when he moved to Wheaton, Minnesota. He practiced there for about 30 years before retiring. He was a member of the AVMA and the MVMA. He was the father of Dr. Robert Rydell, ISU, 1934, who practiced for a time in Minnesota and then moved to Turtle Lake, North Dakota.

SCHWARTZKOFF, Olaf, (Imperial Veterinary College, Berlin, 1880). Born on August 29, 1855, in Ostromzetzko, Germany; died on June 3, 1923, in Wiesbaden, Germany. After receiving his veterinary degree, Dr. Swchwartzkoff practiced in Germany until 1885 when he immigrated to the United States. He took an assistantship with Dr. F.S. Billings, a noted veterinarian in New York City. After about a year, he left Dr. Billings and became a veterinarian with the U.S. 8th Calvary. He was a member of the command when the 8th Calvary went overland a distance of two thousand miles from Fort David, Texas, to Fort Meade, South Dakota. On January 1, 1889, he accepted a position of Professor of Veterinary Science in the College of Agriculture and Experiment Station at the University of Minnesota where he instituted the curriculum in veterinary medicine. He resigned from his post at the University in 1892. Dr. Schwartzkoff went to the McKillip Veterinary College in Chicago and was dean when it opened

in 1894. He remained there until 1897 when he left and became a professor in the American Veterinary College in New York City. In 1900, he was reappointed as an Army veterinarian and was assigned to the 3rd Calvary which spent some time in the Philippines. When the Army was reorganized in 1901, he was appointed Veterinarian of the Calvary. In May of 1918, he was transferred to Fort Snelling, Minnesota, as Post Veterinarian. He remained there until September of 1918 when he was transferred to Fort D.A. Russell in Wyoming. He retired on August 19, 1919, at the rank of major and moved back to Germany. Dr. Schwartzkoff was an early advocate of proper recognition of veterinarians in the Army. He was a prolific writer and a frequent contributor to veterinary periodicals. He did not hesitate to disagree in a forceful manner with the views and beliefs of others. For many years, he was a collaborator on the editorial staff of the American Veterinary Review.

SCRUBY, W.H., (CVC, 1897), St. Cloud, Minnesota. Born in April, 1843 at Oconomowoc, Wisconsin; date and place of death unknown. Dr. Scruby was one of the non-graduate veterinarians appointed to the first Board of Veterinary Medicine on which he served from 1893 to 1896. From his experience on the Board, he saw the importance of formalized training in veterinary medicine. He subsequently attended the Chicago Veterinary College and obtained his veterinary degree in 1897. By the time he received his license to practice, he had relocated to Melrose, Minnesota. He is believed to have practiced at St. Cloud for a time and then moved to Richmond, Minnesota. In the January 13, 1910 issue of the St. Cloud Daily Journal-Press, an article entitled, "Man Found Lying in Snow," appeared that stated Dr. Scruby collapsed while walking through the snow to the Great Northern Depot. He was going to take the train home to Richmond. He was found by a passerby and taken to a hotel where he spent the night. The next morning Dr. Scruby was better but unable to remember what had happened to him. He was eventually able to return home.

SIGMUND, Charles J., (OVC, 1893), Pipestone, Minnesota. Born on February 3, 1867, in Cook County, Illinois; died on January 25, 1955, in Pipestone, Minnesota. Dr. Sigmund started to practice in Duluth, Minnesota, and, after a short time, moved to Austin, Minnesota. He eventually located in Pipestone, Minnesota, where he remained until his death. He retired in 1945 and died after a long illness. He was a member of the MVMA and was president from 1912 to 13.

SONERAL, William, (CVC, 1897), Cambridge, Minnesota. Born on April 10, 1867, in Vastmanland County, Sweden; died on June 11, 1950, in San Francisco, California. Dr. Soneral moved to Ludington, Michigan, with his parents when he was 16 years old. In his early 20s, he ran a grocery store in Chicago for a time and later entered the Chicago Veterinary College. When he graduated in 1897, he started a practice in Cambridge where he practiced until his retirement. He served as mayor of Cambridge and was on the School Board for several years. Dr. Soneral was a large man with tremendous strength. He enjoyed showing his strength by crushing the other person's hand during a handshake and watching them cringe with pain.

SPENCE, Andrew, (OVC, 1893), Hallock, Minnesota. Born on the Orkney Islands on the North Coast of Scotland; died on January 12, 1943, in Hallock. Minnesota. Dr. Spence came to Emerson, Manitoba, Canada, in the 1880's where he worked for a veterinarian. The veterinarian helped finance his schooling at the Ontario Veterinary College. After receiving his veterinary degree, Dr. Spence returned to Emerson to practice. Emerson is located near the Manitoba-Minnesota line, and some of his calls took him to Minnesota. In 1903, he moved to Hallock, Minnesota, which is near Emerson but across the border of the two countries. Dr. Spence continued to take calls in Manitoba as well as in North Dakota. Dr. Spence was noted for his willingness to help needy persons. He also was a great supporter of the Hallock community.

TREACY, Michael J., (Royal Veterinary College, London), St. Paul, Minnesota. Born in New York City, date unknown; died of yellow fever on July 14, 1899; in the District Army Hospital near Puero Principe, Cuba. Dr. Treacy joined the British Calvary after receiving his veterinary degree. He served in India from 1874 to 1879. He practiced in various parts of Western United States until 1883 when he joined the U.S. 7th Calvary. He left the service in August of 1888 to become the first veterinarian on the staff of the University of Minnesota. However, he resigned after only a short time and rejoined the Army. He was assigned to the 8th Calvary where he remained until his death. Dr. Treacy was a strong advocate of reform in the U.S. Army Veterinary Corps. He published a leaflet, "The Defects of the U.S. Army Veterinary Service." This was used for many years as a guide in requesting Army veterinary reform legislation in Congress. Finally, the Army Reorganization Bill was passed which included some of the changes he had proposed, including as an examination for veterinary competency. He had taken and passed the examination just prior to his death.

WARD, Samuel H., (OVC, 1894), St. Paul, Minnesota. Dr. Ward was born in Selkirk, Manitoba, Canada, date unknown; died of influenza on December 14, 1918, in St. Paul, Minnesota. After receiving his veterinary degree, Dr. Ward began a practice in St. Cloud, Minnesota. He stayed there until he was elected secretary and executive officer of the Board of Animal Health in 1903. With the exception of from 1907 to 1908, he held this position until his death in 1918. Dr. Ward was a charter member of the MVMA and president from 1900 to 1901. He was president of the U.S. Animal Health Association in 1912, and secretary from 1915 until his death.

WHITCOMB, Morton S., (CVC, 1892), St. Paul, Minnesota. Born in 1866 in Austin, Minnesota; died on November 30, 1940, in St. Paul, Minnesota. Dr. Whitcomb began practice in Austin, Minnesota, and continued there until 1904 when he accepted a position with the Board of Animal Health in St. Paul. He served as secretary and executive officer for one year. He remained with the Board until he resigned in 1931. He was also a member of the AVMA.

WHITE, Robert, (OVC, 1879), St. Paul, Minnesota. Born on February 19, 1853, in Toronto, Canada; died on March 2, 1941, in St. Paul, Minnesota. After graduation, Dr. White came to St. Paul where he practiced all of his professional life. For 18 years, he was veterinarian for the St. Paul Fire Department and traveled to the various fire stations to care for its horses. He also was a contract veterinarian for the U.S. Calvary at Fort Snelling. In the 1890s, he wrote a veterinary column in the Northwestern Farmer and Breeder. Dr. White was the owner of one of the first automobiles in St. Paul.

WILLYOUNG, Lester Edwin, (McG, 1890), St. Paul, Minnesota. Born on December 10, 1869, in Bowmanville, New York; died on July 11, 1937, in Princeton, West Virginia. Dr. Willyoung practiced in St. Paul from the time of his graduation until 1903 when he became an Army veterinarian. He retired from the Army on January 17, 1917, with the rank of first lieutenant. On May 17, 1917, he was called back to active duty as a captain in the meat inspection service. He retired from the Army in 1919. Dr. Willyoung was a member of the AVMA.

YOUNGBERG, Anton, (CVC, 1892), Lake Park, Minnesota. Born in March of 1861, in Sweden; died in 1907 in California. Dr. Youngberg was a prominent member of the veterinary profession. He often appeared on professional programs both locally and nationally. He was a charter member of the MVMA and served on many committees. Dr. Youngberg was the father of Dr. Stanton Youngberg who received his veterinary degree from Ohio State University in 1911.

KEY TO ABBREVIATIONS FOR VETERINARY SCHOOLS

AmVC	American Veterinary College
CVC	Chicago Veterinary College
ISU	Iowa State Veterinary College
McK	McKillip Veterinary College, Chicago
McG	McGill University Veterinary College, Canada
NWV	Northwestern Veterinary College, Minneapolis
OVC	Ontario Veterinary College, Canada
RVC	Royal Veterinary College, Denmark
UP	University of Pennsylvania Veterinary College
WVC	Western Veterinary College, Kansas City

PRIMARY SOURCES LISTING

CHAPTER I

PIONEER VETERINARY MEDICINE IN MINNESTOA

American Veterinary History; 1891, 1892, 1900
Evolution of Veterinary Art, by J.F. Smithcors, 1957
History of Minnesota, by Val Bjornson, vol. I, 1969
History of Minnesota, by Willaim W. Folwell, vol I, 1921
Men to Remember, by Kenneth D. Ruble, 1947
Minnesota Board of Animal Health Minutes and Records
Minnesota Board of Veterinary Examiners Records
Minnestoa State Board of Health Reports; 1886-1890
Northwestern Farmer and Breeder; 1882,1884,1885,1892
Obituaries in local newspapers, American Veterinary Review and Journal of the American Veterinary Medical Association (JAVMA)
Practice of Veterinary Surgery, by Jno. A.W. Dollar, Vol. I, 1902
Red River Trails, by Rhoda Gilman, Carolyn Gilman and Deborah Gilman, 1979
U.S. Agricultural Census; 1870, 1880
Veterinary Materia Medica and Therapeutics, by Kennels Winslow, 3rd Ed., 1904
Veterinary Military History by Louis A. Merillat and Delwin M. Campbell
Oral Histroies: T.R. Eliason, Leslie Jacobson, M.P. Maher, A.C. Spannaus, and C.H. Wetter
Personal Information: Leslie Jacobson, Fred Gehrman, A.C. Spannaus, and C.H. Wetter

CHAPTER II

BOARD OF VETERINARY EXAMINERS

Journal of Minnesota House of Representatives: 1889-H.F. 113; 1891-H.F. 31; and 1893-H.F. 201
Laws of Minnesota: 1893-Chapter 31; 1901-Chapter 291; 1903-Chapter 149; and 1907-Chapter 419
Minnesota Board of Animal Health Minutes
Minnesota Vaterinary Examiners Board Minutes and Reports
Oral Histories: Griselda (Bee) Hanlon, and Joan Parent
Personal Information: Harold Kircher, Roland Olson, and Glen Nelson

CHAPTER III

CONTROL OF ANIMAL DISEASES

BOARD OF ANIMAL HEALTH

Albert Lea Tribune, Feb. 3, 1959
American Vetrinary Review, Vol 20, 1897
Bricelyn Sentinel, Mar. 3, 1960
Century of Progress, Iowa Veterinary Medical Association, by Ron Lutz, 1979
Ineffectiveness of proprietary remedies and other drugs in the control of Bang's disease with special reference to "3V Tonic and Bowman's," by A.R. Crawford and R.A. Beach, J. Agr. Res., Vol 60, 1940
Grant County Herald, Jan. 3, 1963
Invited and conquered - Historical Sketch of Tuberculosis in
Minnesota, by J. Arthur Myers, 1949
Litchfield Independent: May 2, 1923, Mar. 4, 1925, and Mar. 11, 1925 Minnesota by J. Arthur Myers, 1949
Minnesota Board of Health Annual and Biennial Reports
Minnesota Board of Health Minutes: 1903-1988
Minnesota Senate Journal: 1895
Minnesota State Board of Health Annual and Biennial Reports: 1883-1886
Pope County Tribune, Sept. 2, 1948
Vaccination against Bang's disease in an infected herd with United States Bureau of Animal Industry Brucella abortus strain 19, by C.M. Haring, J.A.V.M.A. Vol 92, 1946
Unpublished material, by Harry Olson
Personal Information: Jack Flint, George Keller, Harold Kircher, Walter Mackey, B.S. Pomeroy, Robert Pyle, C.H. Wetter, and G.F. Yager

CHAPTER IV

STATE AND REGIONAL ASSOCIATIONS

American Veterinary Review: 1892 and 1902
Information from officers and records of regional veterinary associations in Minnesota
J.A.V.M.A. issues with information about Minnesota veterinary associations
Minnesota Academy of Veterinary Medical Practice Records
Minnesota Academy of Veterinary Technicians Records
Minnesota Veterinary Medical Association Records

Proceedings of 19th Yearly Session of Minnesota
Veterinary Association
St. Paul Pioneer Press, Jan. 19, 1897 (and other
issues at time of Annual Meeting of M.V.M.A.)
Women's Auxillary of Minnesota Veterinary
Medical Association Records
Personal Information: W. Clough Cullen, Fred
Gehrman, James Karcher, Walter Mackey, and
B.S. Pomeroy

CHAPTER V

COLLEGE OF VETERINARY MEDICINE

American Veterinary Review, 1888
College of Veterinary Medicine Files
Faribault Daily News, Mar. 3, 1947
Grant County Herald, Jan. 3, 1963
Journal of Minnesota House of Represenatives:
1947-H.F. 420; and H.F. 1573
Journal of Minnesota Senate: 1947-S.F. 1422
Laws of Minnesota: 1947, pages 598, 1039, 1284
Minnesota Daily: Feb. 24, 1947; Feb. 19, 1947;
Feb. 29, 1947; and April 26, 1947
Minnesota Journal of Veterinary Medicine
St. Paul Dispatch, Mar. 13, 1947
St. Paul Pioneer Press, Nov. 29, 1946; Feb. 15,
1947; April 12, 1947; Mar. 12, 1947; Mar. 19,
1947; Mar. 23, 1947; April 18, 1947; April 21,
1947; April 22, 1947; Sept. 30. 1947; and Dec. 17,
1948
University of Minnesota Archives
W.L. Boyd papers
College of Agriculture correspondence regarding
veterinary medicine
College of Agriculture papers and reports
History of School of Agriculture by Andrew Boss
(unpublished)
Information on and photographs of buildings
Letters to Dean Bailey
Letters of Presidents Burton and Coffey
M.H. Reynolds papers
U. of M. Board of Regents Minutes: 1881-80
U. of M. Presidents Annual and Biennial Reports
Oral History: Robert Dunlop, Griselda Hanlon,
William Kehr, Representative August Mueller,
Senator Ancher Nelson, Glen Nelson, JoAnn
Schmidt O"Brien, Arden Ostergaard, Benjamin
S. Pomeroy, Jay Sautter, Dale Sorensen, and
Alvin Weber
Personal Information: Sidney Ewing, Gary
Duke, William Kehr, Glen Nelson, Arden
Ostergaard, and Dale Sorensen

SUBJECT INDEX

INDEX TO NAMES IN TEXT

Butman, Mrs. Leslie (Rosemary), 115
Butters, J.R., 125,230
Button, A.L., 14
Campbell, Mrs. John N., 114
Campbell, John N., 92,105,119,141,142,144,145, 151,156
Campbell, M.R., 117
Cano, Marie Joy, 157
Carey, Senator D.M., 136,137
Carlson, C.R., 118
Carlson, Alfred, 119
Carlson, F.W., 118
Carnes, Norris, 42,105
Carolus, Donna, 23
Carroll, Bill, 30
Carroll, Nellie, 30
Casey, Charles, 105,171
Cashman, Thomas E., 60
Casky, Mike, 45
Cavanaugh, J.L., 119
Chapin, Mrs. G.V. (Mildred), 114
Chase, C.C., 86
Chesley, A.J., 68
Christensen, Patricia (Patti), 86
Christensen, Clyde, 105
Christensen, M.B., 157
Christensen, C.A., 158
Christensen, Mrs. L.T. (Dorothy), 114
Christensen, LeRoy T., 93,105
Christianson, Odell, 86
Christianson, N.A.,125
Christianson, Governor Theodore, 34,167
Christie, Patti, 116
Christison, Thomas M., 142
Christison, M.J., 158
Chute, E.N., 89,231
Clausen, L.E., 71,72
Clauson, Mrs. Wm. E. (Kathy), 115
Clauson, Wm. E., 117
Clifford, Donald, 117,156
Clough, Gov. David Marston, 27
Coffeen, R.J., 18,23,31,32,92,231
Coffey, Walter C., 35,144,167
Coffman, Lotus D., 131,167
Collier, John R., 139
Collins, James, 169
Contag, Carlus H., 86
Contag, Mrs. Carlus H. (Ann), 115
Converse, Clarence, 71
Converse, Clarence, 71
Conway, R.L., 120
Cook, Alvina, 177
Cook, B.L., 92

Cotton, Mrs. Charle E., 108,114
Cotton, Charles E., 17,29,31,34,35,37,47,57,60,61, 65,67,68,71,73,85,89,92,103,125,128,167,231
Covington, Betty L., 156
Covinton, Betty, 116
Cowan, Bertha M., 156
Cox, Paul J., 91,93,140
Coy, George, 45
Crawford, T.E., 74
Crenshaw, Milton, 23
Crimi, Anthony, 116
Cullen, Mrs. W. Clough, 115
Cullen, W. Clough, 93,115,178
Czarnecki, Caroline, 157,160
Dahl, Mrs. V.L., 114
Dahl, Vern L., 93,140
Dallimore, G.A., 88,231
Daniels, Susan, 177
Daun, Representative Joe, 137
Davenport, Representative E.J., 14
Davis Robert D., 103
Davis, Senator Miford, 42,137
Davison, Mrs. J. Robert, 115
DeBoer, Wendell, 105,156
Decosse, Katie, 116
Delaney, Jack, 86
DenBoer, Donna, 177
Detlefson, Kenneth, 108
Dewerff, Karel, 155
Dexheimer, Jeanette, 157
Dial, Gary, 166
Dick, Mrs. J.S.,Jr., 108
Dick, J.S.,Jr,, 93
Dickinson, Barbara, 157
Dickson, William, 14
Diesch, Mrs. Stanley L. (Darlene), 115
Diesch, Stanley L., 157,171
Dietl, Mrs. Robert A. (Mary Ann), 115
Dietl, Robert A., 107
Dietz, Senator William L., 136
Dingle, Joseph H., 19
Dinwoodie, J.T.E., 127
Dirham, Senator Aubrey W., 134
Donaldson, R.R., 92
Donlin, Jenet, 105
Donnistown, Rollin, 105
Dorenthal, Henry, 137
Dorset, M., 52
Douglas, Joseph M., 231
Dovre, O.E., 121
Dowell, A.A., 150
Driver, Fred C., 75,86
Drum, Chris, 116

Dubbe, Ronald F., 107,108
Duke, Gary E., 158,172
Dulles, John Foster, 176
Dunlop, Robert, 105,131,155,163,164,155,169,171
Dunsmore, F.,122
Durand, Claudia, 116
Duschene, Ruth, 105
Dyer, Ernest, 77
Dyer, W.K., 78
Dzuik, Harold, E., 158,160,161
Eaton, R.D., 125
Eckles, Charles E., 232
Ecklund, Mrs. Allen E. (Janice), 115
Eckstein, John, 75,118
Edborg, Carl W., 158
Eddy, H.L., 88
Eder, Mrs. E. Paul, 114
Edgell, Southwell, 155,157
Eisenhauer, President Dwight, 171
Eken, Willis, 46
Elgen, W.F., 121
Ellery, John Cowell, 158
Enge, P.C., 119
Enge, Mrs. C.O., 114
Enge, C.O., 116
England, Reid, 142,145
Englerth, L.S., 69
Eppele, Page E., 46,86
Erb, Nelson S., 88,92,232
Erdahl, Senator L.B., 144
Estey, C.B., 120,121
Evanson, Harry, 56,89,92
Evarts, A.H., 39
Ewald, Charles, 86
Ewing, Sidney Allen, 105,158,160,161,162,164,157, 169,173
Fahning, Melvin, 157
Failing, Mrs. G.S., 108
Failing, G.S., 92,108
Falconer, Thomas, 232
Farnsworth, Ralph J., 157
Feldman, W.H., 119
Fell, David, 115
Fenske, T.M., 150
Fenstermacher, Ruel, 79,93,129,134,139,141,142, 152,167,168,169
Ferden, Ellen, 177
Ferguson, Mrs. T.H., 108
Fetrow, John, 166
Fetters, M.D., 116
Field, Mark, 118
Fields, Lillian R., 156
Filice, Lawrence, 169

Findlay, J.J., 15, 232
Finnegan, Rosemary, 105,154,157
Fisch, H.M., 119
Fitch, Mrs. C.P., 108,114
Fitch, Ernest, 117
Fitch, C.P., 68,86,89,101,108,129,130,131,167
Flanary, W.F., 93,119
Flanary, James B., 86,119
Fleming, Laurie, 116
Fleming, Representative E.A., 14
Fleming, H.G., 121
Fletcher, Thomas F., 157
Fletcher, John, 105
Flint, Jean C., 142
Flint, Jack G., 29,40,45,46,84,85,103
Flynn, John, 118
Fogerty, John, 86,140
Foley, W.T., 77
Foley, E.J., 121
Follstad, Barbara, 177
Forsburg, H.T., 35
Forsythe, Representative R.H., 21
Frank E.T., 92, 232
Frank, L.E., 121
Frank C.C., 56
Fredericksen, Eiler, 75
Frederickson, Norman, 117
French, Mrs. Donald (Isabelle), 115
Fretz, W.J., 60,68,86
Friendshuh, Mrs. Keith, 115
Friendshuh, Keith, 93,108
Frost, Fern, 139,142
Fuglsang, Harold, 105,117
Funk, William, 105,108
Furlong, J.J., 29,85
Gabbert, Mr. & Mrs. Don, 173
Gale, Charles, 168
Gandrud, Linda, 177
Gehrman, Fred, W., 93,103,105,118, 156
Gehrman, Mrs. F.W., 114
Gehrman, Charles, 108
Gelatt, Kirk, 160
Ghostley, G.F., 86
Gibson, Charles, 157
Gilbert, Kathryn, 157
Gillingham, J.E., 57
Girard, Jim, 45
Citis, Toby Lca, 142
Gladisch, William, 140
Glick, David, 140
Gloege, Karen, 157
Gloss, Mrs. Ellis H., 114
Gloss, Ellis H., 18,75,86,93

Glotfelter, C.E., 60
Gluck, Mark, 179
Gochnauer, Mrs. O.B., 114
Gochnauer, O.B., 80
Good, Archie, 155,158
Goodrich, Richard, 105
Gough, Francine, 177
Gould, J,N., 8,15,53,86,88,92,123,125,232
Gould, John Whipple, 232
Grady, Margaret K., 139,142,155,157
Graham, Christofer, 125,233
Graham, Christofer, 125
Graham. L., 122
Gray, Grace, 158
Greaves, H.A., 86,89,92
Gregg, Oren C., 125
Gregorson, Mr., 77
Greiner, Kenneth, 93
Griebe, K.E., 117
Griffiths, Henry J., 105,141,142,152,155,157
Grogan, P.H., 85
Groth, Evelyn, 177
Gustafson, Dorothy, 101
Gustafson, Bonnie, 177
Gute, Russell, 72
Gutman, Dr., 67
Gysland, Verdie, 75,117
Hadlow, William J., 142
Hagen, W.A., 144
Hagen, D.D., 119
Hagerty, T.J., 29,85,93,105
Haggard, C.H., 93
Hakomski, Mildred R., 157
Hall, Jeffrey, 179
Hall, E.A., 121
Hallquist, R.A., 62
Halstad, Representative Charles, 71
Halstenson, Diane C., 157
Halver, D.L., 93
Halverson, Herbert, 86
Hammer, Robert, 157
Hammond, Paul B., 145,155,158,160
Hanish, J.A., 89,233
Hanlon (Wolf), Griselda (Bee), 105,117,158,175,
   176,177
Hansen, F.W., 92
Hansen, Mrs. F.W., 114
Hansen, Mrs. Carl H., 114
Hansen, Carl H., 93
Hanson, Ray L., 75,117
Hanson, Mrs. James O. (Carol), 115
Hanson, James O., 93,101,105,107,108,118,167,
   170,171

Hanson, H.P., 119
Hardy, Robert M., 105,172
Hartle, George G., 93,105,117
Hartle, Mrs. George G., 114
Hartmen, Warren, 117
Hartung, Charles, 86
Hawton, Jerry, 46
Hay, Leopold, 23,53,88,92,101,120,233
Hayden, David, 165
Hayes, Wilma, 142,155,158
Healy, O.W., 86
Heath, Everrett, 157
Held, Stanley E., 93,101,105,118,156
Hemmingway, Allen, 141,142
Hendricks, Mrs. Stanley L., 115
Hendricks, Stanley L., 105
Hennen, Nancy, 116
Henry, John F.,Jr., 142
Henry, John, 118
Henry, Forest, 29,85
Hewitt, Earl A., 178
Hewitt, C.H., 25,26,27,57
Hicks, Donald B., 121,140
Higbee, Myron H., 16,17,92
Higbee, Mrs. John M. (Lucille), 115
Higbee, John M., 17,119,157,168,169
Himes, Wade, 108
Hinman, J., 14
Hobert, Randall, 136
Hobert, E.S., 119
Hohn, Bruce, 119
Hokkanen, Elmer, 75,93,101,102
Holland, Adelaide,, 149
Holland, P.O., 86
Holt, Ann, 177
Hoover, J. Edger, 176
Horita, Kenji, 142
Hormann, Steve, 179
Hormel, Jay, 118,119
Hoskins, H.P., 126,127,128
Hovde, T.C., 86
Howe, John, Jr., 86
Hoyt, Harvey H., 104,142,144,145,146,149,150,156,
   178
Hubbard, Gov. L.F., 26
Huff, T.B., 56
Huffman, Greg, 116
Hughes, E.G., 93
Huisinga, Theodore, 86
Humphrey, U.S. Senator Hubert, 105
Hurley, Sharon, 86
Husby, L.A., 119
Hystad, Janice, 155

Illstrup, F.A., 233
Ingvaldson, Vern, 46
Innes, Donald, 118
Irwin, John B., 60
Jacobberger, Patricia, 165
Jacobi, G.E., 117
Jacobi, Mrs. G.E., 114
Jahn, B.F., 121
Jamison, Robert, 30
Jankus, Edward R., 158
Jasper, Donald E., 131,139
Jegers, Angelika, 155,158
Jenkins, L.E., 38,67,68,77,80,82
Jenkins, Mrs. L.E., 108
Jennings, C.G., 62
Jensen, V.K., 93,105
Jensen, Millard, 142,156
Jergenson, Lawrence, 139
Jessen Carl Roger, 158,160
Johnson, Rodney, 45
Johnson, Linda J., 158
Johnson, Andrea, 116
Johnson, Senator C.E., 137
Johnson, C.A., 20
Johnson, LaRue W., 120,156,157
Johnson, Donald W., 120,156,157,171,178
Johnson, Beverly J., 158
Johnson, Kenneth H., 157,160,161,165
Johnston, Shirley, 165
Jones, Florence, 82,139,142
Jones, J.Senaca, 134,136
Jones, Marion J., 62,121
Joneschild, E.M., 86
Jorgensen, Sally E., 105
Kalb, Edward L., 233
Kallestad, T.E., 116
Kampmeier, Don, 46
Kanning, Herbert H, 105.
Karcher, James N., 93,101,105
Karcher, Mrs. James N., 114
Karlson, Alfred, 119
Karnis, E.K., 86
Kehr, William T., 139,142,157
Keller, George E., 38,75,76,105
Keller, Kenneth, 164
Kelly, J.J., 86,93,105,121
Kempena, J.A., 119
Kenaley, Rose, 107,139,142,154
Kernkamp, H.C.H., 47,53,56,93,101,105,119,127,
    139,140,141,142,150,167,168,178
Kernkamp, Mrs. H.C.H. (Edna), 108,114
Kerr, E.J., 86
Ketchum, F.D., 120

Kiebel, R.W., 120,121
Kind, Gene R., 93,105
Kinzer, Senator John J., 134
Kirby, B.W., 15,234
Kircher, William, 107
Kislingbury, Kent, 46
Kitchell, Ralph L., 131,140,142,150,151,154,155,178
Kjerner, Rudy, 234
Klein, Lyle, 75,121
Klett, Donna M., 142
Knoche, Karl, 119
Knodt, E.H., 86
Koch, Robert, 57
Koepke, George, 120
Koffer, Henry, 162
Kohler, Edmund, 119
Kontz, M.J., 119
Korn, Marlys, 116
Kruger, Ruth, 177
Kuch, Ella K., 157
Kuecker, Ronald D., 23,93,105
Kufrin, R.S., 86,93,105
Kuhns, Walter A,, 234
Kunkel, Al J., 93,120
Kurtz, Harold John, 158,169
Kuschel, August, 71
La Due, Senator Jay, 14
Lacher, Linda, 101,102
Lambrechts, Bernard, 89, 234
Lamphere, Lyle, 107
Landman, John, 47
Landman, Mrs. John, 115
Langevin, H., 89,234
LaPointe, J.T., 234
Larson, Arleen, 177
Larson, Vaughn, 157,160
Larson, Alice L., 177
Larson, George A., 93
Larson, Lester, 172
Larson, Harvard, 75
Larson, Calvert, 155
Lauermann, Leo, 56
Lauritson, Diane, 177
Leary, Robert, 140,168
Lee, J.F., 122
Leech, G. Ed., 16,101,234
Lees, A.F., 53,92,235
Leibbrand, Wilbur, 179
Lein, Ambrose, 142
Leino, Richard L., 167
Leman, Al, 166
Lenker, J.W., 64
Leuck, A.T., 18

LeVander, Governor Harold, 40,42
Lewis, B. Robert, 105,118
Lewis, Jim, 45
Libby, James A.,93,105,157,170
Lieske, Jim, 46
Lilleodden, Joan, 157
Lind, Governor John, 27,28
Lindberg, Lois Elaine, 86
Lindorfer, Robert K., 155,157,160
Ling, Clifford, 169
Linneman, M.C., 121
Lipp, C.C., 126
Locey, David, 107
Loken, Keith, 156,157,160
Long, D.F., 120
Lorenz, Robert, 108
Low, Donald, 118, 142,145,156,157
Lucas, Edith M., 177
Lucast, Barbara, 157
Lucey, Governor Patrick, 162
Luchsinger, Donald, 86
Lund, Mary, 116
Lundgren, Paul, 140
Lupfer, J.R., 120,121
Lyford, C.C., 7,8,14,15,88,92,122,123,235
Lynd, Jim Girard, 45
Lyon, H.C., 32,92
Maas, Donald, 120
Mack, C.A., 92,101
Mackenthun, Merlin, 45
Mackerwith, R.C., 120
Mackey, Edmund, 32
Mackey, Walter J., 32,44,93,105,140
Macy, Harold, 107,139,149,150,151,153
Magnusson, A.B., 86,93,105
Magnusson, Mrs. A.B., 114
Magrath, Peter, 162
Maher, William F., 23
Maher, M.P., 121
Maheswaren, S.K., 157
Malcolm, Peter, 64
Malcomson, Nanette, 115,116
Malmquist, William A., 142
Manthei, D.A., 120
Marsh, C.H., 86, 167
Martens, Robert A. (Bob), 45,105
Martens, Mrs. Robert A., 115
Martin, Frank, 105
Martin, William D., 157
Maruska, Senator Harveydale, 19
Mason, R.C., 122
Mather, George W., 115,117,142,144.145,149,156,
    157,178

Mayo, C.W., 149
McBain, Judy Ann, 177
McBroom, Geo., 121
McBroom, J.D., 26
McBryde, C.M., 52
McCarthy, U.S. Senator Eugene, 56
McCleary, James, 56
McConnell, Richard H., 118
McConnell, W.W.P., 29,85
McCulley, Graydon, 86
McDonald, D.M., 32
McGillivary, George, 92,235
McGinn, H.G., 71,92
McKay, John M., 235
McKee, J.C., 121
McKenzie, K.J., 53,88,92,101,125,235
McLaughlin, William, 89,92
McLellan, B.W., 122
McLeod, Senator Lawrence, 21
McLoughlin, J.J., 235
McMemony, Michael F., 105, 165
McPherson, Charles, 119
McReeve, Representative R.M., 14
Melin, Dale, 46
Melton, Deborah, 101,
Merrill, Robert A., 92,121,141,142,144,156
Merrill, Mrs. Robert A., 103,114
Mersch, Robert, 86
Meyer, Karl F., 175
Michie, Pamela, 156
Miller, C.B., 136
Miller, Garth, 158
Miller, Paul E., 150
Miller, R.E., 35
Mittlestadt, D.W., 120
Mixa, Mr., 83
Moenning, Arno, 45
Mohler, John R., 78,129
Molnau, Ralph, 93,105,120
Montgomery, J.E., 60
Moon, Harley, 168,169
Moore, William E., 156
Morgan, M.T., 35
Morgan, Ora B., 117
Morgan, Robert, 86
Morrill, James L., 136,137,139,142,144,148,149,153
Morrison, Bob, 46
Moscrip, W.S., 69,86,137,167
Moser, Ron, 166
Moulton, Jack E., 142
Mueller, Representative August, 105,134,137
Mueller, Emil, 236
Muns, C.E., 72

Munson, Roy C., 105
Murphy, Cletus, 72
Myers, J. Arthur, 67,105
Myers, Margo, 177
Myers, Victor S.,Jr., 118,158,160
Nankervis, T.P., 93,105
Navarro, Manuel, 118
Neaton, Holly, 108
Nelson, Paul L., 120
Nelson, Mrs. Paul L., 114
Nelson, Myron Henry, 156
Nelson, Sever, 34
Nelson, Senator Ancher, 105,134,136,137
Nelson, C.A., 85,89,92
Nelson, Melvin E,, 134,136,137
Nelson, Glen H., 23,86,93,105,132,137,140,157,169
Nelson, Barbara J,, 155
Nelson, Gov. Knute, 15,27
Nelson, Mrs. Glen H. (Mary), 23
Nesser, Kenneth E., 86
Nesser, Theodore, 71
Neubauer, Gary D., 93
Newman, J.H., 121
Nielsen, N. Ole, 131,155
Niles, W.B., 52
Nolan, M. Eleanor, 71
Northrop, Cyrus, 124
O;Brien (Schmidt), JoAnne, 175,176,177
O'Dell, Thomas E., 142
O'Leary, Barbara, 93
O'Leary, T.P., 105
Oberste, Lawrence, 158,172
Offerman, Alvin, 86
Olson, Vern, 140
Olson, Mrs. Steven (Norma), 115
Olson, William, 172
Olson, Harry R., 82
Olson, James, 105
Olson, Shelia Jo, 157
Olson, Governor Floyd B., 35,68
Olson, Senator John L., 105, ,153
Olson, Roland, 23
Olson, Mary, 101
Olson, Johannes, 63
Olson, Richard, 93,105,108
Olson, Ned, 169
Opstad, Agnes M., 142
Orr, Senator C.N., 131
Osborn, H.D., 77
Osborn, O.H., 120.121
Osborn, Mrs. Orin, 116
Osborne, Carl A., 105,157,161,165
Osterberg, Geraldine, 177

Ostergaard, Arden, 139,142
Palmby, Clarence, 137
Palmer, Richard, 39
Palmer, C.C., 127
Palmer, D.B., 21,23,39,92,105,118
Palmer, Maurice, 75,117
Palmer, Kenneth, 140
Palmer, Mrs. D.B., 114
Parent, Mrs. J.X., 108
Parent, J.X., 92
Parent, Joan, 13
Parker, C.H., 14
Parker, Frank Henry, 157
Paul, G.J., 121
Pearson, Lester, 57
Penkert, R.A., 119
Penning-Pehrson, Kay, 116
Penny, J.C., 147
Perman, Vic, 115,155,165,172
Person, Donald H., 86
Peters, H,C,, 236
Peterson, Lloyd, 105,166
Peterson, Loraine, 139
Peterson, W.E., 134
Petricka, Sandra V., 154
Philip, Mrs. D.R., 114
Phillips, Mary G., 142,155
Philmon, Henry, 179
Phipps, L.H., 119
Pieper, Charles A., 107
Pierce, C.H., 15
Piermattei, Donald, 158
Pierson, Paul, 45,86
Pint, L.H., 86,93,105
Plager, Carol, 105
Poirot, Susan, 23
Pomeroy, Mrs. B.S. (Margaret), 104,114
Pomeroy, B.A., 89,92,236
Pomeroy, B.S., 80,84,92,93,101,104,105,139,140,
    141,142,151,155,157,160,163,168
Pomplum, W.J., 28,30
Porter, Edward, 123,124
Porter, B.J., 117
Porter, Thayer E., 93,118
Poss, Peter, 93
Price, Richard, 14,15,26,27,88,02,122,236
Pritchard, William R., 131,142,144,145,150
Prouse, W.C., 92
Provost, Robert, 102
Pyle, Robert, 140
Quigley, Mrs. Joseph (Eileen), 115
Rabrassier, R.A., 152
Rackliffe, C.L., 121

Radford, Mrs. P.H., 108
Radford, P.H., 92
Rarig, F.M.,Jr., 35
Rasmussen, Marilyn, 156
Rathje, Jane, 116
Redder, Lester, 140
Redig, Patrick, 172
Reed, William M., 158
Reinertson, Richard H., 121
Rempel, William, 105
Resler, Todd, 45
Reynolds, M.H., 8,16,17,23,37,28,30,31,52,65,85,88,
    89,92,103,120,123,126,127,128,130,167,236
Riede, Peter H., 92,119
Riede, Mrs. Peter H., 108
Rieke, R.W., 116
Roback, Richard J., 157
Robert, David, 73
Robinson, Robert A., 157
Rockne, U.S. Senator Knute, 76,119
Roepke, Martin, 76,119,131,139,140,141,142,149,
    150,175
Roper, Judith Faye, 156
Rose, W.M., 117
Roseen, Barbara L., 158
Rosell, Conway, 118,140
Rosin, Eberhard, 158
Routh, Allen, 45,86
Rowell, E., 14
Rud, Betty Rosalie, 158
Ruebke, H.J., 86
Rupp, Robert, 105
Ruth, George, 169
Ryan, T., 19
Ryan, U.S. Representative Elmer J., 73
Ryan, Joseph J., 72
Rydell, Oscar, 237
Rypka, Jerry, 86
Salihotra, 1
Sandberg, Mrs. C.R., 114
Sather, Dandra Sue, 159
Sauber, Collen, 116
Sautter, Mrs. Jay (Peg), 114
Sautter, Jay H., 104,118,139,140,142,155,157
Sayers, A.L., 86
Schaefer, James, 117
Schall, U.S. Senator Thomas D., 73
Schaller, Senator Albert, 16
Scheftel, Joni, 86
Schiefelbein, Frank, 46
Schipper, Ithel, 132,136,137,140
Schladweiler, Mrs. A. J., 114
Schlauderaff, Clarence H., 105

Schlotthauer, Charles, 149
Schlotthauer, John, 149,155,158
Schlotthauer, Mrs. Carl F., 114
Schlotthauer, Carl F., 93,119,149
Schmidt, JoAnne (See O'Brien)
Schmidt, Conrad, 45
Schmidt, A.H., 92
Schmitz, Mary, 175
Schmitz, Henry, 139,149,150,175,176
Schroeder, Wesley G., 93,107,108,118
Schubert, Glen, 75
Schultz, Rebecca, 116
Schultz, Patricia, 177
Schultz, Richard M., 157,160
Schultze, Max, 105
Schwanke, Commissioner, 71
Schwartze, W.F., 102
Schwartzkoff, Olaf, 123,124,125,237
Schweich, Sandy, 116
Schwermann, Henry E., 93,105
Schwermann, Mrs. Henry E., 114
Scott, J.A., 125
Scott, A., 14
Scruby, W.H., 15,237
Seefeld, Carol Lynn, 156
Sellers, Alvin F., 139,142,155,178,
Setzepfandt, A.C., 86,105
Severson, Verner A., 142
Shapiro, Judith Leah, 142
Sharma, Jagdev, 166
Shaw, Daniel, 169
Shears, M.I.V., 35
Shelton, George C., 131
Shepherd, William G., 158
Sherwood, Harrison B., 71
Sholin, Carl, 86
Shope, Richard E.,Jr., 157
Shore, C.S., 92
Short, Everett C., 158,160,161
Siewart, Bernette, 116
Sigmond, C.J., 92,237
Sime, Donald, 105
Sims, P.T., 75
Sinn, Larry, 179
Sloan, R.J., 149
Smith, H.R., 86
Smith, John Day, 30
Smith, C.A., 170
Soderstrom, Judy, 177
Solac, Raymond, 104,120,157,170
Soneral, William, 238
Sook, Ronald M., 121
Sorensen, Mrs. Dale K., 114

INDEX TO NAMES OF PERSONS IN PHOTOGRAPHS

Hammond, Paul, 143
Hanlon Wolf, Bee, 153,154,175
Hansen, F.W., 98
Hansen, Mrs. F.W., 111
Hansen, Mrs. Carl, 111
Hansen, Carl, 98
Hanson, Mrs. James O. (Carol), 113
Hanson, James O., 96,99
Hartle, Mrs. George G., 112
Hartle, George G., 95,96,99
Hartmann, William L., 85
Hay, Leopold, 97
Held, Stanley E., 95.96,99
Hemmingway, Allan, 143
Hendricks, Mrs. Stanley L. (Doris), 112
Henry, John, 143
Henry, Forest, 29
Herschler, Richard, 154
Hess, William, 143
Hewitt, Earl A., 129
Hewitt, Charles N., 25
Higbee, M.R., 97
Higbee, John M., 93,95
Higbee, Mrs. John M., 112
Hohn, Bruce, 90, 135,139
Hokkanen, Elmer, 95.96,99
Hoyt, Harvey, 143,154
Hughes, E.G., 94,99
Huisinga, Ted, 87
Hurley, Sharon, 87
Illustrup, F.A., 3
Imm, Senator Val, 138
Jacobi, Mrs. G.E., 111
Jacobson, L.T., 5
Jensen, V.K., 95,96,99
Jepson, Stanley, 139
Johnson, LaRue, 154
Johnson, Mrs. Donald W. (Rose), 110
Johnson, G.A., 3
Jones, J. Senaca, 139
Karcher, James N. 92,96,99
Karcher, Mrs. James N., 111
Keller, George E., 76
Kelly, J.J., 93,99
Kenaley, Rose, 130
Kent, Marvin, 130
Kernkamp, H.C.H., 94,99,129,130,143,150
Kernkamp. Mrs. H.C.H., 109,111
Kiebel, R.W., 106
Kind, Gene R., 100
King, Lucille Bishop, 130
Kingrey, Dean, 90
Kitchell, Ralph, 143
Knodt, E.H., 40

Kook, Chang Cheong, 154
Korsunsky, Alex, 143
Kuecker, Ronald, 24, 92, 100
Kufrin, R.S., 94, 95, 99
Kummer, J.W., 106
Kunkel, Al, 95,100
Lacher, Linda, 102
Lambert, J.M., 3
Lambrechts, Bernard, 3
Landman, Mrs. John (Marilyn), 112
Landman, John, 85
LaPointe, R., 3
Larson, Mrs. George A., 109
Larson, George A., 94,99
Lawson, W.M., 93
Lees, A.F.97
LeVander, Governor Harold, 76
Libby, James A., 100
Low, Ronnie, 154
Low, Donald, 143,154
Lyford, C.C., 3,97
Lyon, H.C., 3,97
Mack, C.A., 3.97
Mackey, Mrs. Walter J. (Phyllis), 110
Mackey, Walter J., 85,90,100, 135
Madden, Lauren, 154
Magnuson, Kenneth, 95
Magnusson, Mrs. A.B. (Mary), 110,112,114
Magnusson, A.B., 90,91,99
Malmquist, Winston, 143
Martens, Mrs. Robert A. (Carol), 110,112
Mather, George, 143,154,155
McConnell, W.W.P., 29
McDonald, D.M., 3
McGee, Marie, 40
McGillivary, G., 97
McGinn, H.G., 98,106
McKenzie, K.J., 3,97
McLaughlin, W., 98
Merrill, Mrs. Robert A., 109,111
Merrill, Robert A., 98,143
Miller, Emma, 130
Molnau, Ralph G., 100
Mueller, Representative August, 134
Nankervis, T.P., 99
Nelson, C.A., 97
Nelson, Glen H., 90,95,96,99,139
Nelson, Senator Ancher, 135,138,139
Nelson, Senator Ancher,
Nelson, Barbara, 154
Nelson Mrs. P.L., 112
Neubauer, Gary, 100
Nilson, W., 130
O'Brien Schmidt, JoAnne, 174